Controversies in hip surgery

Controversies in hip surgery

Edited by
Robert Bourne

Professor and Chair, Division of Orthopaedic Surgery,
University of Western Ontario, Canada

OXFORD
UNIVERSITY PRESS

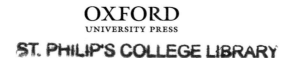

OXFORD

UNIVERSITY PRESS

Great Clarendon Street, Oxford OX2 6DP

Oxford University Press is a department of the University of Oxford.
If furthers the University's objective of excellence in research, scholarship,
and education by publishing worldwide in

Oxford New York

Auckland Bangkok Buenos Aires Cape Town Chennai
Dar es Salaam Delhi Hong Kong Istanbul Karachi Kolkata
Kuala Lumpur Madrid Melbourne Mexico City Mumbai Nairobi
Sao Paulo Shanghai Singapore Taipei Tokyo Toronto

Oxford is a registered trade mark of Oxford University Press
in the UK and in certain other countries

Published in the United States
by Oxford University Press Inc., New York

British Library Cataloguing in Publication Data

(Data available)

Library of Congress Cataloging in Publication Data

ISBN 0 19 263161 6

10 9 8 7 6 5 4 3 2 1

Typeset by Integra Software Services Pvt. Ltd, Pondicherry, India
Printed in Great Britain
on acid-free paper by Biddles Ltd., Guildford

Contents

8

Criteria for implant selection in revision total hip arthroplasty: a North American perspective *181*
David A. Parker and Cecil H. Rorabeck

9

Criteria for implant selection in revision total hip arthroplasty: a European perspective *229*
H. Wagner and M. Wagner

10

Bearing surfaces in total hip replacements: state of the art and future development *249*
Harry A. McKellop

11

Controversies in deep vein thrombosis prophylaxis following total hip arthroplasty: a North American perspective *279*
Clifford W. Colwell and Mary E. Hardwick

12

Management of the infected total hip arthroplasty: a North American perspective *289*
M. Gavan McAlinden, Bassam A. Masri, and Clive P. Duncan

Abbreviations

AAOS	American Academy of Orthopaedic Surgeons
BMD	bone mineral density
BMI	body mass index
CT	computed tomography
DDH	developmental dysplasia of the hip
DVT	deep vein thrombosis
FDA	US Food and Drug Administration
INR	International Normalized Ratio
LMWH	low molecular weight heparin
MEP	motor evoked potential
MRI	magnetic resonance imaging
ORIF	open reduction and internal fixation
PFA	proximal femoral allograft
SCFE	slipped capital femoral epiphysis
SSEP	somatosensory evoked potential
THA	total hip arthroplasty
UHMWPE	ultrahigh molecular weight polyethylene
VTE	venous thromboembolic event

Contributors

George C. Bennet FRCS
Robert B. Bourne MD FRCSC
Clifford W. Colwell Jr MD
Clive P. Duncan MB MSC FRCSC
Mary E. Hardwick RN MSN
J.A. Herring MD
Bassam A. Masri MD FRCSC
M. Gavan McAlinden BSC MPHIL FRCS (TR & ORTH)
Steven J. MacDonald MD FRCSC
Harry A. McKellop PHD
M.D. MacLeod MD FRCSC
Jose A. Morcuende MD PHD
David A. Parker MBBS FRACS
Cecil H. Rorabeck MD FRCSC
Harry Tsigaras MBBS FRACS
H. Wagner MD PHD
M. Wagner MD
Stuart L. Weinstein MD
R. Baxter Willis MD FRCSC

Introduction

We hope that you will enjoy *Controversies in Hip Surgery*. In this volume, we include the contributions of an international array of experts in the field of hip surgery. The purpose of this book is to give an overview in terms of both development and controversies in the field of hip surgery. Contributions cover such important paediatric problems as development dysplasia of the hip, Perthes disease, and slipped capital femoral epiphysis. Hip problems associated with neurological diseases are also covered. Traumatic conditions of the hip, including acetabular fractures and femoral neck fractures, are discussed in detail. Considerable emphasis is given to the field of both primary and revision total hip replacement, particularly with regard to the differences between practice in Europe and North America. Like every other aspect of hip disease, the field of total hip arthroplasty is continuously changing to improve both the quality and the durability of the clinical result. Finally, postoperative complications and their avoidance are covered, particularly deep vein thrombosis and management of the infected total hip arthroplasty. The editor and authors hope that you will enjoy this text and will find it beneficial in managing the hip disorders which face the clinician today.

Special thanks goes to Richard Marley, the Commissioning Editor, and Oxford University Press for supporting this endeavour. It is the hope of the publisher and contributors to this text that our patients will be the beneficiaries.

Robert B. Bourne MD FRSC
A.D. McLachlin Professor,
University of Western Ontario,
London, Ontario, Canada

Developmental dysplasia of the hip: natural history, results of treatment, and controversies

Jose A. Morcuende and Stuart L. Weinstein

Developmental dysplasia of the hip (DDH) is one of the most common problems in paediatric orthopaedics, and one of the most fascinating. DDH represents a spectrum of conditions that range from a simple neonatal instability to an established dislocation. The term **developmental** is now preferred to **congenital** because it is more encompassing as it is taken in the literal sense of organ growth and differentiation, which includes fetal, neonatal, and infantile periods. This terminology includes all cases that are clearly teratological and those that are developmental, and it incorporates dysplasia of the hip, subluxation, and dislocation.

Review of the evolution in our understanding of DDH in the last few decades is very interesting and rewarding. Early diagnosis and treatment, the use of ancillary imaging techniques, more physiological methods of casting, less extensive operative procedures, the use of femoral shortening to prevent femoral head growth disturbances, and improved surgical techniques for correction of residual hip dysplasia signify major advances in this area. However, many issues in the management of DDH are still controversial.

The cause of DDH remains unknown. There is no doubt that genetic and ethnic factors play a key role; the reported incidence of DDH is as high as 50 per 1000 live births in Lapps and North American Indians but it is almost non-existent among Chinese and those of African descent.[1] The ideal management of DDH involves recognition of high-risk infants and early detection of the unstable hip. The introduction of screening programmes based on clinical examination have resulted in improved early detection of unstable hips, but the goal of completely eliminating late cases of dislocation, subluxation, and acetabular dysplasia has not been achieved. Before the introduction of any type of screening, the historical incidence of dislocation was between 0.5 and 1.5 cases per 1000 live births.[2-8] Yet, by clinical testing, 10 to 20 newborns per 1000 are considered to have abnormal hips and therefore require some type of treatment. However, the incidence of a first surgical procedure for DDH in population-based studies has been reported to be very similar to that reported before universal clinical screening was introduced (0.7–2.3 per 1000).[4,9–14] It is important to consider that a large number of these late-diagnosed cases represent loss of follow-up and there is also some evidence that suggests that a very small number of cases of DDH may occur late. Given the variable presentation of DDH, it is therefore extremely important to look for this condition continually after the newborn period and in high-risk infants. The role of parents as well as community health professionals should be recognized, since the largest proportion of children requiring surgery is brought to the attention of the paediatric orthopaedic surgeon by a family member or detected by routine paediatric check ups after 3 to 6 months of age.

Over the last two decades, the ancillary use of ultrasound in the screening, diagnosis, and management of children with DDH has become current practice in many centres.[15–26] Ultrasonographic evaluation has the advantage over clinical testing of allowing objective documentation of the anatomy of the developing hip, and it is safe and non-invasive. Many proponents strongly recommend that ultrasonography should be used as a routine screening tool in the newborn, and others advocate its use for all infants with clinical examination abnormalities and for at-risk patients. However, expensive resources and highly trained operators are required because the technique requires rigorous attention to detail and an understanding of normal and pathological anatomy of the hip. In addition, ultrasonography has a low specificity in the first week of life, so that its use has been associated with overdiagnosis and high follow-up and intervention rates. Debate continues about the appropriate planes and method of evaluation and whether an orthopaedic surgeon, the treating physician, or a radiologist with expertise in ultrasonography should perform the evaluation.[27]

It is now appreciated that a hip with normal anatomy can be unstable, and that one with very abnormal morphology can prove to be stable. Adding ultrasound imaging to clinical examination at birth dramatically increases the number of abnormal hips detected, but most of these 'abnormalities' resolve without treatment; consequently, ultrasonography has been reported not to reduce the prevalence of late-diagnosed cases.[28] Another difficult issue is cost-effectiveness of hip ultrasonography. Marks et al.[24] reported that their screening ultrasound programme required a team of five radiographers to cover daily scanning, and radiographers and physiotherapists to assist at the weekly hip-screening clinic. Davids et al.[29] reviewed the costs and benefits of ultrasonography in different clinical delivery systems (radiology-based, radiology–orthopaedic-based, and orthopaedic-office-based) and found that, once expertise had been gained and start-up costs had been met, the orthopaedic-office-based system was the most convenient, cost-effective, and efficient for patients, families, and treating physicians. Hernandez et al.[30], using the methods of decision analysis, reported that ultrasound is not the preferred strategy for the screening of neonates and high-risk patients since its expected utility is lower than that of physical examination.

Given the variable nature of DDH, it may never be possible to predict outcome, in all cases, based on tests of the status of the hip at birth. Therefore the cornerstone for DDH diagnosis is the clinical examination of all infants by experts on at least two occasions in the first 3 months of life. Until ultrasonography of the hip can distinguish between true dysplasia and the normal variations of anatomy, radiography at 3 to 4 months of age is still the best method of establishing the true diagnosis in a doubtful hip. Further research is required to design studies to understand better the genetic and environmental variations, pathological manifestations, and natural history of infants with DDH to improve the accuracy of prognosis and risk assessment, to establish more accurate methods of case ascertainment, evaluate current screening methods and policies, and develop alternative cost-effective options, and to collaborate in the development of educational programmes to improve the physical examination skills of community health professionals and to increase the awareness and follow-up compliance of parents.

If DDH goes undetected, secondary adaptive changes occur and normal hip joint growth and development is impaired. The secondary changes observed in the joint reflect significant soft-tissue contracture and alterations in normal growth of the femoral head and acetabulum. The longer the femoral head remains out of the acetabulum, the more severe the acetabular dysplasia and the greater the femoral head distortion. Therefore it is important to reduce the hip as soon as possible to improve the results of treatment, decrease the risk of complications, and favourably alter the natural history. Current management of patients with DDH is based on knowledge of the normal acetabular growth and development, the pathology of the hip joint, the natural history of DDH, and the ongoing re-evaluation of past treatment regimes.

Natural history of untreated DDH

During embryonic development the hip components—femoral head and acetabulum—develop from the same primitive mesenchymal cells. At 7 weeks of gestation, a cleft develops defining the femoral head and the acetabulum, and by 11 weeks the hip joint is fully formed. At birth, the femoral head is deeply seated in the acetabulum, and it is difficult to dislocate a normal infant's hip even after division of the joint capsule.[31-33] However, in a dysplastic hip, the tight fit between the femoral head and the acetabulum is lost, and the femoral head can easily be displaced. The degree of hip joint pathology seen in DDH varies from capsular laxity to severe acetabular, femoral head, and femoral neck dysplasia.

For normal hip joint development and growth to occur in the postnatal period, there must be a genetically determined balance of growth of the acetabular and triradiate cartilage, as well as the presence of a well-located femoral head. Experimental studies and clinical findings in humans with unreduced dislocations suggest that the main stimulus for the concave shape of the acetabulum is the presence of a spherical femoral head. Harrison[34] observed that following excision of the femoral head in rats, the acetabulum failed to develop in terms of both area and depth, and there was atrophy and degeneration of the acetabular cartilage. However, the growth plates of the triradiate cartilage remained histologically normal, as did the length of the innominate bone. Similarly, in humans the innominate bone is of normal length in adults with unreduced hip dislocations. Coleman *et al.*[35] also demonstrated that the shape of the femoral head influences the shape of the acetabulum.

If a DDH goes unrecognized, normal development may not occur, leaving the child with a dysplastic hip. The natural history of untreated DDH is quite variable, but the longer hip dysplasia and dislocation goes undetected the greater is the impairment of the femoral head and acetabular development.[1] Barlow[2] reported that one in 60 newborns has instability on clinical examination in the neonatal period, but more than 60 per cent stabilize during the first week of life, and 88 per cent stabilize during the first 2 months without treatment. Yamamuro and Doi[36] followed 52 hips with positive Ortolani's sign over a 2-year period, without treatment for the first 5 months. Of the 12 with 'dislocated' hips, three (25 per cent) were radiographically normal at 5 months of age. Of the 42 of with 'subluxable' hips, 24 (57 per cent) were normal at 5 months. Pratt *et al.*[37] followed 18 'dysplastic' hips in patients younger than 3 months of age for an average of 11.2 years and found that 15 were radiographically normal. Coleman[38] followed 23 untreated DDH patients younger than 3 months of age and found that 26 per cent of the hips remained dislocated, 13 per cent were subluxated, 39 per cent remained located but retained dysplastic radiographic features, and 22 per cent were normal. Unfortunately, there is no method for predicting the outcome of unstable hips; hence all newborn hip 'instability' should be closely followed and treated.

In adults, the natural history of untreated complete dislocations varies and depends on two factors—the presence or absence of a well-developed false acetabulum and bilaterality. Interestingly, societal considerations also influence its natural history. In a study of 420 cases of DDH in the Cree–Ojibwa Island Lake Community population of Manitoba, Walker[39] reported that 'functional disability in everyday life was neither admitted nor observed...People viewed DDH in the same way as urban societies view left-handedness. ...The sole disability admitted by an Island Lake individual (unaffected) was that it was difficult to portage a canoe with a man who limps.' Wedge and Wasylenko[40] observed only a 24 per cent chance of a good clinical result with a well-developed false acetabulum, but with a moderately developed or absent acetabulum patients had a 52 per cent chance of a good clinical result. Milgram[41] reported a case of bilateral DDH discovered at postmortem examination. This 74-year-old man had no hip or thigh pain and only mild backache for 5 years before his death. His femoral head had no articulation with any portion of the ilium. In the absence of a false acetabulum, most patients with complete dislocations do well, maintaining a good range of motion with little disability. Factors that lead to the formation or lack of formation of a false acetabulum remain unknown. Back pain may occur in patients with bilateral dislocations. This is thought to be secondary to associated hyperlordosis of the lumbar spine.

In unilateral hip dislocations, secondary problems of limb-length inequality, deformity of the hip, ipsilateral knee pain, scoliosis, and gait disturbances are common. Limb-length inequalities of 10 cm or more have been reported, and these patients acquire flexion–adduction deformities of the hip which may lead to valgus deformities of the knee with attenuation of the medial collateral ligament and lateral compartment degenerative joint disease. In Wedge and Walsylenko's series,[40] seven of 22 patients with unilateral dislocation had valgus knee deformities, with 60 per cent complaining of some knee pain. The same factors concerning the development of secondary degenerative disease in the false acetabulum with associated clinical disability in bilateral cases also affect unilateral dislocations.

The natural history of subluxation and dysplasia in untreated patients is extremely important because this information may be extrapolated to residual subluxation and dysplasia after treatment. Outside the neonatal period, the term dysplasia has an anatomical and radiographic definition. The anatomical definition of dysplasia refers to inadequate development of the acetabulum, the femoral head, or both. In radiographic dysplasia, Shenton's line is intact. All subluxated hips are by definition anatomically dysplastic. The radiographic definition of subluxation is based on a disrupted Shenton's line and femoral head displacement with respect to the acetabulum superiorly, laterally, or superolaterally. The terms subluxation and dysplasia are often used interchangeably in the DDH literature.

It has become clear through the years that the primary factor in the development of degenerative joint disease of the hip is subluxation. Wedge and Wasylenko[40] reported a three-peak incidence of pain associated with hip subluxation depending on the severity of the the subluxation. Patients with subluxated hips usually have symptom onset at a younger age than those with complete dislocations. Invariably, radiographic subluxation leads to degenerative joint disease. The rate of deterioration is related directly to the

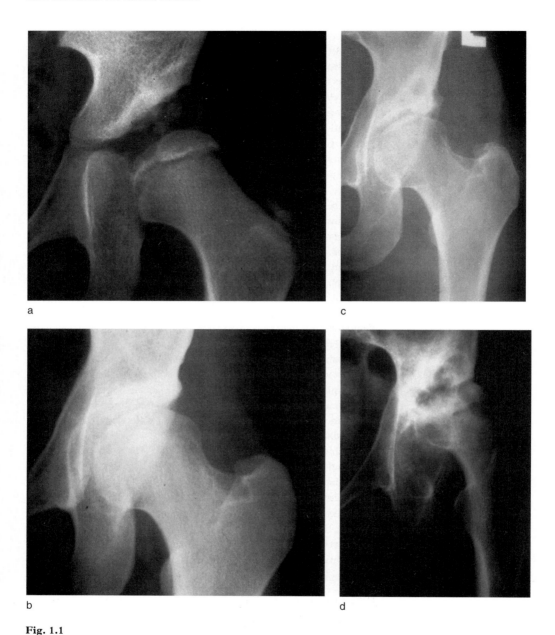

a

c

b

d

Fig. 1.1
Anteroposterior radiographs taken after the closed reduction of developmental dislocation of the hip performed when the patient was aged 2 years and 4 months: (a) 39 months after reduction, when the patient was aged 5 years and 7 months, the accessory centres of ossiification are visible in the acetabular cartilage; (b) 15 years after reduction, when the patient was 17 years old, the Shenton line is intact and there is mild acetabular dysplasia; (c) 42 years after reduction, when the patient was 44 years old, degenerative changes are present; (d) 51 years after reduction, when the patient was 53 years old, the hip is subluxed and has severe degenerative changes (Iowa Hip Rating, 48 of 100 points). The patient subsequently underwent toal hip replacement. (Reproduced with permission from Malvitz TA, Weinstein SL: Closed reduction for congenital dysplasia of the hip: functional and radiographic results after an average of thirty years. *Journal of Bone and Joint Surgery* [Am] **76**: 1777, 1994.)

severity of the subluxation and the age of the patient. Patients with the most severe subluxation usually developed symptoms during the second decade of life. Those with moderate subluxation presented at 30 to 40 years of age, and those with minimal subluxation experienced symptoms usually around menopause. It is rare to see radiographic changes of degenerative joint disease such as joint-space narrowing, osteophyte formation, or subchondral cysts at symptom onset. The only radiographic signs may be subchondral sclerosis in the weight-bearing area. After clinical symptoms and radiographic signs of degenerative joint disease appear, progression is rapid.

The true incidence of hip dysplasia is unknown and its natural history in the absence of subluxation is difficult to predict. Physical signs may be absent, and the diagnosis only established with the onset of symptoms or as an incidental radiographic finding. However, there is considerable evidence that residual radiographic hip dysplasia, particularly in females, leads to secondary degenerative joint disease, although there are no predictive radiographic parameters. Stulberg and Harris[42] observed that 48 per cent of patients in a series of 130 patients evaluated for primary or idiopathic degenerative disease of the hip had evidence of primary acetabular dysplasia and that acetabular dysplasia frequently occurred in females with degenerative joint disease. They also found that 50 per cent of their patients with dysplasia and degenerative joint disease had dysplasia in the opposite hip. Wiberg[43] suggested there was a direct relation between the onset of radiographic degenerative disease and the amount of dysplasia as measured by a decrease in the centre–edge angle. However, Cooperman et al.[44] reviewing 17 cases on which Wiberg based his conclusions, demonstrated that seven were actually subluxated and all had radiographic degenerative changes by the age of 42 years. The other ten hips were dysplastic and developed degenerative joint disease by an average of 57 years. This study demonstrated that the conventional parameters used to describe dysplasia cannot predict the rate at which the hip joint develops degenerative joint disease.

Treatment of DDH and long-term results

The goals in the treatment of DDH are to obtain a concentric reduction and then maintain that reduction to provide an optimal environment for femoral head and acetabular development. Such a reduction will optimize the changes so that the hip will function normally for the patient's lifetime. It involves a reduction between the femoral head and the acetabulum without interposition of soft tissues and with stability in a safe position that does not interfere with the blood supply to the proximal femoral epiphysis. Treatment options will depend primarily upon whether the hip is reducible and the age of the child at diagnosis.

Debate continues concerning which abnormal hips actually require active intervention. In the newborn most 'unstable hips' (those with a positive Ortolani sign) will stabilize in a very short time without treatment. However, a certain percentage of hips will go on to subluxation or dislocation, and some hips may remain located but retain dysplastic features. Unfortunately, even with the use of ultrasonography, it is not possible to know which of these unstable hips will attain spontaneous stability. Therefore it is recommended that all unstable hips in the newborn period are treated to ensure proper development of the hip.

From birth to age 6 months, an abduction device can treat most hips. In this age group, the hip is usually dislocatable or dislocated but capable of being reduced. Positioning of the hip in flexion and abduction often achieves desired stable reduction, but rigid immobilization in forced abduction is to be avoided. The use of triple diapers in the treatment of DDH has demonstrated no improvement in the results compared with no treatment at all in the first 3 weeks of life. A number of devices have been used for the treatment of DDH (Frejka pillow, Craig splint, Ilfeld splint, von Rosen splint, and hip spica casts), but the most widely used method in this age group is the Pavlik harness. This device holds the hips in a flexed ($100°-110°$) and abducted ($50°-70°$) position, allowing a safe range of hip motion. Attention to the principles of positioning the device is important to prevent complications, including loss of reduction, femoral nerve palsy and inferior dislocation, avascular necrosis of the femoral head, brachial plexus palsy, knee subluxation, and skin breakdown.[45-47] Reduction of the hip should be confirmed ultrasonographically or radiographically after reduction because continued use of the harness with a non-concentric reduction can result in further acetabular dysplasia. The Pavlik harness has been shown to be effective in 90 per cent of patients with hip subluxation and in 85 per cent of patients with complete dislocations, and is associated with a low incidence of aseptic necrosis. However, long-term results of Pavlik harness treatment demonstrate that up to approximately 20 per cent of the hips may show acetabular dysplasia at an average age of 12 years.[48] In addition. Borges et al.[49] reported worse prognosis for boys with DDH.

If the diagnosis of DDH is not made early, secondary changes develop that subsequently impair the normal growth and development of the hip and increase the risk for late degenerative joint disease. Therefore attainment and maintenance of a congruent stable joint is critical for normal hip development. Closed reduction is indicated for patients over 6 months of age at diagnosis and those who have failed a trial of Pavlik harness reduction. In most centres, closed reduction and spica cast immobilization is usually preceded by a period of traction.[50-60] The use of pre-reduction traction is one of the most controversial topics in DDH. Traction is advocated to facilitate closed reduction, to decrease the need for open reduction, and to decrease the incidence of femoral growth disturbances. In theory, traction facilitates reduction by stretching the soft tissues and contracted muscles, allowing reduction without excessive force, but the effect of traction on all these structures depends on the direction and magnitude with which the force is applied.

Traction regimes vary considerably. In North America most clinicians apply traction in a modified overhead position with the hips in some degree of flexion.[61,62] In this position the iliopsoas is relaxed, but unless the hips are significantly abducted, no effect can be expected on the adductor muscles. Salter et al.[63] demonstrated the importance of avoiding the hyperabducted position. In the European literature there are reports of success with prolonged (weeks to months) use of various traction regimes in hip extension with progressive abduction and varying degrees of internal rotation. However, these regimes require hospitalization and careful supervision, and are probably prohibitive in the context of today's health care environment and patient expectations.

The amount of weight that can be applied also depends on whether skin or skeletal traction is used. Importantly, the use of significant traction to the skin and soft tissues (as much as one-third of body weight) is not without risks, including neurovascular compromise to the extremity, compartment syndrome, skin slough, and even aseptic necrosis. Skeletal traction is used infrequently and carries the associated risks of pin-tract infection, fracture, growth-plate injuries, and necrosis.[64]

Despite widespread popularity, there is no objective evidence for the effectiveness of traction in isolation from other treatment variations. Even among proponents of pre-reduction traction, there is disagreement as to the most beneficial type (skin versus skeletal), direction of the pull (overhead versus longitudinal and amount of abduction), amount of weight, duration of treatment, or whether traction can be applied effectively in the home or should be used in the hospital setting under careful physician supervision. In addition, there is no objective evidence in the medical literature that traction affects any of these obstacles to reduction. Moreover, it is extremely doubtful that traction, as it is most commonly applied (to the skin and with minimum weight), has any effect whatsoever. The effect of traction on the need for open reduction is also controversial. Zionts and MacEwen[65] reported successful closed reduction in 75 per cent of their patients after the use of traction, and DeRosa and Feller[61] reported a 91 per cent success rate. However, several recent studies have shown no difference in the rates of femoral head growth disturbances or in successful closed reduction in comparable groups of infants treated with and without traction.[66-74]

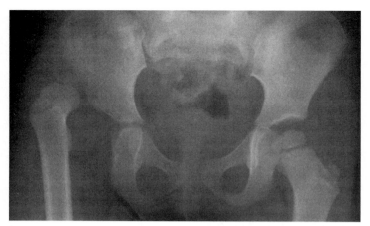

a

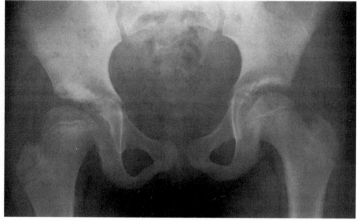

b

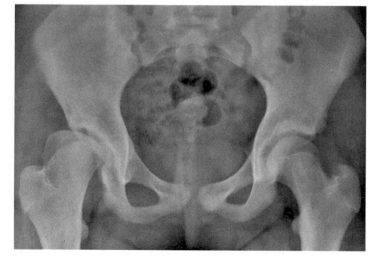

c

Fig. 1.2

(a) Posterior radiograph of the pelvis and hips of a 45-month-old child with a high right hip dislocation. The patient was treated by adductor tenotomy and closed reduction. (b) Anteroposterior radiograph at 9 years of age. There is lateral tilting of the proximal femoral epiphysis on the neck with a bone bar located on the superolateral aspect of the neck. Shenton's line is broken, the head is slightly flattened, and the acetabulum is dysplastic. (c) Anteroposterior radiograph at 11 years of age. There is severe valgus deformity of the femoral head on the neck with residual acetabular dysplasia, poor development of the teardrop figure, and subluxation of the right hip. (Reproduced with permission from Kim H, Morcuende JA, Dolan LA, Weinstein SL: Lateral growth disturbance of the proximal end of the femur after reduction of CDH. *Journal of Bone and Joint Surgery* [Am] **82**: 1692, 2000.)

The authors' general recommendation for treatment in the late-diagnosed DDH is to take the patient to the operating room and attempt a closed reduction under general anaesthesia with arthrographic control. The extra-articular obstacles to reduction are released surgically as necessary, including the adductor longus and iliopsoas. If the reduction is anatomical, the patient is casted. If the reduction is not anatomical, the hip is openly reduced to address the intraarticular obstacles, and subsequently a cast is applied in the appropriate human position. The authors prefer to avoid using the femoral head as a dilating sound to overcome the intra-articular obstacles to reduction. The reduction is maintained in a well-moulded plaster cast, specifically dorsal to the greater trochanters to prevent redislocation. The 'human position' of hyperflexion and limited abduction is the preferred. Wide forced abduction or abduction with internal rotation should be avoided because these approaches are associated with an increased incidence of proximal femoral head growth disturbances. The length of time in the plaster cast varies considerably, as does the subsequent use of abduction orthoses.

An area of continued debate in the treatment of DDH is the surgical approach to open reduction. Open reduction of a dislocated hip can be accomplished through a variety of approaches, including medial, anterior, anterolateral, and lateral. The choice of approach tends to depend on surgical training and experience. The most commonly used approach is the anterolateral Smith–Petersen approach with a modified 'bikini' incision, as described by Salter.[75] The advantage of this approach is that it avoids the medial circumflex vessels and allows capsular plication and a concomitant pelvic osteotomy. However, the disadvantages may include greater blood loss, possible damage to the iliac crest apophysis and hip abductors, and postoperative stiffness. The various medial and anteromedial approaches[73,76-78] have the advantage of approaching the hip joint directly over the site of the obstacles to reduction, requiring minimal soft-tissue dissection, avoidance of the iliac apophysis, minimal blood loss, and excellent cosmesis. The disadvantages include poor access to the acetabulum and inability to plicate the capsule.

The management of the neolimbus during open reduction is not widely agreed upon. Ponseti[33] demonstrated that the neolimbus as seen on arthrogram is frequently a ridge in the articular cartilage of the acetabulum created by pressure of the femoral head rather than a true inverted labrum. In those rare instances that the neolimbus is an obstacle to reduction, it should be everted following radial cuts around its circumference. A long-term follow-up after neolimbus excision demonstrated that 44 per cent of the hips had radiographic degenerative joint changes and 17 per cent had severe arthrosis. This group of patients had been treated between the ages of 1 and 3, and followed to the ages of 16 to 31.[58,79] It is considered prudent in most cases to leave the limbus in place and allow remodelling to occur through superiorly directed pressure from the reduced femoral head.

Open reduction of the hip may be combined with femoral shortening, femoral derotation osteotomy, and pelvic osteotomy. A secondary acetabular and femoral procedure is rarely indicated in children younger than 2 years. The potential for acetabular development after closed and/or open reduction is excellent and continues for 4 to 8 years after the index procedure.[65,80-84] The age range of 2 to 3 years of age at diagnosis is considered a 'grey zone', with some surgeons advocating a concomitant femoral shortening and an acetabular procedure. In children older than 3 years, femoral shortening to avoid excessive pressure on the proximal femur gives far lower rates of avascular necrosis than does preliminary traction followed by open reduction.[85-87]

Derotation osteotomy is almost always combined with femoral shortening in older children. Some authors have advocated the use of derotational osteotomy with almost all open reductions, as excessive femoral anteversion very often accompanies the dislocation. Nevertheless, many surgeons elect simply to perform open reduction since femoral natural derotation will be spontaneously corrected with growth. Specific criteria for derotational osteotomy have yet to be established. Pelvic osteotomy combined with open reduction is used to increase the stable zone of the hip and it is thought that it accelerates the development of the acetabulum. However, no long-term follow-up studies are available to provide evidence of the effectiveness of this osteotomy. Some authors have reported an increased risk of avascular necrosis with the use of concomitant acetabular osteotomies.[88,89]

If a concentric stable reduction is maintained, the acetabulum has the potential for recovery and resumption of normal growth and development. However, when primary treatment fails and residual acetabular dysplasia persists, long-term function is threatened by an increased prevalence of early degenerative joint disease and clinical disability.[1,40,42,43,90-93] However, it is not clear at what point dysplastic changes become irreversible and why this phenomenon occurs. The resumption and adequacy of acetabular development is multifactorial and depends on the age at which the reduction is obtained and on whether the growth potential of the acetabular cartilage and proximal femur is normal. In addition, the biological and mechanical effects of failure to attain a stable congruent joint or the loss of such a joint are also unknown.

Several reconstructive acetabular and femoral osteotomies have been developed to reverse residual hip dysplasia, each with its own degree of technical difficulty, advantages, and disadvantages. Unfortunately, while the orthopaedic literature is replete with studies of the technique and outcomes of these procedures, there is no evidence-based protocol dictating the need for them. Several authors have proposed preventing residual acetabular dysplasia through early operative intervention,[16,94] including femoral osteotomy[90,95-97] or acetabuloplasty.[75,98-100] On the other hand, several studies have described spontaneous remodelling of the acetabulum after initial reduction, indicating that secondary operative procedures may not be routinely necessary.[80,82,101] However, it remains to be established which of the secondary procedures provides long-term beneficial effects and which criteria to use for the optimal matching of patient, procedure, and timing. Systematic clinical studies and animal models could help to answer these questions and provide a better understanding of the effects of these different procedures on the long-term outcomes.

Finally, the most disastrous complications associated with the treatment of DDH are the various degrees of growth disturbances of the proximal femur. They are seen following every method of treatment for DDH, including the Pavlik harness, and can also occur in the contralateral non-affected hip. The growth disturbances may be caused by a vascular insult or by pressure injury to the epiphysis or growth plate. The reported prevalence of growth disturbances after treatment of DDH ranges from zero to 73 per cent. Different opinions exist about the reasons for this large variation. The age at reduction, high dislocations, the use of pre-reduction traction, inadequate reduction, and postoperative immobilization have been implicated. However, a factor in this variation is the question of what exactly is classified as growth disturbance, and many authors think that the incidence may be much less variable than the means by which it is assessed. Several classification schemes have been published including those of Salter et al.[63] Bucholz and Ogden,[102] and Kalamchi and MacEwen.[103] However, there are few studies documenting the inter- and intra-observer reliability of these classifications, and as many as 25 per cent of hips may not fit in a particular classification. In addition, the lateral physeal arrest pattern, which is the most common type of growth disturbance, may not be evident until the patient is more than 10 to 12 years old. Therefore any follow-up study with a duration of less than 12 years may not reflect the actual prevalence of proximal femoral growth disturbances and must be regarded as preliminary.[69,104]

In the treatment of the residual effects of necrosis, reduction must be maintained by corrective femoral and/or acetabular procedures. With arrest of the proximal femoral growth plate, trochanteric overgrowth ensues, producing abductor lurch. A trochanteric physeal plate arrest may maintain the articulotrochanteric distance if performed in children less than 8 years of age; otherwise, distal transfer of the greater trochanter may be necessary. Long-term follow-up studies of patients suffering a femoral head growth disturbance indicate an increased prevalence of early arthritis.[71,105,106]

References

1   Weinstein SL: Natural history of congenital hip dislocation (CDH) and hip dysplasia. *Clinical Orthopaedics and Related Research* **225**: 62–76, 1987.

2   Barlow TG: Early diagnosis and treatment of congenital dislocation of the hip. *Journal of Bone and Joint Surgery* [Br] **44**: 292–301, 1962.

3   Jones D: An assessment of the value of examination of the hip in the newborn. *Journal of Bone and Joint Surgery* [Br] **59**: 318–22, 1977.

4   McKenzie IG (1972). Congenital dislocation of the hip: the development of a regional service. *Journal of Bone and Joint Surgery* [Br] **51**: 18–39, 1972.

5   Noble TC, Pullan CR, Craft AW: Difficulties in diagnosing and managing congenital dislocation of the hip. *British Medical Journal* ii: 620–3, 1978.

6   Ortolani M: Congenital hip dysplasia in the light of early and very early diagnosis. *Clinical Orthopaedics and Related Research* **119**: 6–10, 1976.

7   von Rosen S: Early diagnosis and treatment of congenital dislocation of the hip joint. *Acta Orthopaedica Scandinavica* **26**: 136–55, 1956.

8   Walker G: Problems in the early recognition of congenital hip dislocation. *British Medical Journal* iii: 147–8, 1971.

9   Bjerkreim I, Arseth PH: Congenital dislocation of the hip in Norway: late diagnosis CDH in the years 1970–4. *Acta Paediatrica Scandinavica* **67**: 329–32, 1978.

10 Bjerkreim I, Hagen OH, Ikonomou N, Kase T, Kristiansen T, Arseth PH: Late diagnosis of developmental dislocation of the hip in Norway during the years 1980–1989. *Journal of Pediatric Orthopedics* [Part B] **2**: 112–11, 1993.

11 Catford JC, Bennet GC, Wilkinson JA: Congenital dislocation of the hip: an increasing and still uncontrolled disability? *British Medical Journal* **285**: 1527–30, 1982.

12 Godward S, Dezateux C: Surgery for congenital dislocation of the hip in the UK as a measure of outcome of screening. *Lancet* **351**: 1149–52, 1998.

13 Jones DA, Powell N: Ultrasound and neonatal hip screening: a prospective study of 'high risk' babies. *Journal of Bone and Joint Surgery* [Br] **72**: 457–9, 1990.

14 Williamson J: Difficulties of early diagnosis and treatment of congenital dislocation of the hip in Northern Ireland. *Journal of Bone and Joint Surgery* [Br] **54**: 13–17, 1972.

15 Berman L, Klenerman L: Ultrasound screening for hip abnormalities: preliminary findings in 1001 neonates. *British Medical Journal* **293**: 719–22, 1986.

16 Bialik V, Benyamini O: Developmental dysplasia of the hip: pathophysiology and surgical indications in the first two years of life. *Journal of Pediatric Orthopaedics* [B] **3**: 1–4, 1994.

17 Bialik V, Bialik GM, Wiener F: Prevention of overtreatment of neonatal hip dysplasia by the use of ultrasonography. *Journal of Pediatric Orthopaedics* [B] **7**: 39–42, 1998.

18 Boeree NR, Clarke NMP: Ultrasound imaging and secondary screening for congential dislocation of the hip. *Journal of Bone and Joint Surgery* [Br] **76**: 525–33, 1994.

19 Castelein RM, Sauter AJM: Ultrasound screening for congenital dislocation of the hip in neonates: its value. *Journal of Pediatric Orthopaedics* **18**: 666–70, 1988.

20   Castelein RM, Sauter AJM, de Vlieger M, van Linge B: Natural history of ultrasound hip abnormalities in clinically normal newborns. *Journal of Pediatric Orthopaedics* **12**: 423–7, 1992.

21   Engesaeter LB, Wilson DJ, Nag D, Benson MKD: Ultrasound and congenital dislocation of the hip: the importance of dynamic assessment. *Journal of Bone and Joint Surgery* [Br] **72**: 197–201.

22   Graf R: The diagnosis of congenital hip-joint dislocation by the ultrasonic combound treatment. *Archives of Orthopaedic and Traumatic Surgery* **97**: 117–33, 1980.

23   Harcke HT, Kumar SJ: The role of ultrasound in the diagnosis and management of congenital dislocation and dysplasia of the hip. *Journal of Bone and Joint Surgery* [Am] **73**: 622–8, 1991.

24   Marks DS, Clegg J, Al-Chalabi AN: Routine ultrasound screening for neonatal hip instability. *Journal of Bone and Joint Surgery* [Br] **76**: 534–8, 1994.

25   Terjesen T, Bredland T, Berg V: Ultrasound for hip assessment in the newborn. *Journal of Bone and Joint Surgery* [Br] **71**: 767–73, 1989.

26   Tonnis D, Storch K, Ulbrich H: Results of newborn screening for CDH with and without sonography and correlation of risks factors. *Journal of Pediatric Orthopaedics* **10**: 145–52, 1990.

27   Weintroub S, Grill F: Ultrasonography in developmental dysplasia of the hip. *Journal of Bone and Joint Surgery* [Am] **82**: 1004–18, 2000.

28   Clarke NMP, Clegg J, Al-Chalabi AN: Ultrasound screening of hips at risk for CDH: failure to reduce the incidence of late cases. *Journal of Bone and Joint Surgery* [Br] **71**: 9–12, 1989.

29   Davids JR, Benson LJ, Mubarak SJ, McNeil N: Ultrasonography and developmental dysplasia of the hip: a cost-benefit analysis of three delivery systems. *Journal of Pediatric Orthopaedics* **15**: 325–9, 1995.

30   Hernandez RJ, Cornell RG, Hensinger RN: Ultrasound diagnosis of neonatal congenital dislocation of the hip. A decision analysis assessment. *Journal of Bone and Joint Surgery* [Br] **76**: 539–43, 1994.

31   Dunn PM: Congenital dislocation of the hip (CDH): necropsy studies at birth. *Journal of the Royal Society of Medicine* **62**: 1035–7, 1969.

32   Ponseti IV: Growth and development of the acetabulum in the normal child: anatomical, histological and roentgenographic studies. *Journal of Bone and Joint Surgery* [Am] **60**: 575–9, 1978.

33   Ponseti IV: Morphology of the acetabulum in congenital dislocation of the hip. Gross, histological and roentgenographic studies. *Journal of Bone and Joint Surgery* [Am] **60**: 580–5, 1978.

34   Harrison TJ: The influence of the femoral head on pelvic growth and acetabular form in the rat. *Journal of Anatomy* **95**: 127–32, 1961.

35   Coleman CR, Slager RF, Sith WS: The effect of environmental influence on acetabular development. *Surgical Forum* **9**: 775–80, 1958.

36   Yamamuro T, Doi H: Diagnosis and treatment of congenital dislocation of the hip in newborns. *Journal of the Japanese Orthopaedic Association* **39**: 492, 1965.

37   Pratt WB, Freiberger RH, Arnold WD: Untreated congenital hip dysplasia in the Navajo. *Clinical Orthopaedics and Related Research* **162**: 69–77, 1982.

38   Coleman SS: Congenital dysplasia of the hip in the Navajo infant. *Clinical Orthopaedics and Related Research* **56**: 179–93, 1968.

39   Walker JM: Congenital hip disease in a Cree–Ojibwa population: a retrospective study. *Canadian Medical Association Journal* **116**: 501–4, 1977.

40   Wedge JH, Wasylenko MJ: The natural history of congenital dislocation of the hip: a critical review. *Clinical Orthopaedics and Related Research* **137**: 154–62, 1978.

41   Milgram JW: Morphology of untreated bilateral congenital dislocation of the hips in a seventy-four-year-old man. *Clinical Orthopaedics and Related Research* **119**: 112–15, 1976.

42   Stulberg SD, Harris WH (1974). Acetabular dysplasia and development of osteoarthritis of the hip. In *The Hip: Proceedings of the Open Scientific Meeting Hip Society*, p. 82. CV Mosby, St Louis, MO, 1974.

43   Wiberg G: Studies on dysplastic acetabula and congenital subluxation of the hip joint. *Acta Chirurgica Scandinavica, Supplementum* **58**, 1939.

44   Cooperman DR, Wallensten R, Stulberg SD: Post-reduction avascular necrosis in congenital dislocation of the hip. *Journal of Bone and Joint Surgery* [Am] **62**: 247–58, 1980.

45   Mubarak S, Garfin S, Vance R, McKinnon B, Sutherland D: Pitfalls in the use of Pavlik harness for the treatment of congenital dysplasia, subluxation and dislocation of the hip. *Journal of Bone and Joint Surgery* [Am] **63**: 1239–48, 1981.

46   McHale KA, Corbett D: Parental noncompliance with Pavlik harness treatment of infantile hip problems. *Journal of Pediatric Orthopaedics* **9**: 649–52, 1989.

47   Viere RG, Birch JG, Herring JA *et al.*: Use of the Pavlik harness in congenital dislocation of the hip. Analysis of failures of treatment. *Journal of Bone and Joint Surgery* [Am] **72**: 238–44, 1990.

48   Tucci JJ, Kumar SJ, Guille JT, Rubbo ER: Late acetabular dysplasia following early successful Pavlik harness treatment of congenital dislocation of the hip. *Journal of Pediatric Orthopaedics* **11**: 502–5, 1991.

49   Borges JL, Kumar SJ, Guille JT: Congenital dislocation of the hip in boys. *Journal of Bone and Joint Surgery* [Am] **77**: 975–84, 1995.

50   Camp J, Herring JA, Dworezynski C: Comparison of inpatient and outpatient traction in developmental dislocation of the hip. *Journal of Pediatric Orthopaedics* **14**: 9–12, 1994.

51   Gage JR, Winter RB: Avascular necrosis of the capital femoral epiphysis as a complication of closed reduction of congenital dislocation of the hip. *Journal of Bone and Joint Surgery* [Am] **54**: 373–88, 1972.

52   Crego CH, Schwarzmaan JR: Follow-up study of the early treatment of congential dislocation of the hip. *Journal of Bone and Joint Surgery* [Am] **30**: 428–42, 1948.

53   Esteve R: Congenital dislocation of the hip. A review and assessment of results of treatment with special reference to frame reduction as compared with manipulative reduction. *Journal of Bone and Joint Surgery* [Br] **42**: 253–63, 1960.

54   Kramer J, Schleberger R, Steffen R: Closed reduction by two-phase skin traction and functional splinting in mitigated abduction for treatment of congenital dislocation of the hip. *Clinical Orthopaedics and Related Research* **258**: 27–32, 1990.

55   Mau H, Dorr WM, Henkel L, Lutsche J: Open reduction of congenital dislocation of the hip by Ludloff's method. *Journal of Bone and Joint Surgery* [Am] **53**: 1281–8, 1971.

56   Morel G: The treatment of congenital dislocation and subluxation of the hip in the older child. *Acta Orthopaedica Scandinavica* **46**: 364–99, 1975.

57   Petit P, Queneau P, Borde J: Traitement des luxations et subluxations congenitales de la hanche dans le premiere enfance. *Revue Chirurgie Orthopedique* **48**: 148–86, 1962.

58   Somerville EW: A long term follow-up of congenital dislocation of the hip. *Journal of Bone and Joint Surgery* [Br] **60**: 25–30, 1978.

59 Tavares JO, Gottward DH, Rochelle JR: Guided abduction traction in the treatment of congenital hip dislocation. *Journal of Pediatric Orthopaedics* **14**: 643–9, 1994.

60 Weiner DS, Hoyt WA Jr, Odell HW: Congenital dislocation of the hip. The relationship of premanipulation traction and age to avascular necrosis of the femoral head. *Journal of Bone and Joint Surgery* [Am] **59**: 306–11, 1977.

61 DeRosa GP, Feller N: Treatment of congenital dislocation of the hip. Management before walking age. *Clinical Orthopaedics and Related Research* **225**: 77–85, 1987.

62 Fish DN, Hezenberg JE, Hensinger RN: Current practice in the use of prerreduction traction for congenital dislocation of the hip. *Journal of Pediatric Orthopaedics* **11**: 149–53, 1991.

63 Salter RB, Kostiuk J, Dallas S: Avascular necrosis of the femoral head as a complication of treatment for congenital dislocation of the hip in young children: a clinical and experimental investigation. *Canadian Journal of Surgery* **12**: 44–61, 1969.

64 Kruse RW, Bowen JR: Complications in the treatment of developmental dysplasia of the hip. In *Complications in pediatric orthopaedic surgery* (ed. CH Epps Jr and JR Bowen), pp. 337–61. JB Lippincott, Philadelphia, PA, 1995.

65 Zionts LE, MacEwen GD: Treatment of congenital dislocation of the hip in children between the ages pf one and three years. *Journal of Bone and Joint Surgery* [Am] **68**: 829–46, 1986.

66 Brougham DI, Broughton NS, Cole WG, Menelaus MB: Avascular necrosis following closed reduction of congenital dislocation of the hip. Review of influencing factors and long-term follow-up. *Journal of Bone and Joint Surgery* [Br] **72**: 557–62, 1990.

67 Coleman S: A critical analysis of the value of preliminary traction in the treatment of CDH. *Orthopaedic Transactions* **13**: 180, 1987.

68 Kahle WK, Anderson MB, Alpert J, Stevens PM, Coleman SS: The value of preliminary traction in the treatment of congenital dislocation of the hip. *Journal of Bone and Joint Surgery* [Am] **72**: 1043–7, 1990.

69 Morcuende JA, Meyer MD, Dolan LA, Weinstein SL: Long-term outcome after open reduction through an anteromedial approach for congenital dislocation of the hip. *Journal of Bone and Joint Surgery* [Am] **79**: 810–17, 1997.

70 Quinn RH, Renshaw TS, DeLuca PA: Preliminary traction in the treatment of developmental dislocation of the hip. *Journal of Pediatric Orthopaedics*, **14**: 636–42, 1994.

71 Thomas IH, Dunin AAJ, Cole WG, Menelaus MB: Avascular necrosis after open reduction for congenital dislocation of the hip: analysis of causative factors and natural history. *Journal of Pediatric Orthopaedics* **9**: 525–31, 1989.

72 Tumer Y, Ward WT, Grudziak J: Medial open reduction in the treatment of developmental dislocation of the hip. *Journal of Pediatric Orthopaedics* **17**: 176–80, 1997.

73 Weinstein SL, Ponseti IV: Congenital dislocation of the hip. *Journal of Bone and Joint Surgery* [Am] **61**: 119–24, 1979.

74 Weinstein SL: Traction in developmental dislocation of the hip. Is its use justified? *Clinical Orthopaedics and Related Research* **338**: 79–85, 1997.

75 Salter RB: Innominate osteotomy in the treatment of developmental hip dysplasia and subluxation of the hip. *Journal of Bone and Joint Surgery* [Br] **43**: 518–39, 1961.

76 Ludloff K: The open reduction of the congenital hip dislocation by an anterior incision. *American Journal of Orthopaedic Surgery* **10**: 438–54, 1913.

77 Ferguson AB Jr: Primary open reduction of congenital dislocation of the hip using a median adductor approach. *Journal of Bone and Joint Surgery* [Am] **55**: 671–89, 1973.

78 Weinstein SL: Closed versus open reduction of congenital dislocation in patients under 2 years of age. *Orthopaedics* **13**: 221–7, 1990.

79 Gibson PH, Benson MKD: Congenital dislocation of the hip. Review at maturity of 147 hips treated by excision of the limbus and derotation osteotomy. *Journal of Bone and Joint Surgery* [Br] **64**, 169–75, 1982.

80 Cherney DL, Westin GW: Acetabular development in the infant's dysplastic hips. *Clinical Orthopaedics and Related Research* **242**: 98–103, Janson-RomanOsF.

81 Heyman CH: Long-term results following a bone-shelf operation for congenital and some other dislocations of the hip in children. *Journal of Bone and Joint Surgery* [Am] **45**: 1113–46, 1963.

82 Lindstrom JR, Ponseti IV, Wenger D: Acetabular development after reduction in congenital dislocation of the hip. *Journal of Bone and Joint Surgery* [Am] **61**: 112–18, 1979.

83 Weintroub S, Green I, Terdiman R, Weissman SL: Growth and development of congenitally dysplastic hips reduced in early infancy. *Journal of Bone and Joint Surgery* [Am] **61**: 125–30, 1979.

84 Williamson DM, Glover SD, Benson MKD: Congenital dislocation of the hip presenting after the age of three years. *Journal of Bone and Joint Surgery* [Br] **71**: 745–51, 1989.

85 Dimitriou IX, Cavadias AX: One-stage surgical procedure for congenital dislocation of the hip in older children. Long-term results. *Clinical Orthopaedics and Related Research* **246**: 148–56, 1989.

86 Galpin RD, Roach IW, Wenger DR, Herring IA, Birch IG: One-stage treatment of congenital dislocation of the hip in older children, including femoral shortening. *Journal of Bone and Joint Surgery* [Am] **71**: 734–41, 1989.

87 Schoenecker PL, Strecker WB: Congenital dislocation of the hip in children. Comparison of the effects of femoral shortening and skeletal traction in treatment. *Journal of Bone and Joint Surgery* [Am] **66**: 21–7, 1984.

88 Marden-Bey TH, MacEwen GD: Congenital hip dislocation after walking age. *Journal of Pediatric Orthopaedics* **2**: 478–86, 1982.

89 Powell EN, Gerratana FJ, Gage JR: Open reduction for congenital hip dislocation: the risk of avascular necrosis with three different approaches. *Journal of Pediatric Orthopaedics* **6**: 127–32, 1986.

90 Lloyd-Roberts GC: The role of femoral osteotomy in the treatment of congenital dislocation of the hip. In *Congenital dislocation of the hip* (ed. MO Tachdjian), pp. 427–35. Churchill Livingstone, New York, 1982.

91 Tasnavites A, Murray DW, Benson MKD: Improvement in acetabular index after reduction of hips with developmental. *Journal of Bone and Joint Surgery* [Br] **75**: 755–9, 1993.

92 Tonnis D: Normal values of the hip joint for evaluation of X-rays in children and adults. *Clinical Orthopaedics and Related Research* **119**: 39–47, 1976.

93 Weinstein SL: Congenital dislocation of the hip. Long-range problems, residual signs, and symptoms after successful treatment. *Clinical Orthopaedics and Related Research* **281**: 69–74, 1992.

94 Barrett WP, Staheli LT, Chew DE: The effectiveness of the Salter innominate osteotomy in the treatment of congenital dysplasia of the hip. *Journal of Bone and Joint Surgery* [Am] **68**: 79–87, 1986.

95 Kasser JR, Bowen JR, MacEwen GD: Varus derotation osteotomy in the treatment of persistent dysplasia in developmental hip dysplasia of the hip. *Journal of Bone and Joint Surgery* [Am] **67**: 195–202, 1985.

96 Schoenecker PL, Anderson DJ, Capelli AM: The acetabular response to proximal femoral varus rotational osteotomy: Results after failure of post-reduction abduction splinting in patients who had congenital dislocation of the hip. *Journal of Bone and Joint Surgery* [Am] **77**: 990–7, 1995.

97 Somerville EW, Scott JC: The direct approach to congenital dislocation of the hip. *Journal of Bone and Joint Surgery* [Br] **39**: 623–40, 1957.

98 Fasciszewski T, Kiefer GN, Coleman SS: Pemberton osteotomy for residual acetabular dysplasia. *Journal of Bone and Joint Surgery* [Am] **75**: 643–9, 1993.

99 Pemberton PA: Pericapsular osteotomy of the ilium for the treatment of congenital subluxation and dislocation of the hip. *Journal of Bone and Joint Surgery* [Am] **47**: 65–86, 1965.

100 Salter RB, Dubos JP: The first fifteen years' experience with innominate osteotomy in the treatment of developmental hip dysplasia and subluxation of the hip. *Clinical Orthopaedics and Related Research* **98**: 72–103, 1974.

101 Harris NH, Lloyd-Roberts GC, Gallien R: Acetabular development in congenital dislocation of the hip, with special reference to the indications for acetabuloplasty and pelvic or femoral realignment osteotomy. *Journal of Bone and Joint Surgery* [Br] **57**: 46–52, 1975.

102 Bucholz RW, Ogden IA: Patterns of ischemic necrosis of the proximal femur in nonoperatively treated congenital hip disease. In *The Hip: Proceedings of the 6th Open Scientific Meeting of the Hip Society*, pp. 43–63. CV Mosby, St. Louis, MO, 1978.

103 Kalamchi A, MacEwen GD: Avascular necrosis following treatment of congenital dislocation of the hip. *Journal of Bone and Joint Surgery* [Am] **62**: 876–888, 1980.

104 Kim H, Morcuende JA, Dolan LA, Weinstein SL: Lateral growth disturbance of the proximal end of the femur after reduction of CDH. *Journal of Bone and Joint Surgery* [Am] **82**: 1692–1700, 2000.

105 Cooperman DR, Wallensten R, Stulberg SD: Acetabular dysplasia in the adult. *Clinical Orthopaedics and Related Research* **175**: 79–85, 1983.

106 Tonnis D: *Congenital hip dislocation: avascular necrosis*. Thieme-Stratton, New York, 1982.

2

Perthes disease: natural history, results of treatment, and controversies

J.A. Herring

Introduction

It is not difficult to discuss controversies concerning Legg–Perthes disease—in fact, it is hard to find a topic which is not controversial! The natural history of the disorder has long been considered to be one of benign resolution in the majority of hips, with only a few having long-term disability. With modern studies the picture has changed and we now know that about half the patients will develop degenerative disease by their sixth decade of life. Methods of classification have evolved and will continue to do so. Currently we use the lateral pillar classification which is useful in predicting likely outcome. An additional dimension has emerged with the addition of serial technetium scanning which evaluates the loss and return of perfusion of the femoral head.

Treatment has always been controversial and continues to be so. Long and arduous methods of bracing and immobilization have been replaced by both operative and non-operative approaches. The treatment camps fall into three categories: those who never operate, those who almost always operate, and those who pick and choose.

Natural history

The first 'Perthes enigma' is that of the natural history. Compared with other disorders such as untreated hip sepsis, tuberculosis of the hip, and rheumatoid arthritis, Legg–Perthes disease is relatively benign. The affected children present with a limp and experience mild pain which is exacerbated with activity. As the femoral head softens, primarily during the stage of fragmentation, pain and stiffness increase and the child becomes less active. Once reossification begins in the femoral head, which can occur as early as 6 months or as late as several years after onset, symptoms gradually resolve and the child will return to previous activities. Thus, by most standards, it is a benign disease.

On the other hand, for some this disorder is a more debilitating process. For example, an active 10-year-old boy begins to feel pain in his hip and is found to have Legg–Perthes disease. For that individual the process may be one of persistent hip pain and disability with only partial relief when the head is healed. Treatment may or may not alter this outcome.

From a third viewpoint, the long-term natural history is also controversial. Many studies have shown that most patients are doing very well in adulthood. Ratliff[1] followed 34 hips for an average of 30 years and found that four of five were fully active and pain free. However, only two of five had good results radiographically. Englehardt[2] reported 55 patients followed for an average of 42 years, noting that only nine hips had disabling arthritis. Saito et al.[3] reported an 18-year follow-up of 56 hips, with 13 having coxarthrosis. Perpich et al.[4] reported 40 patients with an average follow-up of 30 years and found only 10 per cent with poor outcomes. Factors which these various authors found predicted a poor outcome included age at onset, lateral calcification of the femoral head, a steep slope to the acetabulum, and loss of sphericity of the femoral head.

In a classic review by Stulberg et al.[5], the shape of the femoral head at maturity was classified and shown to have a strong prognostic influence. Heads which were within 2 mm of a circle (groups I and II) did not develop degenerative changes. Those which were ovoid and congruent (group III) did well but showed degenerative changes radiographically. Those which were flattened (group IV) showed more extensive degenerative changes. Group V, which were of older onset with collapse of the femoral head without acetabular remodelling, i.e. a square peg in a round hole, did the worst, with early symptomatic degenerative disease.

In 1971, Gower and Johnston[6] reported a follow-up of 36 patients at 36 years and found good results in most of them. The average Iowa Hip Score was 91 and only three patients required surgery for degenerative hip disease. McAndrew and Weinstein[7] followed this group of patients again at 47.7 years and found a major shift in outcome as they reached the fifth and sixth decades. Half of the group had either had a hip replacement or were disabled enough to have such surgery recommended.

Studies performed in the last 10 years continue to show divergent results. In 1992, Chigwanda[8] reported 30 untreated hips from Wales with 60 per cent good, 23 per cent fair, and only 3 per cent poor results. On the other hand, Norlin et al.[9] followed 20 hips, all untreated, after 19 years of age. Only six had no pain, and only two reached 100 points on the Iowa Hip Scale. None were spherical on radiographs.

From this information, we can conclude that Legg–Perthes disease is not the worst disease that can occur, but it does cause a year or two of disability during childhood and there is a fifty–fifty chance of symptomatic hip disease in later adulthood. A treatment which can be shown to improve femoral head sphericity should improve that later prognosis.

Classification

The remarkable variability of the Legg–Perthes syndrome is such that clinicians have searched from the outset for a reliable way to predict the likely course of the disease. Radiographic classifications began with Legg,[10] who proposed a mushroom type and a cap type. Waldenstrom[11] suggested a three-part classification and rather nicely described some of the findings later termed risk signs. Catterall[12] proposed his four-part classification in 1971 and noted that the presence of risk factors was an essential feature of the prognostic information available on radiographs. Subsequently, Herring et al.[13] developed the lateral pillar classification to assess the likelihood of femoral head collapse more specifically. Recently, Conway[14] has proposed classifying severity based on serial technetium scans of the femoral head. We may ask why there are so many different approaches and which is most useful.

Some of the confusion about classification has to do with terminology. A commonly used term is femoral head 'involvement'. What does this mean? In the early 'avascular' phase of the disease an MRI or a bone scan will show the entire femoral head to be ischaemic. Radiographs in the initial phase usually show uniform increased density throughout the femoral head. Total head involvement would be a safe conclusion (Fig. 2.1). However, as the femoral head begins to fragment, several different patterns emerge. Some heads have a central density which collapses relative to the medial and lateral portions of the head on the anteroposterior radiograph. Others have collapse which includes the lateral and central portions, while still others have collapse of the entire head. In this stage of the disease, 'involvement' could mean the collapsed segment. (Catterall[12] used the term 'sequestrated'.) Serial technetium scans show several patterns of returning blood supply. A rapid return which portends a good result is called recanalization, while a slow process which indicates a poor outcome is called neovascularization.[14] Perhaps the whole head is 'involved' somehow, but the physiological events vary considerably. I suggest that we avoid this ambiguous term 'involvement' altogether in favor of terms like 'collapse' and 'extrusion' which specify femoral head morphology.

For two decades the Catterall classification was almost exclusively used to stratify involvement of the femoral head. During that time several studies questioned the ability of various orthopaedists to reproduce the classification. Christensen et al.[15] and Hardcastle et al.[16], in separate studies, found unacceptable inter-observer agreement in its use. Our group of orthopaedists in the Legg–Perthes Multicenter Study were also unable to find enough inter-observer

23

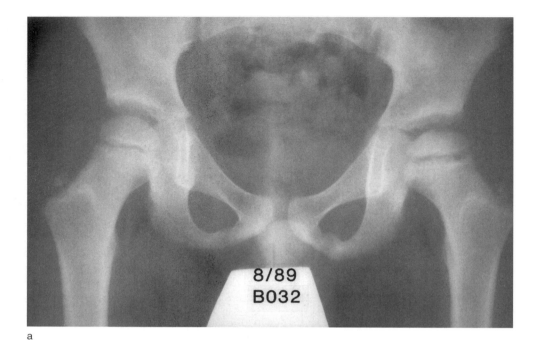

a

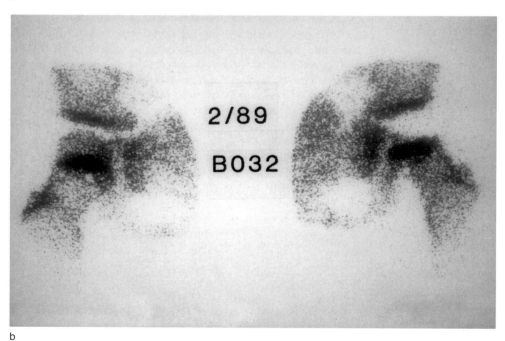

b

Fig. 2.1

A patient with Legg–Perthes disease and a misleading bone scan. (a) The earliest radiograph showing widening of the joint and mildly increased density throughout the femoral head. (b) A technetium scan showing almost total absence of blood flow. Is this total head 'involvement'?

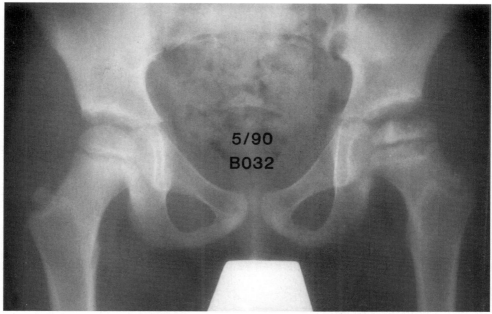

c

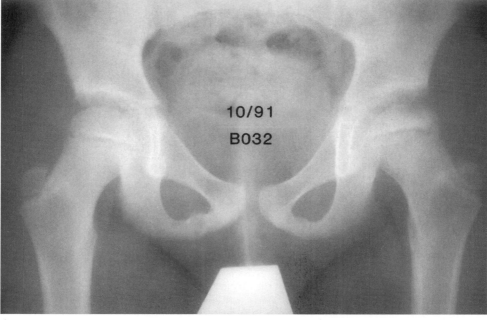

d

Fig. 2.1 *(continued)*

(c) Radiograph at maximal fragmentation showing a central area of collapse with preserved lateral and medial pillars of the head. (d) Radiograph taken several years later showing healing with no deformity. This case illustrates how the term 'involvement' is misleading.

25

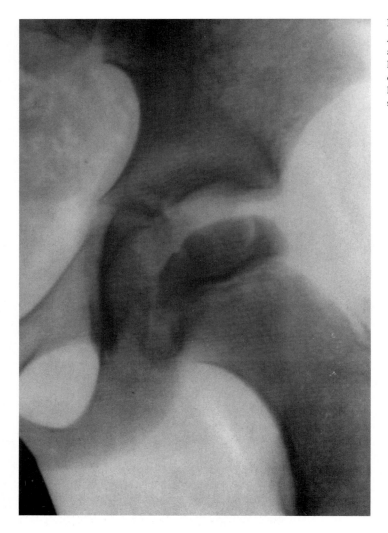

Fig. 2.2
An example of a hip classified as lateral pillar type A. The lateral pillar is clearly demarcated and there is no lucency or collapse of that segment of the head.

agreement to use the Catterall classification as the basis of the study. Consequently, we developed the lateral pillar classification.[13] Several subsequent studies[17-19] have shown better inter-observer agreement and strong correlation of classification with outcome with this system.

The lateral pillar classification is based on changes within the lateral portion of the femoral head. Specifically, we evaluate the degree of collapse in the early fragmentation stage. In a group A hip there is no collapse of the lateral pillar, and usually no density changes (Fig. 2.2). In group B hips there are density changes in the lateral pillar and a loss of height up to but not exceeding 50 per cent of the original height of the pillar (Fig. 2.3). In group C hips the collapse of the lateral column exceeds 50 per cent of the original height

Fig. 2.3

An example of a lateral pillar type B hip. There are density changes in the lateral pillar and it has lost some height, yet retains more than half its original height.

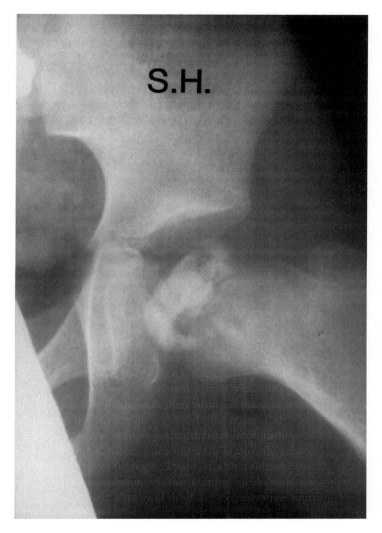

S.H.

(Fig. 2.4). Actual measurement of these degrees of collapse are difficult. One can compare with the uninvolved hip in unilateral cases, but the designation is usually an estimate rather than a measured difference.

In addition, certain patterns emerge in the lateral pillar system. In group B there is often early depression of the central portion of the femoral head with a demarcation between the central and lateral portions. Conversely, when there is early collapse of the lateral pillar relative to the central portion, a type C pattern subsequently evolves.

At present the lateral pillar classification is used widely and is useful in predicting likely outcome. When the classification is considered relative to the maturity of the patient, its predictive value improves. Because most children with Legg–Perthes disease are skeletally immature, we find that skeletal age, assessed by either

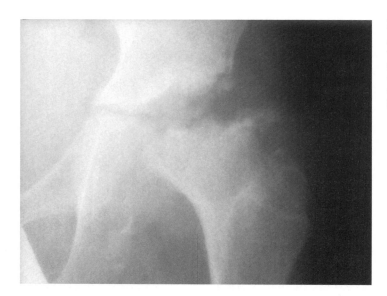

Fig. 2.4

An example of a lateral pillar type C hip. The lateral segment of the head has collapsed beyond half its original height, and in this case has extruded laterally.

wrist or pelvic films, is more useful than chronological age as a prognostic factor. In our experience, all group A hips do well without treatment. Group B hips have a good prognosis in children with a bone age of 6 years or less. Those with a bone age between 6 and 9 years have an intermediate prognosis, while those over 10 years have a higher incidence of poor results. Hips in group C risk a poor outcome at any age, even 4 or 5 years, with the older hips faring the worst. As we move forward, greater use of more physiological studies such as bone scan and MRI may add to our prognostic armamentarium.

Results of treatment

Now for the real controversy. The treatment of Legg–Perthes disease remains the most controversial area within paediatric orthopaedics today. Many of my colleagues feel that it is usually a benign disease and that the more severe cases will not be improved by treatment. Their philosophy usually results in symptomatic treatment such as rest, traction, anti-inflamatory agents, and an occasional intervention to improve range of motion. A second philosophy is that which focuses on range of motion. With this philosophy, the range of motion is the indicator of success or failure. If a 'good' range of motion can be maintained, all will be well. Methods to improve motion in stiff hips include traction, muscle releases, Petrie cast wear, and bracing.

Many orthopaedists subscribe to the containment approach, even though Rab[20] has shown that true containment of the femoral head is impossible. Salter[21] showed in pig experiments that avascular heads which were 'contained' within the acetabulum by abduction plasters, and were allowed to move in flexion and extension, stayed round. (Hips left alone or placed in abduction flattened.) Containment may be obtained by casts, braces, or by surgery which repositions the femoral head (varus osteotomy) or the acetabulum (innominate osteotomy) or both. Shelf arthroplasty is also considered by some to contain the femoral head.

The wide diversity of opinion among the paediatric orthopaedic community led to the formation of a multicenter study. Five treatment groups have been studied: no treatment, range-of-motion treatment, Atlanta Scottish Rite brace treatment, femoral varus osteotomy, and Salter innominate osteotomy. The results of the study await the skeletal maturity of the patients. Based on certain early patterns of outcome we have adopted a strategy of management which we continue to evaluate. We believe that hips in lateral pillar group A need only minimal symptomatic management. Hips in group B in children with a skeletal age of 6 years or less also receive only symptomatic treatment. Group B hips in children with skeletal ages of greater than 6 years are treated with surgical containment. Group C hips in all children over 6 years are also treated surgically. Currently, we prefer the Salter procedure for children up to age 10. After age 10 we prefer combined mild varus femoral osteotomy with the Salter procedure. We also prefer to initiate surgical treatment in the early phases of the disease, i.e. the stage of increased density or early fragmentation. We find that the remodelling ability of the femoral head is reduced in the later stages of the process.[22]

Conclusion

I continue to be mesmerized by the problems of Legg–Perthes disease. I have read and re-read the literature, carefully studied hundreds of patients both treated and untreated, and have seen clear differences in outcome which may be due to treatment. Yet I still find it hard to pick the right treatment for each patient that I see. Hopefully, as our studies mature, definitive answers will emerge so that our treatment will be based on solid evidence and not prior habit patterns.

References

1 Ratliff AH: Perthes' disease. A study of thirty-four hips observed for thirty years. *Journal of Bone and Joint Surgery* [Br] **49**: 102, 1967.

2 Englehardt P: Late prognosis of Perthes' disease. Which factors determine arthritis risk? *Zeitschrift für Orthopädie* **123**: 168, 1985.

3 Saito S, Takaoka K, Ono K *et al.*: Residual deformities related to arthrotic change after Perthes' disease. A long-term follow-up of fifty-one cases. *Archives of Orthopaedic and Traumatic Surgery* **104**: 7, 1985.

4 Perpich M, McBeath A, Kruse D: Long-term follow-up of Perthes disease treated with spica casts. *Journal of Pediatric Orthopaedics* **3**: 160, 1983.

5 Stulberg SD, Cooperman DR, Wallensten R: The natural history of Legg–Calvé–Perthes disease. *Journal of Bone and Joint Surgery* [Am] **63**: 1095, 1981.

6 Gower WE, Johnston RC: Legg–Perthes disease: long-term follow-up of thirty-six patients. *Journal of Bone and Joint Surgery* [Am] **53**: 759, 1971.

7 McAndrew MP, Weinstein SL: A long-term follow-up of Legg–Calvé–Perthes disease. *Journal of Bone and Joint Surgery* [Am] **66**: 860, 1984.

8 Chigwanda PC: Early natural history of untreated Perthes' disease. *Central African Journal of Medicine* **38**: 334, 1992.

9 Norlin R, Hammerby S, Tkaczuk H: The natural history of Perthes' disease. *International Orthopaedics* **15**: 13, 1991.

10 Legg A: Osteochondral trophopathy of the hip joint. *Surgery, Gynecology and Obstetrics* **22**: 307, 1916.

11 Waldenstrom H: The definite form of coxa plana. *Acta Radiologica* **1**: 384, 1922.

12 Catterall A: The natural history of Perthes' disease. *Journal of Bone and Joint Surgery* [Br] **53**: 37, 1971.

13 Herring JA, Neustadt JB, Williams JJ *et al.*: The lateral pillar classification of Legg–Calvé–Perthes disease. *Journal of Pediatric Orthopaedics* **12**: 143, 1992.

14 Conway JJ: A scintigraphic classification of Legg–Calvé–Perthes disease. *Seminars in Nuclear Medicine* **23**: 274, 1993.

15 Christensen F, Soballe K, Ejsted R *et al.*: The Catterall classification of Perthes' disease: an assessment of reliability. *Journal of Bone and Joint Surgery* [Br] **68**: 614, 1986.

16 Hardcastle PH, Ross R, Hamalainen M *et al.*: Catterall grouping of Perthes' disease. An assessment of observer error and prognosis using the Catterall classification. *Journal of Bone and Joint Surgery* [Br] **62**: 428, 1980.

17 Farsetti P, Tudisco D, Caterini R *et al.*: The Herring lateral pillar classification for prognosis in Perthes disease: late results in 49 patients treated conservatively. *Journal of Bone and Joint Surgery* [Br] **77**: 739, 1995.

18 Ismail A, Macnicol M: Prognosis in Perthes disease. *Journal of Bone and Joint Surgery* [Br] **80**: 310, 1998.

19 Ritterbusch JF, Shantharam SS, Gelinas C: Comparison of lateral pillar classification and Catterall classification of Legg–Calvé–Perthes disease. *Journal of Pediatric Orthopaedics* **13**: 200, 1993.

20 Rab GT: Determination of femoral head containment during gait. *Biomaterials, Medical Devices and Artificial Organs* **11**: 31, 1983.

21 Salter R: Experimental and clinical aspects of Perthes' disease. *Journal of Bone and Joint Surgery* [Br] **48**: 393, 1966.

22 Herring J: *Legg–Calvé–Perthes disease*. AAOS, Rosemont, IL, 1996.

3

Slipped capital femoral epiphysis: natural history, results of treatment, and controversies

R. Baxter Willis

Introduction

Slipped capital femoral epiphysis (SCFE) is a condition which occurs during a period of rapid growth in adolescence. Owing to a weakening of the proximal femoral growth plate and increased shear stress most commonly associated with obesity, the capital femoral epiphysis displaces posteriorly and medially, resulting in a deformity of the hip which alters normal hip motion, causes pain, and may eventually lead to degenerative joint disease.

In recent years, owing to increased understanding of the anatomy of SCFE and improved imaging techniques, the incidence of major complications such as pin penetration and chondrolysis have been reduced to near zero. However, the problem of avascular necrosis related to unstable slipped epiphysis remains a serious challenge.

Etiology

Many theories have been proposed to account for SCFE. In all likelihood, its etiology is multifactorial,[1-6] with the major factors responsible being mechanical[1-3,7-10] and biochemical,[6,11-17] but heredity[18] and pathological alterations[19-22] in the physis of the proximal femur also play a role.

Mechanical factors

The majority of patients who develop slipped epiphysis are obese.[1,4-6,8,23] A number of studies have demonstrated that more than 50 per cent of patients with SCFE are greater than the 95th percentile for weight for their age.[5,6,8,23] In addition to increased body weight, there are anatomical variations in the hip joint which support the concept that mechanical factors are responsible. Femoral retroversion is a more frequent finding in children with

SCFE.[1,7,24] Normal-weight adolescents average 10.6° of femoral neck anteversion, while obese adolescents have an average of 0.4° anteversion.[1] In addition, children with SCFE have an increase of 8°–11° in physeal slope compared with the normal hip.[24] Acetabular coverage is also increased from a normal value of 33°–37° when one compares Wiberg's centre–edge angle.[25] This increased containment may allow for increased shear stresses to be transmitted to the proximal femoral physis.

Biochemical and hormonal factors

A number of studies have examined the relationship of oestrogens and androgens to physeal strength.[5] SCFE is a disease of puberty. At puberty, overall physeal strength or resistance to shear stresses is reduced because of the increased width of the hypertrophic zone and the zone of provisional calcification.[10,16] Oestrogens also increase the resistance to shear stresses whereas androgens decrease physeal strength.[5]

SCFE is known to occur in children with certain endocrinopathies.[5,14,15,17,26] Of all the endocrine disorders, hypothyroidism is probably the most common.[10,11,14] Hypothyroidism in the growing child is associated with growth retardation and can often be recognized on the presenting plain radiographs. By the age of approximately 10 years, the capital femoral epiphysis tends to overlap the femoral neck metaphysis on the anteroposterior radiograph. Because of the growth-retardation effect in hypothyroidism, the capital femoral epiphysis is narrower than the femoral neck. When this combination of changes is noted in a child with a slip, the diagnosis of hypothyroidism should be strongly considered.[5]

Other endocrinopathies associated with SCFE include children taking growth hormone supplementation[17] and children with hypogonadism.[14]

Although most children with SCFE do not have a demonstrable endocrinopathy, it should be seriously considered in the child younger or older than the standard age presentation curve.[5,14]

Heredity

Heredity also plays a role in SCFE.[18] If one child presents with a slip, the chance of a second child in the family being affected is approximately 7 per cent. Of all children presenting with a slip, 14.5 per cent have a family member who shares the same diagnosis.

Histopathology of the proximal femoral growth plate

Some pathological specimens of the growth plate have been obtained at the time of open bone graft epiphyseodesis.[5,19,20,22] Standard haematoxylin and eosin stains have demonstrated clustering of the chondrocytes and a generalized disorder and disarray in the otherwise ordered hypertrophic zone. In the provisional zone, there are glycoprotein/proteoglycan changes when stains are employed to enhance or visualize proteoglycans.[5,19,20]

The ultrastructure of the hypertrophic zone has been examined under high-power electron microscopy. These studies have demonstrated defective collagen fibrils and collagen banding. In summary, the histopathological studies by routine and electron microscopy have shown consistent alterations in the collagen–proteoglycan framework of the physis.[20] The same changes are seen in the proximal tibial physis in adolescent Blount's disease. Whether these changes are cause or effect remains controversial.

Epidemiology and demographics

Incidence

The incidence of SCFE varies widely by geographical location, with incidences of 10.08 per 100 000[3,23] in the northeast United States, 2.13 per 100 000 in the southwest United States,[23] and 0.2 per 100 000 in eastern Japan.[23]

Demographics

SCFE is a disease of obese males. The male-to-female ratio of involvement is 60 per cent male to 40 per cent female.[3] It occurs bilaterally in 18–50 per cent of cases depending on the particular study.[3,27,28] The incidence of bilaterality increases with a younger age of presentation for the first hip. If the child is 12 years of age at initial presentation, there is a great likelihood of the other hip being involved. Approximately 50 per cent of hips in bilateral cases are diagnosed simultaneously, while 50 per cent are diagnosed subsequently. The average age of presentation is 13.5 years for boys and 12.0 years for girls, with an age range of 9–16 years.

If the child presents with a slip at 13 years or older, there is a decreased likelihood of the other hip being involved. Loder et al.[29] found that 82 per cent of the second slipped epiphyses occurred within 18 months of the first slip.

The age at presentation decreases with obesity, with an age of presentation of 12.4 years if the child is above the 95th percentile for weight but of 14.3 years if the child is below the 10th percentile.[3]

The relative racial frequencies of SCFE were investigated in an international multicentre study.[4] Whites were assigned a relative mean frequency of 1.0; Polynesians had the highest frequency at 4.5, followed by blacks (2.2), Amerindians (1.05), and Indonesian-Malays (0.5), with the lowest frequency being found in the Indo-Mediterranean race (0.1).[4] This relative racial frequency coincides with average body weights among the same racial groups.

There is a seasonal variation in the incidence of slipped epiphysis in the northern hemisphere.[30] North of latitude 40° N, the highest incidence occurs in summer and autumn which may coincide with the period of highest physical activity in the age groups involved.[30]

Classification

There are a number of classifications of slipped epiphysis. The widely used and traditional temporal system classifies SCFE in relation to the duration of symptoms: an **acute** slipped epiphysis has a symptom duration of less than 3 weeks,[31] a **chronic** slip has a symptom duration greater than 3 weeks, and an **acute-on-chronic** slip has symptoms of duration greater than 3 weeks with a recent sudden increase in symptom severity.[5]

Loder *et al*.[32] have advocated a newer and more practical classification based on physeal stability: in a **stable** slip the patient is able to ambulate with or without crutches, usually without, and in an **unstable** slip the patient is unable to ambulate even with crutches (Figs 3.1 and 3.2). Kallio *et al*.[33,34] reported on the sonographic findings of the hip in stable and unstable slips. They demonstrated that the characteristic findings in an unstable slip are the presence of a hip joint effusion in association with the absence of femoral neck or metaphyseal remodelling. This can be an important diagnostic tool prior to treatment in unstable slips because it implies that

Fig. 3.1

Anteroposterior radiograph of pelvis of an 11-year-old boy with unstable (acute) SCFE of left hip.

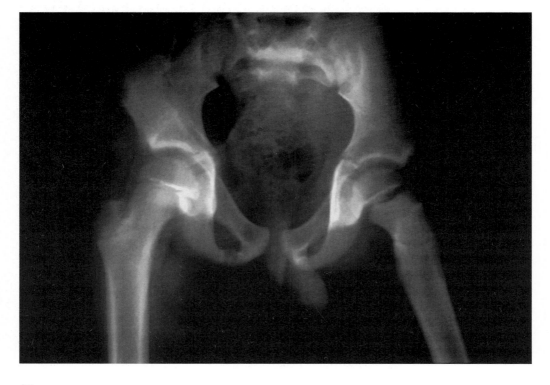

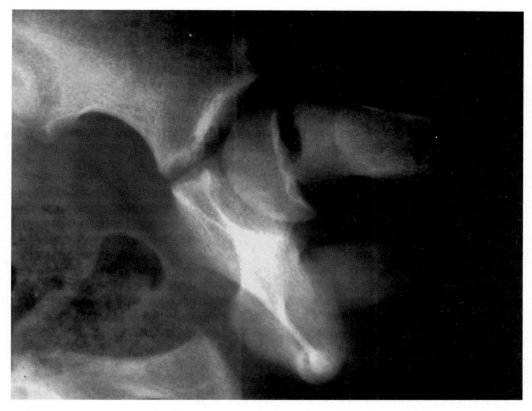

Fig. 3.2
True lateral radiograph of the patient in Fig. 3.1. Note the lack of remodelling of the femoral neck and the absence of new bone formation on the inferior aspect of the neck seen in stable (chronic) slips.

a 'reduction' or 'gentle manipulation' may be safe. Exactly opposite ultrasound findings are noted in stable slips, i.e. no hip joint effusion is seen but evidence of femoral neck remodelling is visualized.

Loder's classification scheme is widely employed today because it provides a definite prognosis depending on the type. The complications of avascular necrosis and chondrolysis are virtually unheard of in stable slips as long as the appropriate surgical technique is used. However, in unstable slips the incidence of avascular necrosis is markedly increased, approaching 50 per cent even if appropriate surgery is performed.[6,31,32,35-43]

Radiographic classification systems are also used to characterize the severity of the slip. The first method employs the degree of epiphyseal displacement as a percentage of the width of the metaphysis. In a mild slip the displacement is less than one-third of the femoral neck metaphysis, in a moderate slip the displacement is up to half the width of the femoral neck, and in a severe slip the displacement is more than half the width of the femoral neck.[5]

Southwick[44] devised another radiographic classification based on the lateral epiphyseal shaft angle. A mild slip has an angle of 30°, a moderate slip has an angle of 30°–50°, and a severe has an angle of more than 50°. A lateral epiphyseal shaft angle of up to 12° is considered normal.

Natural history

The true natural history of slipped epiphysis remains an enigma because of the paucity of true natural history studies and long-term follow-up investigations.[6,10,45-49] Stulberg et al.[26] described the 'pistol grip deformity' in approximately 40 per cent of patients without known prior hip disease who were undergoing total hip replacement. He hypothesized that this deformity was secondary to old, healed, and unrecognized SCFE. Murray[50] described a 'tilt deformity' similar to the 'pistol grip deformity' in 40 per cent of 200 patients thought to have primary degenerative joint disease. Resnick[51] demonstrated that the 'tilt deformity' was related to remodelling changes from osteoarthritis and not from SCFE.

Carney and Weinstein[52] reported on the natural history of untreated chronic SCFE. They evaluated 28 patients with 31 involved hips at a mean follow-up of 41 years: 17 hips were classified as mild slips, 11 as moderate, and three as severe. The mean age of the patients at follow-up was 54 years. Complications occurred in four of the hips: two displaced further to become severe slips, one mild slip developed chondrolysis, and one severe slip developed avascular necrosis. None of these hips had undergone surgical stabilization. The mean Iowa Hip Ratings (out of a possible 100 points) were 89 in the group as a whole, 92 in the mild slips, 87 in the moderate slips, and 75 in the three severe slips.

In another long-term study from Iowa,[46] 35 cases were observed for a period of time prior to treatment. Six of the 35 (17 per cent) displaced further, five of these to the severe category. Eleven of the 35 cases (31 per cent) had an acute episode superimposed on chronic symptoms (acute-on-chronic slip), and all of these patients progressed to severe slips prior to surgical treatment.

In a long-term study performed in Sweden, Ordeberg et al.[22] evaluated 49 patients 20–40 years after their diagnosis. These patients had no prior treatment or only symptomatic primary treatment. Interestingly, few patients were restricted in any work-related activity or in their social life. Only two of the patients had required surgery for degenerative joint disease.

From these reports it is apparent that the natural history of stable slips is favourable provided that the displacement is mild or moderate and the complications associated with slipped epiphysis, i.e. avascular necrosis and chondrolysis, are avoided.[6,10,45,46,48,52,53] Stable but severely displaced slips will undergo mild deterioration to degenerative joint disease (Fig. 3.3). The degree of deterioration is related to the severity of the slip and any complications of treatment.[22,45,46,52]

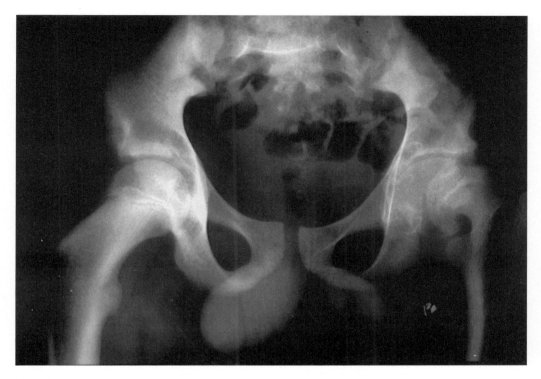

Fig. 3.3

Anteroposterior radiograph of the pelvis of a 14-year-old boy with stable SCFE of the left hip. The patient had had symptoms for approximately 12–18 months prior to seeking medical attention. Note the remodelling and rounding off of the superior aspect of the femoral neck and new bone formation on the inferior aspect of the femoral neck.

The major complications of SCFE are avascular necrosis and chondrolysis. Factors known to be associated with the onset of avascular necrosis are acute and unstable slips, reduction or vigorous manipulation of an unstable slip, attempts to reduce a chronic slip or over-reduce an acute-on-chronic slip, pins placed in the superolateral quadrant of the epiphysis,[36] and reconstructive osteotomies of the femoral neck.[5,38,44,54] The natural history of avascular necrosis in association with slipped epiphysis is universally dismal, with rapid development of degenerative joint disease. Recent delineation of the factors responsible for this complication have resulted in a marked decrease in the incidence of avascular necrosis.[36] Rates ranging from zero to 5 per cent for all types of slipped epiphysis are to be expected,[32,41,42] with the majority of these in the unstable group where an avascular necrosis incidence of 25–50 per cent has recently been reported.[35] For the most part avascular necrosis is a complication of treatment and the surgeon should be aware of the risk factors. Avoidance of forced reduction manoeuvres in unstable slips, over-reduction of unstable slips, attempts to reduce chronic slips, and placing screws or pins in the superolateral quadrant of the epiphysis will reduce the incidence of this dreaded complication. Recognition that this complication is most associated with the treatment of the unstable slip should make the surgeon more aware of the risks.[32,35,42]

The natural history of avascular necrosis following SCFE was evaluated in a long-term follow-up study by Krahn et al.[41] They found that, out of a total of 264 patients, 36 (14 per cent) had developed avascular necrosis following treatment. Twenty-two of these were evaluated at an average follow-up of 31 years. Nine had undergone reconstructive surgery, four during the adolescent period and five as adults. The remaining 13 patients with 15 involved hips had significant degenerative joint disease but had not yet undergone reconstructive surgery. The natural history of this complication is the development of gradual joint degeneration. Reconstructive surgery is often necessary to alleviate symptoms, but can usually be delayed until adulthood. Pretreatment bone scan may be a sensitive method of predicting the development of avascular necrosis in unstable slips.[43]

The second major complication seen in SCFE is the phenomenon known as chondrolysis which is defined as the dissolution of the articular cartilage in association with rapid progressive joint stiffness and pain.[5,12,55–61] Chondrolysis is known to be associated to some degree with cast immobilization,[62,63] persistent pin penetration,[64] severe slips,[56,57] long duration of symptoms prior to treatment,[5,6] and autoimmune phenomena.[5,6,12]

The incidence of chondrolysis varies widely from a low of 1.8 per cent to a high of 55 per cent depending on the type of slip, the method of treatment, and the historical time period.[5,6,12,55–58] Overall, the incidence may be as high as 15–20 per cent. The incidence is known to be higher in females, in acute or unstable slips, in more severe slips, and in patients of African-American and Polynesian ancestry.[5,6,65]

Chondrolysis is diagnosed clinically by postoperative pain and stiffness which is progressive. Plain radiographs demonstrate joint-space narrowing to less than 3 mm. A septic process (septic arthritis) should be excluded by appropriate blood tests including complete blood count with white blood cell count and differential, erythrocyte sedimentation rate, and C-reactive protein. If indicated, an ultrasound scan should be performed to detect the presence of a hip joint effusion. An aspiration may be undertaken if an effusion is detected. Treatment factors contributing to the incidence of chondrolysis which can be controlled are the use of manipulative reduction, prolonged immobilization in a hip spica, and persistent pin penetration.[60]

The natural history of chondrolysis is for eventual arthrofibrosis and joint ankylosis in approximately two-thirds of patients.[26,55–57,59,60,66–68] The ankylosis and joint stiffness gradually increase over time. However, for unknown reasons, there is spontaneous resolution in approximately 33 per cent of patients which may occur slowly over 2–3 years.[57] There have been anecdotal reports of improvement with non-steroidal anti-inflammatory drugs and systemic steroids.[57]

Clinical presentation

The diagnosis of SCFE is not difficult to make if it is considered on physical examination and appropriate anteroposterior and frog lateral radiographs of both hips are taken. SCFE should be suspected in any child between 9 and 16 years of age who presents with a limp and hip, groin, thigh, or knee pain. Remember that hip pain is often referred to the distal thigh or knee region and that children do not usually 'pull' muscles in the region of the hip.

In an unstable slip, the child presents much like an individual with a fractured hip. The child is in severe pain and is unable to bear weight or walk without great difficulty.

Stable slips present in an entirely different manner. The onset of pain is gradual and not severe. The patient is able to weight bear but ambulates with an antalgic and Trendelenburg gait. When placed supine, the hip falls into external rotation as it is passively flexed. This positive physical finding is virtually pathognomonic of SCFE and is due to the posterior slippage of the epiphysis on the femoral neck.[69] This results in impingement of the femoral head as the hip is flexed, which can be avoided by external rotation which allows for further flexion. In almost all cases, the patients will be obese, with more than 50 per cent above the 95th percentile for weight for their age. All these factors should raise a high index of suspicion and call for appropriate radiographs (Fig. 3.4).

Radiographic examination

The radiographic signs of a slipped epiphysis are numerous and easy to recognize if the slip has progressed beyond a mild degree and comparative radiographs of the opposite hip are obtained. If a slipped epiphysis is suspected, an anteroposterior radiograph of the pelvis (including both hips) and a frog lateral radiograph of both hips should be requested.

Radiographic signs of a slipped epiphysis include loss of epiphyseal height due to posterior slipping of the epiphysis on the neck, widening and relative radiolucency of the physis which is more predominant on the metaphyseal side, and a radiodense area in the femoral neck (the so-called Blanch sign) due to overlap of the posteriorly displaced epiphysis and the metaphysis.[49] In a normal hip a line drawn along the superior aspect of the femoral neck should intersect a corner of the epiphysis. This is known as Klein's line.[5] In slipped epiphysis, Klein's line may not transect the epiphysis at all or considerably less than the opposite hip.

CT may be employed as a teaching tool to demonstrate the degree of posterior displacement of the epiphysis on the femoral neck (Fig. 3.5). CT scans do not need to be ordered routinely if one understands the anatomy of a SCFE. In the acute situation there may be a need for preoperative bone scans to assess the

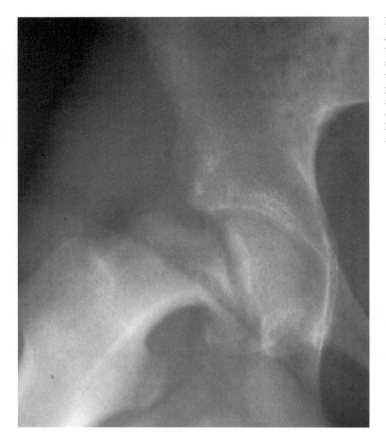

Fig. 3.4
Anteroposterior radiograph of the right hip of a patient with acute-on-chronic SCFE. Note the remodelling as described previously. The patient had an acute episode superimposed on chronic symptoms which had been present for approximately 9 months.

vascularity of the capital femoral epiphysis as a predictor of ischaemia and avascular necrosis.[43]

Treatment

The goals of treatment of SCFE are to prevent progression of the slippage and to avoid the complications of avascular necrosis and chondrolysis which lead to degenerative joint disease.

A number of treatment modalities to prevent progression of the slippage have been recommended over the past 25 years. Historically, multiple pins were placed across the physis into the capital femoral epiphysis to prevent progression. However, significant complications arose, with avascular necrosis and chondrolysis occurring in 20–40 per cent of cases where multiple pins were used (Fig. 3.6).[6,64] An important contribution to the understanding of the etiology of chondrolysis and its relationship to pin penetration of the hip joint was made by Walters and Simon.[64] They eloquently demonstrated that a pin may actually be penetrating the femoral head while appearing radiographically to be within the head. They showed that persistent pin penetration leads to a higher incidence of

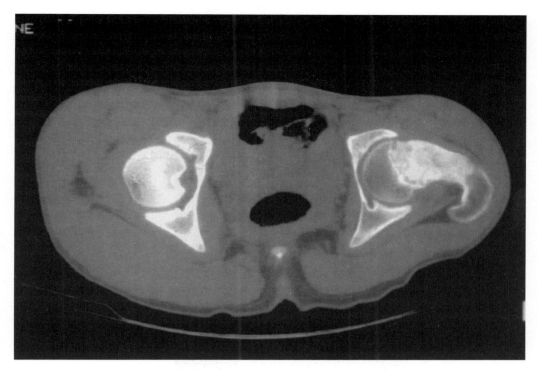

Fig. 3.5
CT scan through the femoral neck and head of a patient with SCFE. Note the posterior displacement of the femoral head on the neck. In order to place a screw across the physis into the centre of the head, the starting point of the screw must be on the anterior neck.

chondrolysis, although some cases of chondrolysis are seen before treatment of slipped epiphysis and some are not associated with slipped epiphysis at all. In another important paper, Brodetti[36] demonstrated that the lateral epiphyseal vessels enter the postero-superior quadrant of the femoral head. These vessels are the main blood supply to the epiphysis, and pins or screws in the supero-lateral quadrant may disrupt them and lead to avascular necrosis. These two studies led to the concept of single-screw fixation in the centre of the epiphysis inserted at right angles to the physis as the treatment of choice.[5,35,68,70–72]

The concept of single-screw fixation in the centre of the epiphysis in conjunction with image intensification has been a major advance in the management of SCFE. Pin penetration and the resultant chondrolysis have virtually been eliminated as complications.[5,35,68,70,71] With this technique, the patient is best managed on a fracture table. The leg is gently positioned with the knee in a neutral or anterior position with no formal attempt to 'reduce' the slip. Chronic slips are pinned *in situ*.

Fluoroscopy is used and an anteroposterior image is obtained first. A guidewire is used to draw a line on the skin coinciding with the centre of the femoral neck and epiphysis. The image intensifier is then positioned for a lateral radiograph and a line is drawn on the skin superimposed over the direction of the guidewire starting anterior on the neck and ending in the centre of the head. A small

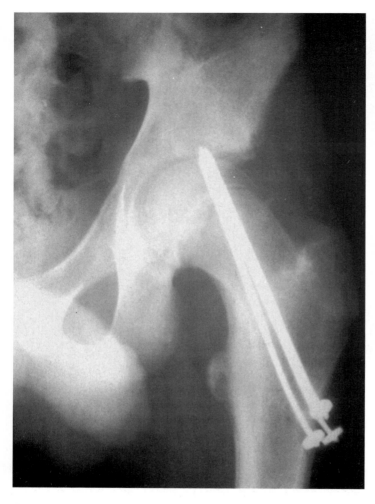

Fig. 3.6
Anteroposterior radiograph of a patient with SCFE of the left hip treated by multiple *in situ* pinning prior to the era of fluoroscopic imaging techniques. Note the protrusion of the pins into the joint and the resultant chondrolysis.

(1–2 cm) skin incision is made at the point of intersection of the two lines drawn on the skin.

A guidewire is inserted with its entry point usually on the anterior aspect of the neck rather than the lateral cortex as is the case with a subcapital fracture. Radiographs are taken in the anteroposterior and lateral planes to ensure that the guidewire ends in the centre of the epiphysis. A cannulated drill is used to drill over the guidewire and a 7.3-mm cannulated screw of the appropriate length is inserted. At least five or six threads should cross the physis and be in the epiphysis with the tip of the screw being about 4–5 mm from the edge of the subchondral bone. This is not a true compression screw but is used to 'stabilize' the epiphysis. Therefore not all the threads have to cross the physis, and in fact a 32-mm thread length has advantages over a 16-mm thread length. The head of the screw should approximate the femoral neck and not be left too long (Figs 3.7 and 3.8). There is no need

Fig. 3.7
Anteroposterior radiograph of
mild chronic slip (SCFE).
Note the position of the screw
in the centre of the femoral
head and the starting point of
the screw on the anterior
femoral neck.

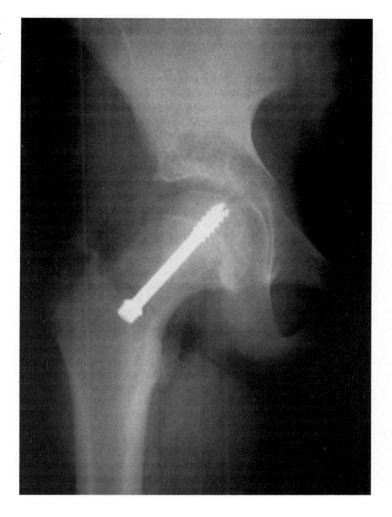

to remove the screws subsequently as they do not cause pain or
interfere with hip joint function.[73]

Postoperatively, the patient is managed on crutches for 4–6
weeks. If the slip is unstable, weight-bearing should be partial for
at least 8–12 weeks until the epiphysis has 'stabilized'. Contact
sports are not permitted until the surgeon is able to show that an
epiphyseodesis has occurred, which takes 9–12 months in most
cases.

Ward *et al.*[68] reported on 42 patients with 53 involved hips.
Ninety-two per cent of the hips went on to uneventful physeal
fusion and participated in full activities. In the vast majority of
cases a single 7.3-mm cannulated screw is sufficient for both stable
and unstable slips. If a second screw is necessary it should be
placed inferior to the first screw to avoid the superior and posterior
quadrants.[36]

43

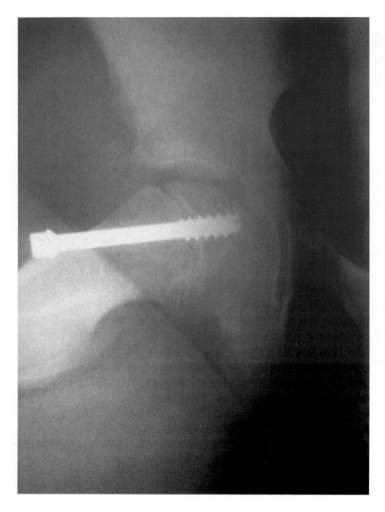

Fig. 3.8
Frog lateral radiograph of the patient in Fig. 3.7. Note the entry point used to achieve the position of the screw in the femoral head.

Single-screw fixation has become the gold standard in the treatment of SCFE. Other treatment methods have been advocated but for the most part have little or no role to play in SCFE (Fig. 3.9).

Open bone graft epiphyseodesis has been advocated by Weiner et al.[74] because of its low rate of avascular necrosis and chondrolysis. It has the advantages of no pin protrusion (no chondrolysis) and no hardware failure. However, it requires an extensive anterior approach, opening of the capsule and bone graft from the iliac crest to be placed in a drill hole across the physis. No internal fixation is employed and so a postoperative hip spica is necessary.

The disadvantages of open bone graft epiphyseodesis are a more extensive operative approach with increased risk of blood loss and further epiphyseal slippage. Rao et al.[18], in a study of 43 patients with 64 involved hips, found that progression occurred in 27 (42 per cent),

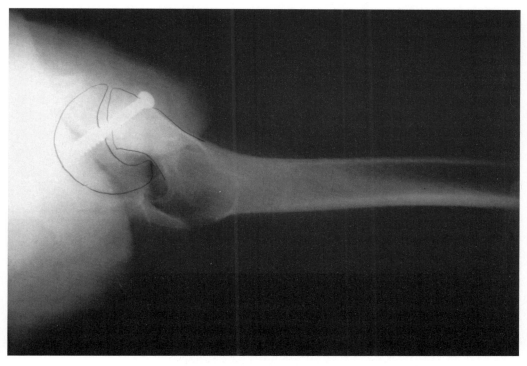

Fig. 3.9
True lateral radiograph of
a patient with severe posterior
SCFE. Again the entry point
is well anterior on the femoral
neck.

avascular necrosis in four (6 per cent), and chondrolysis in three
(5 per cent). However, Weiner et al.[74], reporting on 159 patients with
185 involved hips, found slip progression in four (2 per cent), avascular necrosis in two (1 per cent), and chondrolysis in none.

As a result of the complications of operative treatment, non-
operative immobilization in a hip spica cast was proposed.[62,63] The
theory was that a stable slipped epiphysis was similar to a stable
Salter–Harris type I physeal injury and therefore stability would
occur if the hip was immobilized. Betz et al.[62] reported on 32
patients (37 involved hips) who were managed in a hip spica cast
for 12 weeks. Progression of the slip occurred in two (5 per cent),
chondrolysis in nine (19 per cent), and avascular necrosis in none.
Despite its perceived advantages, application and maintenance of a
hip spica is not a benign procedure in an obese adolescent. Slip
progression and chondrolysis are also realistic disadvantages.

Multiple pins in situ were the procedure of choice until approximately 15–20 years ago. The increased risks of pin penetration,
chondrolysis, and avascular necrosis led to the concept of single-
screw fixation crossing the physis at right angles into the centre of
the epiphysis.[72] With proper fluoroscopic imaging pin penetration
should not occur. After the pin or cannulated screw has been
placed, the hip should be taken through a complete range of
motion. With the image intensifier in the anteroposterior position,
the hip is taken from maximal external rotation to internal rotation.

The image intensifier is kept on throughout the complete arc of rotation and the position of the screw in relation to the joint noted at all times. The image intensifier is then placed to obtain a lateral view and the hip is taken through a complete arc of rotation while a constant fluoroscopic image is obtained. The relationship of the screw to the joint is again noted. If any of the images show the screw to be impinging or penetrating the joint it must be backed out and the process repeated until no joint penetration is observed. In a recent series of stable and unstable slips, Loder et al.[32] showed satisfactory results in 96 per cent with no cases of avascular necrosis or chondrolysis.

Complications

Residual deformity

Despite the fact that an epiphyseodesis of the proximal femoral physis occurs 6–12 months after screw fixation, remodelling of the proximal femur occurs. The metaphysis of the anterior and lateral femoral neck is resorbed to some extent, resulting in an improved range of hip motion.[24,69,75,76]

However, in certain individuals with severe slips (lateral head shaft angle greater than 60°) not enough remodelling occurs to allow for normal hip function.[24,69,76] As a result the hip is limited in flexion, internal rotation, and abduction, which renders certain activities of daily living difficult, including sitting if there is severe posterior slipping, riding a bicycle, and ascending stairs. Rab[69] has shown in computer-generated models that there is impingement of the anterior femoral neck, the amount of which is directly related to the degree of posterior slippage. There is also evidence that this impingement or articulation of the femoral neck with the acetabulum in less severe slips will lead to degenerative joint disease (Fig. 3.10).[26,46,48,52,69,76]

In an attempt to improve hip joint motion and function and to prevent osteoarthritis of the hip joint, a number of osteotomies have been advocated.[9,18,38–40,42,44,54,66,77–79]

Femoral neck osteotomies have been performed with the principle that the osteotomy is done at the site of the deformity.[38–40,42,54,77,78] However, this procedure has a high rate of significant complications, including avascular necrosis and chondrolysis, unless performed by a very experienced surgeon. Fish[40] reported the results in 61 patients (68 involved hips): 55 hips (83 per cent) were evaluated as excellent, six (9 per cent) as good, and five (8 per cent) as fair or poor.

Abraham et al.[54] have advocated a corrective osteotomy at the base of the femoral neck at the time of pinning the slip. The complications of avascular necrosis and chondrolysis are less with a more distal osteotomy, but are still potentially significant.

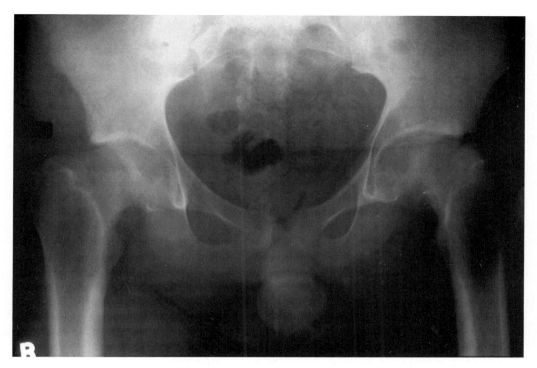

Fig. 3.10

Anteroposterior radiograph of the pelvis of a 16-year-old boy with untreated severe stable slips. The patient complained of loss of hip flexion and severe external rotation gait.

Southwick[44] proposed an intertrochanteric osteotomy based on correction of the extension deformity (posterior slippage), varus deformity (medial slippage), and external rotation deformity. This triplane osteotomy is a flexion, valgus, and internal rotation osteotomy. Its advantage is improved range of motion with relative little risk of avascular necrosis. This procedure was performed on 28 hips in 26 patients with excellent results reported in 21, good in five, and fair in two.[44] There were no cases of avascular necrosis and a shortening of 1–2.5 cm was noted. The disadvantages of an intertrochanteric osteotomy are limited correction (45° flexion, 60° valgus), limb shortening, and chondrolysis. Jerre et al.[80] reported on a mixed group of patients (37 involved hips) who had undergone corrective osteotomies for residual deformity following slipped epiphysis.[75] The average follow-up was 34 years and significant complications were noted in 32 per cent of cuneiform osteotomies and 27 per cent of intertrochanteric osteotomies.

Avascular necrosis

Avascular necrosis is seen most commonly in acute and unstable slips.[31,32,35] It is a rare complication in stable slipped epiphyses as long as the fixation device is kept out of the posterior and lateral quadrant, thus avoiding the branch of the epiphyseal vessels which enters the head at a constant anatomical location.[36]

Loder *et al.*[32] analysed the results of 58 slips: 25 were stable and none went on to develop avascular necrosis; the remaining 33 were unstable and avascular necrosis was seen in 16 of them (47 per cent). Interestingly, if stabilization was undertaken within 48 hours, the rate of avascular necrosis was 88 per cent, whereas if it was delayed to later than 48 hours the rate fell to 32 per cent. However, there were not enough cases to allow statistical analysis. In a study by Peterson *et al.*[42] 42 hips underwent gentle closed reduction and stabilization with three (7 per cent) developing avascular necrosis. Forty-nine hips underwent gentle manipulation after 24 hours with 10 (20 per cent) developing avascular necrosis. Much work remains to be done to determine the critical factors necessary to lower the incidence of this dreaded complication which inevitably leads to degenerative joint disease.[41,46,52,81] If a screw which was originally in good position appears at risk of penetrating the joint, it should be removed. Usually, the epiphysis has become stable by the time that this is necessary.

If patients with this complication remain symptomatic with significant pain, hip arthrodesis should be considered (Figs 3.11 and 3.12).

Chondrolysis

Prior to the development of proper fluoroscopic radiographic equipment, the incidence of chondrolysis was significant because of

Fig. 3.11
Anteroposterior radiograph of the right hip of a patient with unstable SCFE treated with 'gentle' manipulation and pinning. The patient went on to develop avascular necrosis with segmental collapse.

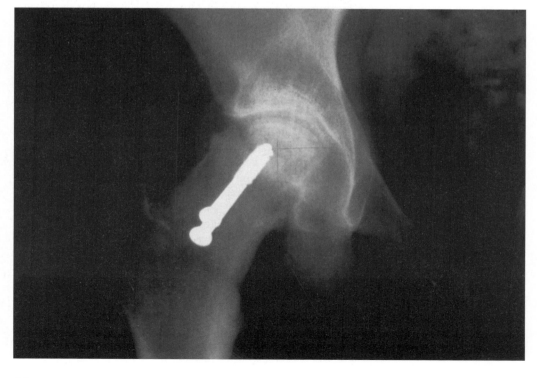

Fig. 3.12
The patient in Fig. 3.11,
6 months later. Note the
severe collapse and
deformity.

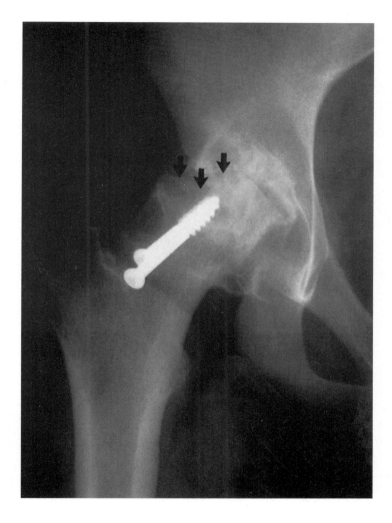

the 'blind spot', described in the classic paper by Walters and Simon,[64] which often occurred when plain radiographs were used. The relationship between the screw and the joint can now be visualized by the surgeon, utilizing the image intensifier and putting the hip through a range of motion at the time of surgery. If at any time during treatment, the tip of the screw is visualized in the joint (pin penetration) the screw needs to be withdrawn immediately.[82] Chondrolysis is defined as joint-space narrowing to less than 3 mm.[5,55,56] Once it has occurred there are few treatment options, but sepsis should be ruled out if there is no evidence of pin penetration. About one-third of these patients will spontaneously resolve over 6–12 months.[57,59] However, approximately two-thirds go on to develop significant pain, joint stiffness, and fibrous ankylosis.[57,59]

Controversies in SCFE

General agreement exists as to the etiology, patho-anatomy, and pathogenesis of slipped epiphysis. *In situ* fixation with a single screw is recognized as the treatment of choice in stable slipped epiphyses.[5,35,68,70-72]

However, there is still controversy regarding the management of unstable slips and the prevention of avascular necrosis, in the role of prophylactic pinning of the contralateral hip, and in the role and type of corrective osteotomy for malposition after severe slips.

Management of unstable slips and prevention of avascular necrosis

The goals of treatment in SCFE are to stabilize the epiphysis and to avoid complications, especially avascular necrosis and chondrolysis. Avascular necrosis is common in unstable slips with an incidence approaching 50 per cent.[35,32] The etiology of the avascular necrosis has not been conclusively proved, but is in part due to the acute displacement of the capital femoral epiphysis with disruption of its tenuous blood supply, the tense effusion in the hip joint producing a vascular tamponade, and the possibility of a manipulative reduction causing vascular compromise.[32,35,41-43]

What is the most appropriate method of treatment when one encounters an unstable slip? Loder *et al.*[32] reported an incidence of avascular necrosis of 88 per cent if the stabilization occurred in the first 48 hours, but only 32 per cent if the stabilization occurred after 48 hours. They proposed waiting to allow for subsidence of the effusion. Peterson *et al.*[42] reported an avascular necrosis rate of 7 per cent (three of 42 hips) if gentle reduction and stabilization were carried out in less than 24 hours, but a rate of 20 per cent if reduction and stabilization occurred after 24 hours.

This question will only be answered with a large multicentre controlled study, but the best approach seems to be an urgent, gentle, and often incidental reduction and stabilization with a single screw within 24 hours.

Prophylactic pinning

In the era of multiple pinning, prophylactic stabilization of the contralateral hip fell into disfavour due to the relatively high rate of complications including chondrolysis secondary to unrecognized pin penetration. With the advent of single-screw fixation and markedly improved imaging techniques, the incidence of pin penetration and chondrolysis has fallen to very acceptable levels of 1-5 per cent. Given the low incidence of complications, is there a role for prophylactic fixation of the contralateral asymptomatic hip? This is a controversial question without a definite answer. However, prophylactic fixation or stabilization should be strongly considered in the following circumstances:

- endocrine or metabolic disorders such as hypothyroidism or hypopituitarism
- young age at presentation (e.g. under 10 years)
- high-risk patient group (very obese) and unreliable family or social situation who may not seek medical attention if the hip becomes symptomatic (relative indication)

Corrective osteotomy for malposition

Some patients with moderate to severe slipped epiphysis have loss of functional range of motion due to healed malposition of the epiphysis.[69,76] In most cases, patients experience enough remodelling after severe slips that corrective realignment osteotomy is not required.[75,76] However, a small percentage of patients have a significant loss of hip motion and function due to impingement of the femoral neck against the acetabular margin.[69,76] In particular, this group of patients complain of loss of hip flexion, internal rotation, and abduction.[44] A certain percentage go on to develop degenerative joint disease due to the impingement and articulation of non-articular femoral neck against the acetabulum.[45,46,52] The concept of corrective osteotomy to correct deformity caused by severe posterior displacement of the epiphysis is an old and controversial topic. Most paediatric orthopaedists agree that corrective osteotomy should only be done after sufficient time for remodelling has been allotted, i.e. at least a year.

If indicated by significant disability and severe posterior slippage, an osteotomy may be performed but the site is highly controversial. The cuneiform or proximal femoral neck osteotomy popularized by Fish, Kramer, and others corrects the deformity at its site but should only be performed by an experienced surgeon.[39,40,77,78] The complication rates of avascular necrosis and chondrolysis are relatively high, ranging from approximately 5 per cent to 30 per cent or more for avascular necrosis and from 7 to 30 per cent for chondrolysis. There is also a base of neck osteotomy with relatively high rates of avascular necrosis and chondrolysis.[54]

Southwick[44] popularized a triplane intertrochanteric osteotomy to correct deformity, with 26 of 28 hips being rated excellent or good and no cases of avascular necrosis. This is a technically demanding operation and should only be performed by an experienced hip surgeon (Figs 3.13 and 3.14).

Another unknown and controversial question which remains to be answered is whether corrective osteotomy will prevent the development of degenerative joint disease. There is a definite mild deterioration over time which is related to the severity of the original slip and any complications of treatment.[80]

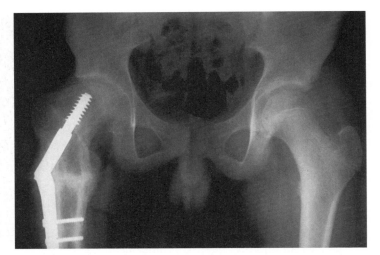

Fig. 3.13
Anteroposterior radiograph of
a patient similar to the patient
in Fig. 3.10. Because of loss
of flexion, abduction, and
internal rotation, a Southwick
intertrochanteric osteotomy
was performed to reposition
the femoral head in a more
functional location.

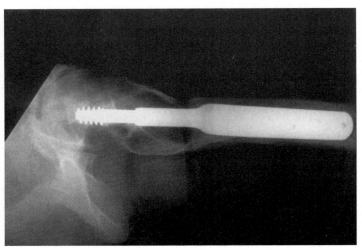

Fig. 3.14
True lateral radiograph of the
patient in Fig. 3.13. Note the
flexion aspect of the osteotomy
at the intertrochanteric area.

Summary

SCFE is a common hip disorder in adolescence. Once diagnosed,
the treatment of a stable slip is urgent *in situ* fixation of the slipped
epiphysis with insertion of a single 7.3-mm cannulated screw to
stabilize the epiphysis. Excellent results should be expected.

The management of an unstable slip is more controversial, but
emergency treatment is necessary. Gentle manipulation is permitted
while placing the leg in the leg holder on the fracture table. Gentle
traction and internal rotation are permitted, but care should be
taken not to over-reduce the slip. If the slip is not totally reduced, it
should be pinned *in situ* using a 7.3-mm cannulated screw.

If the anatomy of the SCFE is understood, the concept of single-
screw fixation into the centre of the epiphysis should be equally
well understood.

References

1 Galbraith RT, Gelberman RH, Hajek PC *et al.*: Obesity and decreased femoral anteversion in adolescence. *Journal of Orthopaedic Research* **5**: 523–8, 1987.

2 Hägglaund G, Hansson II, Ordeberg G: Epidemiology of slipped capital femoral epiphysis in southern Sweden. *Clinical Orthopaedics and Related Research* **191**: 82–94, 1984.

3 Loder RT, Aronsson DD, Greenfield ML: The epidemiology of bilateral slipped capital femoral epiphysis. A study of children in Michigan. *Journal of Bone and Joint Surgery* [Am] **75**: 1141–7, 1993.

4 Loder RT: The demographics of slipped capital femoral epiphysis. An international multi-center study. *Clinical Orthopaedics and Related Research*, **322**: 8–27, 1996.

5 Morrissy RT: Slipped capital femoral epiphysis. In *Lovell and Winter's pediatric orthopedics* (3rd edn) (ed. RT Morrissy), pp. 885–904. JB Lippincott, Philadelphia, PA, 1990.

6 Weinstein SL: Slipped capital femoral epiphysis. I: Background on slipped capital femoral epiphysis. *Instructional Course Lectures* **33**: 310–18, 1984.

7 Gelberman RH, Cohen MS, Shaw BA, Kasser JR, Griffin PP, Wilkinson RH: The association of femoral retroversion with slipped capital femoral epiphysis. *Journal of Bone and Joint Surgery* [Am] **68**: 1000–7, 1986.

8 Kelsey JL, Acheson RM, Keggi KJ: The body build of patients with slipped capital femoral epiphysis. *American Journal of Diseases of Children* **124**: 276–81, 1972.

9 Pritchett JW, Perdue KD: Mechanical factors in slipped capital femoral epiphysis. *Journal of Pediatric Orthopaedics* **8**: 385–8, 1988.

10 Weiner DS: Pathogenesis of slipped capital femoral epiphysis: current concepts. *Journal of Pediatric Orthopaedics, Series B* **5**: 67–73, 1996.

11 Brenkel IJ, Dias JJ, Iqbal SJ, Gregg PJ: Thyroid hormone levels in patients with slipped capital femoral epiphysis. *Journal of Pediatric Orthopaedics* **8**: 22–5, 1988.

12 Eisenstein A, Rothschild S: Biochemical abnormalities in patients with slipped capital femoral epiphysis and chondrolysis. *Journal of Bone and Joint Surgery* [Am] **58**: 459–67, 1976.

13 Exner GU: Growth and pubertal development in slipped capital femoral epiphysis: a longitudinal study. *Journal of Pediatric Orthopaedics* **6**: 403–9, 1986.

14 Loder RT, Wittenberg B, DeSilva G. Slipped capital femoral epiphysis associated with endocrine disorders. *Journal of Pediatric Orthopaedics* **15**: 349–56, 1995.

15 Mann DC, Weddington J, Richton S: Hormonal studies in patients with slipped capital femoral epiphysis without evidence of endocrinopathy. *Journal of Pediatric Orthopaedics* **8**: 268–73, 1988.

16 Morscher E: Strength and morphology of growth cartilage under hormonal influence of puberty. *Reconstructive Surgery in Trauma* **10**: 1–103, 1968.

17 Razzano CD, Nelson C, Eversman J: Growth hormone levels in slipped capital femoral epiphysis. *Journal of Bone and Joint Surgery* [Am] **54**: 1224–6, 1972.

18 Rao J, Francis A, Siwek C: The treatment of chronic slipped capital femoral epiphysis by biplane osteotomy. *Journal of Bone and Joint Surgery* [Am] **66**: 1169–75, 1984.

19 Agamanolis DP, Weiner DS, Lloyd JK: Slipped capital femoral epiphysis: a pathological study I: A light microscopic and histochemical study of 21 cases. *Journal of Pediatric Orthopaedics* **5**: 40–6, 1985.

20 Agamanolis DP, Weiner DS, Lloyd JK: Slipped capital femoral epiphysis: a pathological study. II: An ultrastructural study of 23 cases. *Journal of Pediatric Orthopaedics* **5**: 47–58, 1985.

21 Ippolito E, Mickelson MR, Ponseti IV. A histochemical study of slipped capital femoral epiphysis. *Journal of Bone and Joint Surgery* [Am] **63**: 1109–13, 1981.

22 Ordeberg G, Hansson LI, Sandstrom S: Slipped capital femoral epiphysis in southern Sweden. Long-term result with no treatment or symptomatic primary treatment. *Clinical Orthopaedics and Related Research* **191**: 95–104, 1984.

23 Kelsey JL, Keggi KJ, Southwick WO: The incidence and distribution of slipped capital femoral epiphysis in Connecticut and southwestern United States. *Journal of Bone and Joint Surgery* [Am] **52**: 1202–16, 1970.

24 Mirkopulos N, Weiner DS, Askew M: The evolving slope of the proximal femoral growth plate relationship to slipped capital femoral epiphysis. *Journal of Pediatric Orthopaedics* **8**: 268–73, 1988.

25 Kitadai HK, Milani C, Nery CAS, Filho JL: Wiberg's center–edge angle in patients with slipped capital femoral epiphysis. *Journal of Pediatric Orthopaedics* **19**: 97–105, 1999.

26 Stulberg SD, Cordell LD, Harris WH, Ramsey PL, MacEwen GD: Unrecognized childhood hip disease: a major cause of idiopathic arthritis of the hip. In *The hip. Proceedings of the 3rd Open Scientific Meeting of the Hip Society*, pp. 3–22. CV Mosby, St. Louis, 1980.

27 Hurley JM, Betz RR, Loder RT, Davidson RS, Alberger PD, Steel HH: Slipped capital femoral epiphysis. The prevalence of late contralateral slip. *Journal of Bone and Joint Surgery* [Am] **78**: 226–30, 1996.

28 Stasikelis PJ, Sullivan CM, Phillips WA, Polard JA: Slipped capital femoral epiphysis. Prediction of contralateral involvement. *Journal of Bone and Joint Surgery* [Am] **78**: 1149–55, 1996.

29 Loder RT, Farley FA, Herzenberg JE, Hensinger RN, Kuhn JL: Narrow window of bone age in children with slipped capital femoral epiphysis. *Journal of Pediatric Orthopaedics* **13**: 290–3, 1993.

30 Loder RT: A worldwide study on the seasonal variation of slipped capital femoral epiphysis. *Clinical Orthopaedics and Related Research* **322**: 28–36, 1996.

31 Aadelen RJ, Weiner DS, Hoyt W, Herndon CH: Acute slipped capital femoral epiphysis. *Journal of Bone and Joint Surgery* [Am] **56**: 1473–87, 1974.

32 Loder RT, Richards BS, Shapiro PS, Reznick LR, Aronsson DD: Acute slipped capital femoral epiphysis: the importance of physeal stability. *Journal of Bone and Joint Surgery* [Am] **75**: 1134–40, 1993.

33 Kallio PE, Mah ET, Foster BK, Paterson DC, LeQuesne GW: Slipped capital femoral epiphysis. Incidence and assessment of physeal instability. *Journal of Bone and Joint Surgery* [Br] **77**: 752–5, 1995.

34 Kallio PE, Paterson DC, Foster BK, LeQuesne GW: Classification in slipped capital femoral epiphysis. Sonographic assessment of stability and remodelling. *Clinical Orthopaedics and Related Research* **294**: 196–203, 1993.

35 Aronsson DD, Loder RT: Treatment of the unstable (acute) slipped capital femoral epiphysis. *Clinical Orthopaedics and Related Research* **322**: 99–110, 1996.

36 Brodetti A: The blood supply of the femoral neck and head in relation to the damaging effects of nails and screws. *Journal of Bone and Joint Surgery* [Br] **42**: 794–801, 1960.

37 Casey BH, Hamilton HW, Bobechko WP: Reduction of acutely slipped upper femoral epiphysis. *Journal of Bone and Joint Surgery* [Br] **54**: 607–14, 1972.

38 Dunn DM, Angel JC: Replacement of the femoral head by open reduction in severe adolescent slipping of the upper femoral epiphysis. *Journal of Bone and Joint Surgery* [Br] **60**: 394–403, 1978.

39 Fish JB: Cuneiform osteotomy of the femoral neck in the treatment of slipped capital femoral epiphysis. *Journal of Bone and Joint Surgery* [Am] **66**: 1153–68.

40 Fish JB: Cuneiform osteotomy of the femoral neck in the treatment of slipped capital femoral epiphysis. A follow-up note. *Journal of Bone and Joint Surgery* [Am] **76**: 46–59, 1994.

41 Krahn TH, Canale ST, Beaty JH, Warner WC, Lourenco P: Long-term follow-up with patients with avascular necrosis after treatment of slipped capital femoral epiphysis. *Journal of Pediatric Orthopaedics* **13**: 154–8, 1993.

42 Peterson MD, Weiner DS, Green NE, Terry CL: Acute slipped capital femoral epiphysis: the value and safety of urgent manipulative reduction. *Journal of Pediatric Orthopaedics* **17**: 648–54, 1997.

43 Rhoad RC, Davidson RS, Heyman S, Dormans JP, Drummond DS: Pretreatment bone scan in SCFE: a predictor of ischemia and avascular necrosis. *Journal of Pediatric Orthopaedics* **19**: 164–8, 1999.

44 Southwick WO: Osteotomy through the lesser trochanter for slipped capital femoral epiphysis. *Journal of Bone and Joint Surgery* [Am] **49**: 807–35, 1967.

45 Boyer DW, Mickelson MR, Ponseti IV: Slipped capital femoral epiphysis. Long-term follow-up of one hundred and twenty one patients. *Journal of Bone and Joint Surgery* [Am] **63**: 85–95, 1981.

46 Carney BT, Weinstein SL, Noble J: Long-term follow-up of slipped capital femoral epiphysis. *Journal of Bone and Joint Surgery* [Am] **73**: 667–74, 1991.

47 Hansson G, Billing L, Hogstedt B, Jerre R, Wallin J: Long-term results after nailing in situ of slipped upper femoral epiphysis. A 30-year follow-up of 59 hips. *Journal of Bone and Joint Surgery* [Br] **80**: 70–7, 1998.

48 Ros PM, Lyne ED, Morawa LG: Slipped capital femoral epiphysis: long-term results after 10–38 years. *Clinical Orthopaedics and Related Research* **141**: 176–80, 1979.

49 Steel HH: The metaphyseal blanch sign of slipped capital femoral epiphysis. *Journal of Bone and Joint Surgery* [Am] **68**: 920–2, 1986.

50 Murray RO: The etiology of primary osteoarthritis of the hip. *British Journal of Radiology* **38**: 810–24, 1965.

51 Resnick D: The 'tilt deformity' of the femoral head in osteoarthritis of the hip, a poor indicator of previous epiphyseolysis. *Clinical Radiology* **27**: 355, 1976.

52 Carney BT, Weinstein SL: The natural history of untreated slipped capital femoral epiphysis. *Clinical Orthopaedics and Related Research* **322**: 43–7, 1996.

53 Ponseti IV, McClintock R: Pathology of slipping of the upper femoral epiphysis. Journal of Bone and Joint Surgery [Am] **38**: 71–83, 1956.

54 Abraham E, Garst J, Barmada R: Treatment of moderate to severe slipped capital femoral epiphysis with extracapsular base-of-neck osteotomy. *Journal of Pediatric Orthopaedics* **13**: 294–302, 1993.

55 El-Khoury G, Mickelson M: Chondrolysis following slipped capital femoral epiphysis. *Radiology* **123**: 327–30, 1977.
56 Ingram AJ, Clarke MS, Clarke CS Jr, Marshall RW: Chondrolysis complicating slipped capital femoral epiphysis. *Clinical Orthopaedics and Related Research* **165**: 99–109, 1982.
57 Lowe HG: Necrosis of articular cartilage after slipping of the capital femoral epiphysis. Report of six cases with recovery. *Journal of Bone and Joint Surgery* [Br] **52**: 108–18, 1970.
58 Maurer R, Larsen I: Acute necrosis of cartilage in slipped capital femoral epiphysis. *Journal of Bone and Joint Surgery* [Am] **52**: 39–50, 1970.
59 Tudisco C, Caterini R, Farsetti P, Potezna V: Chondrolysis of the hip complicating slipped capital femoral epiphysis: long-term follow-up of nine patients. *Journal of Pediatric Orthopaedics, Series B* **8**: 107–11, 1999.
60 Vrettos BC, Hoffman EB: Chondrolysis in slipped upper femoral epiphysis: long-term study of the aetiology and natural history. *Journal of Bone and Joint Surgery* [Br] **75**: 956–61, 1993.
61 Warner WC, Beaty JH, Canal ST: Chondrolysis after slipped capital femoral epiphysis. *Journal of Pediatric Orthopaedics, Series B* **5**: 168–72, 1996.
62 Betz RR, Steel HH, Emper WD, Huss GK, Clancy M: Treatment of slipped capital femoral epiphysis. Spica cast immobilization. *Journal of Bone and Joint Surgery* [Am] **72**: 587–600, 1990.
63 Meier MC, Meyer LC, Ferguson RL: Treatment of slipped capital femoral epiphysis with a spica cast. *Journal of Bone and Joint Surgery* [Am] **74**: 1522–9, 1992.
64 Walters R, Simon S: Joint destruction—a sequel of unrecognized pin penetration in patients with slipped femoral epiphyses. In *The hip: Proceedings of the 8th Open Scientific Meeting of the Hip Society*, pp. 145–64. CV Mosby, St. Louis, MO, 1980.
65 Kennedy JP, Weiner DS: Results of slipped capital femoral epiphysis in the black population. *Journal of Pediatric Orthopaedics* **10**: 224–7, 1990.
66 Frymoyer J: Chondrolysis of the hip following Southwick osteotomy for severe slipped capital femoral epiphysis. *Clinical Orthopaedics and Related Research* **99**: 120–4, 1974.
67 Hartman J, Gates D: Recovery from cartilage necrosis following slipped capital femoral epiphysis. *Orthopaedic Review* **1**: 33–7, 1972.
68 Ward WT, Stefko J, Wood KB, Stanitski CL: Fixation with a single screw for slipped capital femoral epiphysis. *Journal of Bone and Joint Surgery* [Am] **74**: 799–809, 1992.
69 Rab GT: The geometry of slipped capital femoral epiphysis: implications for movement, impingement and corrective osteotomy. *Journal of Pediatric Orthopaedics* **19**: 419–29, 1999.
70 Aronsson DD, Carlson WE: Slipped capital femoral epiphysis: a prospective study of fixation with a single screw. *Journal of Bone and Joint Surgery* [Am] **74**: 810–19, 1992.
71 Blanco JS, Taylor B, Johnston CE: Comparison of single pin versus multiple pin fixation in treatment of slipped capital femoral epiphysis. *Journal of Pediatric Orthopaedics* **12**: 384–9, 1992.
72 Nguyen D, Morrissy RT: Slipped capital femoral epiphysis: rationale for the technique of percutaneous *in situ* fixation. *Journal of Pediatric Orthopaedics* **10**: 341–6, 1990.
73 Bellemens J, Fabry G, Molenaers G, Lammens J, Moens P: Pin removal after *in situ* pinning for slipped capital femoral epiphysis. *Acta Orthopaedica Belgica* **60**: 170–2, 1994.

74 Weiner DS, Weiner S, Melby A, Hoyt WA: A 30 year experience with bone graft epiphyseodesis in the treatment of slipped capital femoral epiphysis. *Journal of Pediatric Surgery* **4**: 145–52, 1984.

75 Jones JR, Paterson DC, Hillier TM, Foster BK: Remodelling after pinning for slipped capital femoral epiphysis. *Journal of Bone and Joint Surgery* [Br] **72**: 568–73, 1990.

76 Siegel DB, Kasser JR, Sponseller P, Gelberman RH: Slipped capital femoral epiphysis. A quantitative analysis of motion, gait and femoral remodelling after *in situ* fixation. *Journal of Bone and Joint Surgery* [Am] **73**: 659–66, 1991.

77 Kramer WG, Craig WA, Noel S: Compensatory osteotomy at the base of the femoral neck for slipped capital femoral epiphysis. *Journal of Bone and Joint Surgery* [Am] **58**: 796–800, 1976.

78 Masuda T, Matsuno T, Hasegawa I *et al.*: Transtrochanteric anterior rotational osteotomy for slipped capital femoral epiphysis: a report of five cases. *Journal of Pediatric Orthopaedics* **6**: 18–23, 1986.

79 Salvati EA, Robinson JH Jr, O'Dowd TJ: Southwick osteotomy for severe chronic slipped capital femoral epiphysis: results and complications. *Journal of Bone and Joint Surgery* [Am] **62**: 561–70, 1980.

80 Jerre R, Hansson G, Wallin J, Karlsson J: Long-term results after realignment operations for slipped upper femoral epiphysis. *Journal of Bone and Joint Surgery* [Br] **78**: 745–50, 1996.

81 Lowe HG: Avascular necrosis after slipping of the upper femoral epiphysis. *Journal of Bone and Joint Surgery* [Br] **43**: 688–99, 1961.

82 Zionts LE, Simonian PT, Harvey JP: Transient penetration of the hip joint during *in situ* cannulated screw fixation of slipped capital femoral epiphysis. *Journal of Bone and Joint Surgery* [Am] **73**: 1054–60, 1991.

Additional bibliography for slipped capital femoral epiphysis

Herman MJ, Dormans JP, Davidson RS, Drummond DS, Gregg JR: Screw fixation of Grade III slipped capital femoral epiphysis. *Clinical Orthopaedics and Related Research* **322**: 77–85, 1996.

Herndon CH, Heyman CH, Bell DM: Treatment of slipped capital femoral epiphysis by epiphyseodesis and osteoplasty of the femoral neck. *Journal of Bone and Joint Surgery* [Am] **45**: 999–1012, 1963.

Jerre R, Billing L, Hansson G, Karlsson J, Wallin J: Bilaterality in slipped capital femoral epiphysis: importance of a reliable radiographic method. *Journal of Pediatric Orthopaedics, Series B* **5**: 80–4, 1996.

Jerre R, Billing L, Hansson G, Wallin J: The contralateral hip in patients primarily treated for unilateral slipped upper femoral epiphysis. *Journal of Bone and Joint Surgery* [Br] **76**: 563–7, 1994.

O'Brien ET, Fahey JJ: Remodelling of the femoral neck after in situ pinning for slipped capital femoral epiphysis. *Journal of Bone and Joint Surgery* [Am] **59**: 62–8, 1977.

Pearl AJ, Woodward B, Kelley RP: Cuneiform osteotomy in the treatment of slipped capital femoral epiphysis. *Journal of Bone and Joint Surgery* [Am] **43**: 947–54, 1961.

Rennie AM: The inheritance of slipped upper femoral epiphysis. *Journal of Bone and Joint Surgery* [Br] **64**: 180–4, 1982.

Wells D, King JD, Roe TF, Kaufman FR: Review of slipped capital femoral epiphysis associated with endocrine disease. *Journal of Pediatric Orthopaedics* **13**: 610–14, 1993.

4

The hip in neurological diseases

George C. Bennet

Cerebral palsy

In any condition one must measure the results of treatment by
their effect upon the natural history of the condition. However,
present therapy for cerebral palsy is based upon incomplete knowledge. It is only when one reviews the literature in a short time for
a project such as this that one realizes how deficient it is. The
scientific standard of papers is low. There are no prospective trials.
The typical paper has a snappy title and then goes on to describe
something other than that which the title suggests; for example, the
results of femoral osteotomy are described in a series of patients
of mixed functional ability, half of whom will also have had an
acetabuloplasty. Latterly the gait laboratory has perhaps provided
a scientific sheen. Here we try, by obtaining a series of objective
measurements, to make surgery less unpredictable. However, there
are no prospective trials comparing the results of surgery based
upon gait laboratory data with those based upon clinical observation. All we may have done is to attach numbers to subjective
observations.[1]

Despite all our advances and studies, we still do not know the
best way to manage most, if not all, aspects of cerebral palsy. Are
we making cerebral palsy patients better or merely different?

There is no doubt that this is a complicated subject. Unlike most
of the conditions considered in this book, the primary pathology
is not in the hip. A cerebral abnormality causes a change in
muscle control affecting the tension and growth of muscle, which
in turn leads to contracture and deformity.[2] Habitual malposture
and persistent primitive and pathological reflexes may aggravate
any deformities so produced. All these features are most marked in
the most severely affected children and, as a consequence, so too
are hip deformities. They are aggravated by non-weight-bearing
which affects the structural development of the hip. Even in this
group the hip is initially anatomically normal.

Whilst abnormal tone, muscle imbalance, contracture, and
deformity may all be amenable to treatment, the basic cerebral

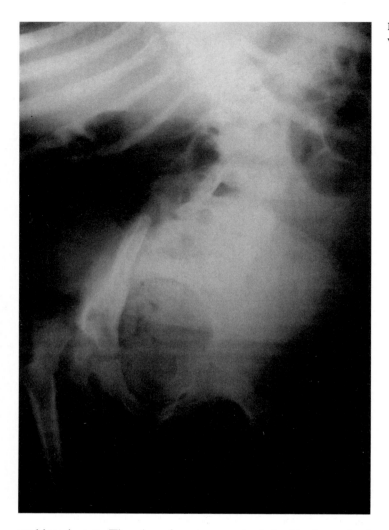

Fig. 4.1
Windswept deformity.

problem is not. The aim of management of the hip in cerebral palsy is to produce a located, painless, and mobile joint. In general, this can be achieved by balancing the muscle groups across it. If this is done early, the development of secondary bony deformity may be prevented. If not, this will also require correction.

The windswept hip

The hip cannot be considered in isolation. It is affected by the overall disturbance of motor control. The severity of hip deformity is related to the severity of spasticity. The combination of hip adduction, pelvic obliquity, and scoliosis is referred to as a windswept deformity (Fig. 4.1). This causes problems of perineal hygiene, sitting, and ultimately pain.

Such a deformity is common in the non-ambulant child with total body involvement. In a study of institutionalized patients,

Samilson et al.[3] found hip dislocation in 28 per cent, pelvic obliquity in 45 per cent, and scoliosis in 45 per cent. Howard et al.[4] found that 59 per cent of quadriplegics had windswept hips.

For some time the combination of hip dislocation, pelvic obliquity, and scoliosis was believed to be related. It is an attractive, and one might say obvious, theory that pelvic obliquity develops, or is caused by, scoliosis and as a result the hip on the high side of the pelvis dislocates.

This view was supported by Letts et al.[5] who found that all of 22 patients with windswept hips had their subluxation on the high side of the pelvis. They also found a temporal relationship between the development of adduction and dysplasia of the hip, pelvic obliquity, and scoliosis. Cooperman et al.[6] studied 21 children with dislocations, 14 unilateral and seven bilateral. In eight of the 14 unilateral cases the dislocation was on the high side of the pelvis. In the rest, the pelvis was level. Cooperman et al. felt that the relationship between dislocated hip, pelvic obliquity, and scoliosis was complex. They were of the opinion that, whilst dislocation did not cause the other deformities, its development was in some way linked. This view was shared by Lonstein and Beck,[7] who hypothesised that, if there were a causal relationship, the dislocation should invariably be found on the high side of the pelvis and opposite the convexity of the scoliosis. They did not find this, and concluded that pelvic obliquity was unrelated to hip location, that the high side of the pelvis did not relate to which hip was dislocated, and that the number of dislocations did not increase with increasing pelvic obliquity.

The patterns of deformity were examined by Nwaobi and Sussman.[8] They studied 13 children with windswept deformities using surface electromyograms and force data from the thigh. One group was passively correctable and the other was not. In both groups the response to passive abduction was mechanical and electrical activity in the adductors. In the abducted hip there was increased electromyographic activity in the abductors when the hip was adducted. In the adducted hip the abductors showed minimal activity in any position. They concluded that muscle imbalance is the cause. However, we know that if a muscle is chronically stretched, it will become electrically silent. It is possible that these authors were studying the effect rather than the cause.

Treatment is difficult. Prophylactic seating systems have been advocated to prevent the development of the deformity but there is no evidence that they work.[8] Robb[9] was of the opinion that adductor tenotomy and anterior branch obturator neurectomy was usually treatment enough, provided that symmetry of abduction could be obtained.

The dislocated hip

Dislocation is variously reported as affecting 60 per cent of dependent sitters,[7] 77 per cent of those aged more than 10 years

with total body involvement,[4] and 28 per cent of institutionalized
patients.[3] The incidence increases with increasing disability. The
vast majority are posterior; only 1.5 per cent of all dislocations are
anterior.[10] It is almost invariably developmental rather than congenital.[11] Samilson et al.[3] reported the mean age of dislocation to
be 7 years.

Dislocation develops because failure of muscle growth, particularly in the iliopsoas and medial hamstrings, produces a shift in the
axis of rotation from the acetabulum to the lesser trochanter. Fetal
anteversion and a deficiency of the posterior acetabulum aggravate
the tendency. The natural history is progression from lateral
subluxation to dysplasia to dislocation. As this gradual process can
be interrupted, the possibility of prevention exists.

Cooke et al.[11] found that the only predictive factor was the
acetabular index. Dysplasia always preceded dislocation, and its
presence in every patient who dislocated suggests that it is a prerequisite for its occurrence. Neither adductor spasm nor scoliosis
seemed to cause dislocation when the acetabulum was normal.
Where the dislocation preceded the development of a scoliosis,
Cooke et al. felt that it might cause the scoliosis or alternatively
both events might reflect increased muscle tone and imbalance. In
other patients scoliosis developed first and, although it did not necessarily cause the dislocation, it seemed to potentiate it and allow it
to occur in the presence of less severe acetabular dysplasia than
would otherwise have been the case.

Anterior dislocation may be spontaneous, presumably caused by
the same factors as above, or iatrogenic following surgical release of
the hip flexors or adductors.[10]

Symptoms

The significance of this deformity is the difficulty that it produces
in the provision of comfortable seating and, more importantly, as
a cause of pain. Hoffer[12] was of the opinion that, by the time the
hip had dislocated, most patients would already have degenerative
joint disease.

Pritchett[13] considered that 62 per cent had pain but admitted
that the nature of the patient population made an accurate assessment difficult. Cooperman et al.[6] believed that the figure was
around 50 per cent. Ultimately most will become painful. Most
affected children cannot communicate and so we rely upon parents and carers reporting general signs of distress. Localization
may be difficult. Is there pain on changing diapers? Can the child
be seated comfortably and remain so? Do not forget that pain may
be due to something other than the hip. Reflux is common. Check
it out!

Bilateral dislocations where the pelvis is level seem less likely to
give rise to pain.[6]

Management

Splintage may remove excessive stretch from weaker muscles (e.g. hip abductors), allowing them to strengthen. Abduction seating will not prevent progression, although it may delay it.

Soft-tissue procedures are not always successful.[14] Banks and Green[15] found that 33 per cent of adductor releases failed to prevent dislocation. Samilson *et al.*[3] reported a 25 per cent dislocation rate after soft-tissue surgery. Patients will inevitably continue to present with established dislocations.

Degenerative changes soon follow dislocation (Fig. 4.2) That said, it would seem reasonable to attempt to reduce a radiologically undeformed hip seen early, perhaps within a year of dislocation. Reduction and correction of the acetabular and femoral defects is then indicated.[16] However, failed bony surgery is a major source of pain. Brunner and Baumann[17] appear to favour reduction even for long-standing dislocations. They mix together both subluxed and dislocated hips and make no mention of the state of the femoral head at the time of operation. That said, they obtained pain relief in a significant number of cases. In Baumann's opinion (personal communication), degenerative changes of the femoral head tended to regress after reduction.

In the case of the longer-standing painful dislocation, the options are more limited. Arthrodesis has little to offer. Proximal femoral resection is an effective procedure in relieving pain and allowing comfortable seating. Cooperman *et al.*[6] reviewed the results of 12 such resections. They reported good results, provided that the resection was done distal to the lesser trochanter. The results obtained by Castle and Schneider[18] were in broad agreement.

This procedure should only be performed in the skeletally mature patient. In younger children one should play for time. The technique of the operation is important. Heterotopic bone formation resulting in stiffness has led many to be reluctant to undertake the procedure. Historically, the results have been dismal because of both this and proximal migration.[18]

McCarthy *et al.*[19] described resection of 56 hips in 34 patients. To minimize the risk of heterotopic bone formation they stressed the need for extraperiosteal dissection, resection more than 3 cm distal to the lesser trochanter, excision of the periosteum, and washout. This technique produced satisfactory results. Twenty-two patients could sit comfortably all day, and the rest could sit for at least 2 hours. Preoperatively 11 had been unable to sit and rest for more than a few hours. Three developed painful heterotopic bone spikes and had to have a more distal resection. Castle and Schneider[18] recommended skeletal 90/90 traction until the soft tissues had healed as an effective method of minimizing the risk of heterotopic bone formation.

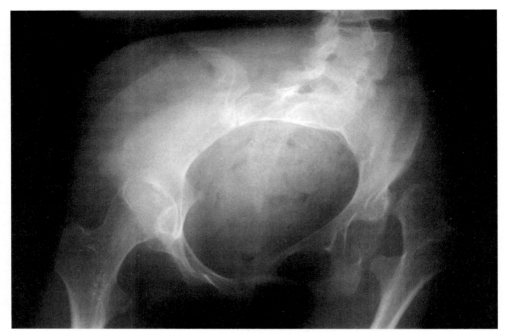

a

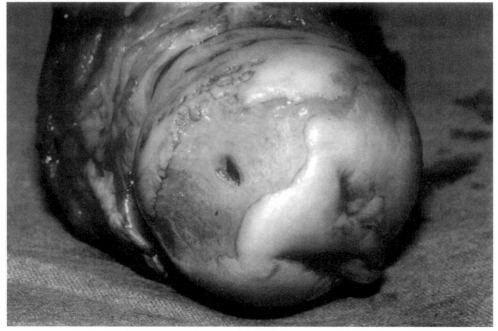

b

Fig. 4.2

(a) Dislocated painful hip in a 13-year-old child with total body involvement cerebral palsy; (b) the resected head showing extensive loss of articular cartilage.

McHale et al.[20] reported satisfactory results in a small number of patients where the excision was performed proximal to the lesser trochanter. This was combined with a subtrochanteric abduction osteotomy to allow 45° of abduction. The iliopsoas was then sutured to the ligamentum teres to anchor the lesser trochanter in the acetabulum. They obtained a good range of movement in all their patients and all had pain-free sitting. No proximal migration occurred.

Root and Mendes[21] described arthrodesis and total hip replacement for the painful dislocated hip. Arthrodesis was chosen before hip replacement was an available option. Six of the eight arthrodeses united primarily. Two required revision. All had relief of pain and those who had been able to walk preoperatively did so again. There were technical problems with total hip replacement. Six dislocated and seven subluxed. Despite this, all but one patient obtained pain relief. Using the same procedure, Cabanala and Weber[22] reported generally good pain relief and improved walking ability (only two of their patients were quadriplegic).

The subluxing hip

Gradually increasing deformity caused by muscle imbalance around the hip has led to an attempt to seek out those at risk and to offer early intervention. The principle of prevention of progression of deformity is universally accepted. The methods by which it should be obtained are not. Any child with delayed weight-bearing and stereotypical posture can be thought of as being at risk.[23]

The aim of clinical testing is to identify those children who require a radiograph to assess the amount of subluxation present. Increasing subluxation portends dislocation.[24] This is done by measuring the amount of abduction in extension at the hips, this being presumed to reflect the amount of subluxation of the hip. Subluxation is quantified by measuring the amount of the femoral head, expressed as a percentage of the whole, which lies lateral to the edge of the acetabulum.[25] Unfortunately, clinical examination is not entirely satisfactory.[24]

Data on the natural history of subluxation of the hip in children with cerebral palsy are sparse.[26] Renshaw[16] agreed, pointing out that it was not possible to predict the natural history of every hip thought to be at risk. This means that some children are being treated unnecessarily as their subluxed hips would not have progressed to dislocation.

Useful data have been provided by Miller and Bagg.[27] They found that hips with a migration index of 30–60 per cent had a 25 per cent risk of further subluxation, and those at a level of 60–90 per cent all progressed to dislocation irrespective of age. Banks and Green[15] confirmed the adverse effect of a significant migration index. Annual progression was never more than 20 per cent so that annual radiographs constituted adequate monitoring.[27]

Children in whom subluxation starts early—specifically before the age of 4—are particularly at risk of progression.[28]

Pathology

The primary deforming force is abnormal muscle tone and growth. Flexion and adduction at the hip overpowers the weaker abductors and extensors. This moves the centre of rotation of the hip to the lesser trochanter and forces the femoral head against the posterosuperior rim of the acetabulum, resulting in deformation. The capsule is stretched, and subluxation and dislocation can then occur.[29,30] This concept of the acetabular deformity was confirmed by Buckley et al.[31] who, using CT reconstructions, found it to be shallow with a defect posteriorly. There was no abnormal version. Dysplasia, which was invariably found, was greater in non-ambulatory children. In contrast, femoral anteversion was most marked in ambulatory children.[32] Using the same technique of CT scanning, Zimmermann and Sturm[33] came to the opposite conclusion. They found that the acetabular defect was anterior. This view received support from Pope et al.[34] who used arthrograms which they claim demonstrated anterolateral insufficiency of the acetabulum. They believed that the genesis of this deformity was probably increased femoral anteversion.

When the basic deformity cannot be agreed upon, it is difficult to have a logical basis for treatment.

There is general agreement that an early release is more effective than waiting until the subluxation is more advanced.[23,24,35,36] It should certainly be done before the development of acetabular dysplasia.

Miller et al.[26] express the majority view that the standard releases should include the prime movers, namely adductor longus, adductor brevis, and gracilis. Less often the iliopsoas and hamstrings are also released.[36] However, Renshaw[16] is of the opinion that the psoas, sparing the iliacus, should be part of the routine release

Anterior branch obturator neurectomy was previously often performed but is now less so as there are doubts as to whether it produces a better result and it certainly leads to an increased risk of the development of a postoperative abduction contracture.[30]

Results of surgery

As has been stated previously, soft-tissue surgery does not necessarily prevent dislocation. It is vital that the population being studied is known. The results of soft-tissue surgery in ambulatory children are uniformly successful.

Bagg et al.[28] found no difference in the amount of subluxation in those who had had a soft-tissue release and those who had not. Femoral osteotomy led to less subluxation. Turker and Lee[36] reported similarly poor results, with 26 of 45 patients being considered failures after soft-tissue release.

The greater the preoperative subluxation, the less is the chance of success. Cornell[37] found that all patients with more than 60 per cent preoperative subluxation had dislocated hips at follow-up. Of those with a migration index of less than 40 per cent, 83 per cent were reduced at follow-up. The preoperative migration index was the only significant predictor of the final result. Onimus et al.[38] did not feel that soft-tissue surgery was effective if the hip was subluxed by more than 30 per cent. Bleck[39] was of the same opinion, reporting that adductor release failed in between 30 and 75 per cent of patients. His conclusion was that this procedure was not the answer. Houkim et al.[30] found that no child older than 6 years had a good result from soft-tissue surgery alone. Banks and Green[15] went further, suggesting that soft-tissue release was not effective in children with total body involvement, i.e. those at most risk of dislocating.

The failure rate of soft-tissue surgery led to attempts by Houkim et al.[30] to improve the results by using bony procedures. They suggested that, after the age of 5, a femoral osteotomy should be performed. If there is acetabular dysplasia, this should be corrected by an augmentation procedure such as a Pemberton or Chiari osteotomy.

The place of the pelvic procedure is ill defined. In the non-ambulatory group the defect is presumably posterosuperior, whereas in ambulatory patients it is less marked and more lateral rather than posterior. The precise indications for acetabuloplasty or Chiari osteotomy, or indeed some other form of pelvic osteotomy, are still not known. A Chiari procedure may be useful where there is global acetabular deficiency not amenable to reconstruction. In less severe cases an acetabuloplasty may be preferable.[40]

There is logic in attempting to correct the anatomy of the proximal femur by combining femoral and pelvic procedures. Song and Carroll[41] found fewer redislocations when femoral osteotomy was combined with acetabuloplasty rather than when it was performed alone. Miller et al.[26] reported similar experience.

Spina bifida

No prospective controlled trial of any surgical procedure in myelomeningocele has ever been performed.[42]

Spina bifida is a developmental defect, affecting 1–5 children per 1000 live births,[43] in which the vertebral arches are not fused and the spinal cord and its membranes are dysplastic. The dura and the arachnoid protrude through the bony defect. Affected children have multiple handicaps. As well as paralysis, they may also be affected by Arnold–Chiari malformation, hydrocephalus, cerebellar hypoplasia, and diastematomyelia. Bladder and bowel incontinence and sensory loss resulting in a predisposition to pressure sores are almost inevitable. Around half will be of normal intelligence.

Potential capabilities

These patients have differing functional goals depending upon their neurosegmental level as this largely dictates their potential mobility, both in childhood and as adults. When they were originally given the potential for survival with the development of effective drainage systems for hydrocephalus, treatment was often not related to the likely outcome and the aim then was to keep all children walking. It gradually became apparent that this was not a realistic goal. Those with an upper-lumbar neurosegmental level will not walk at maturity,[44] whereas all of those with a sacral level will be walking at age 15. However, 30 per cent of these will lose this ability by the age of 30.[42] There is a slow neurological deterioration, even after skeletal maturity.

Genesis of deformity

The aim of othopaedic treatment in the management of spina bifida is to keep the child free of significant deformities so as to allow the fitting of orthoses and thus the most efficient ambulation possible. Traditionally, surgery has been aimed at balancing muscle power across joints, the presumption being that imbalance was the cause of deformity.[45] Indeed, prophylactic surgery was often performed to prevent what was felt to be the inevitable development of deformity if a certain pattern of muscle imbalance was present, for example iliopsoas transfer to prevent hip dislocation in a child with an upper-lumbar lesion, i.e. functioning flexors and adductors and paralysed extensors and abductors. However, Shurtleff et al.[46] raised doubts as to whether this was indeed the case as often the most severe deformities were found in patients with flail hips. Wright et al.[47] were of the same opinion.

Clearly, muscle imbalance is at least a partial explanation as there is a definite correlation between the lowest neurosegmental level and the limb posture. However, it is probably less important than was previously thought. Thus there is no rationale for prophylactic treatment.

Other factors play a part. Wright et al.[47] looked at fixed flexion deformities of the knee. Fifty-five per cent of those children with a deformity of more than 20° had no flexor power. Indeed, the most severe deformities were found in children with a thoracic neurosegmental level despite a total lack of muscle activity. Spasticity was rare and probably not significant in the genesis of deformity.

Treatment is not a matter of what can be done but rather what should be done. The mere presence of deformity is not an indication for surgery. The aim is to maximize the child's potential in achieving mobility, not necessarily walking, and to prevent deterioration in function. This means establishing a stable posture with the centre of gravity over the feet and minimal hip and knee flexion deformity.[45] Although many children will not walk at maturity, it is still desirable for them to do so in childhood. Mazur *et al.*[48] compared two matched groups of children with upper-lumbar or thoracic neuroseg-mental levels. One group was encouraged to walk and the other was taught to adapt to a wheelchair existence. They found that children who were encouraged to walk had fewer fractures and hospital admissions. This advantage carried over into adult life where those who had been walkers in childhood tended to be more independent. The conclusion is that walking should be encouraged.

Surgery should be planned so as to have the least possible effect on the child's life. The principles upon which planning should be based were laid down by Menelaus.[43] He tried to rationalize treatment by operating only on those children who could derive significant benefit, and to condense management so that all procedures were over in a short time and repeated admissions to hospital avoided.

Hips

Some 30–50 per cent of children with myelomeningocele will have a dislocated hip. Historically, the management of dislocated hips in spina bifida was based on the work of Sharrard.[49] He was of the opinion that muscle imbalance caused dislocation and that, by correcting it, dislocation could be prevented and walking ability improved. He based this belief on the fact that dislocations were not found in thoracic-level children with no muscle power across the joint. He felt that most upper-lumbar-level children would develop dislocation and so advocated transfer of the iliopsoas to balance muscle power across the joint. He considered that 're-education of the muscle was rapid' and that independent abduction at the hip could be reliably demonstrated and, as a consequence, dislocation could be prevented.

This is no longer accepted. Why has our view changed? Fiewell[50] found that posterolateral iliopsoas transfers, even when being selective and restricting the procedure to potential ambulators, had a high fail-ure rate. More significantly, he found that some of the failures could still walk and conversely some walkers were worse postoperatively. This led him to question whether hip dislocation was a cause of disability. He concluded that the ability to walk was predomi-nantly determined by the neurosegmental level and not by hip loca-tion. Furthermore, he suggested that neither the reduction nor the muscle transfer improved the lurching abductor gait or changed bracing requirements. Indeed, there may be significant complications that could impair the ability to walk.[51] Fraser *et al.*[52] were of the same opinion. They added that they could find no evidence that chronic dislocation led to osteoarthritic changes.

Broughton and Menelaus[53] concurred with this view, agreeing that hip dislocation had little effect on child's ability to walk. They pointed out that the maximum muscle imbalance was to be found at the L4 level yet the rate of dislocation is lower here than at higher levels. A level pelvis and a good range of motion at the hip are far more important prerequisites for ambulatory function than a reduced hip.

Broughton et al.[54] felt that hip dislocation was not as common as had been previously thought and that the development of deformity could not be accurately predicted on a neurosegmental basis. For this reason they believed that there was no indication for prophylactic operation. A complicating factor is that there may be less than full power in muscle groups which receive their innervation up to three segments higher than the lowest functioning muscle.

As unilateral dislocations in high-level lesions produce few functional problems and there is a significant risk of failure if operative correction is undertaken, this should seldom be done. A unilateral dislocation in a low-level lesion causing limb-length discrepancy, pelvic obliquity, and scoliosis should probably be reduced, but, other than that, there is a strong case for accepting the dislocation. Indeed, Alman et al.[55] did not feel that these deformities were caused by dislocation. Lee and Carroll[45] expressed the opinion that all unilateral dislocations should be reduced to avoid the above complications as well as altered sitting balance and trophic ulceration of the buttock. However, others did not feel that any of these were influenced by unilateral dislocation. Fraser et al.[56] studied 16 patients with limb-length discrepancies of up to 3 cm and found that they had no real effect on gait, did not require a raise, and had no effect on seating. The same authors found that there was a much higher risk of complications in patients with high-level lesions when reduction was attempted, whereas in patients with low-level lesions reduction was always successful and there were fewer postoperative problems. Alman et al.[55] felt that the benefit of operation in children with a low-level lesion was marginal.

There is little to be gained by attempting reduction in the bilateral case. It does not seem to improve function. This view was reinforced in a study from Toronto,[56] where the results of failed surgery were found to be worse than those who had had no surgery. The results of successful surgery were better than those treated conservatively, but this did not reach statistical significance. They concluded that the benefit of surgical relocation was marginal.

Indeed, there may be drawbacks. Stillwell and Menelaus[57] found a significant loss of hip flexion that led to functional impairment. In low-level lesions, radical surgery may be indicated if it is needed to release hip contractures, particularly fixed flexion.[58] Heeg et al.[58] also pointed out that the transferred tendons do not function adequately in gait and the procedure is only effective because of the removal of a deforming force.

It is accepted wisdom that the bony anatomy of the hip should be improved if necessary by femoral or pelvic procedures to improve stability.[59,60]

Complications of attempted reduction are reported at widely varying rates. Redislocation varies from 4 per cent[45] to 40 per cent.[50]

We must conclude that the jury is still out and that the benefits of surgical correction of the dislocated hip in myelomeningocele are marginal.

Abduction deformity

This is usually found in a child with a high neurosegmental level. Such children habitually lie in abduction and external rotation and deformity results. It can be prevented, or at least minimized, by proper positioning and splintage. If it does not lead to a functional problem, then it can safely be ignored. If it does, and that usually means repeated breakage of the hip hinges in hip–knee–ankle–foot orthoses, it can be corrected by a soft-tissue release of tensor fascia lata and any other tight bands anteriorly and laterally. Prolonged stretching will be needed post-operatively to prevent recurrence. If the abduction deformity is severe, the posterior capsule and short external rotators will also need division.

Adduction deformity

This is associated with high-level lesions. If it is causing problems with either sitting or toileting, it can be managed by adductor release.

Fixed flexion deformity

Stillwell and Menelaus[57] found a strong correlation between a fixed flexion deformity of more than 10° and loss of ambulation. It is a significant problem.

Fixed flexion is, of course, physiological in the neonatal period. It does not resolve in thoracic neurosegmental levels, although it does in sacral levels.[53] It averages 22° in children with thoracic neurosegmental levels at age 11, and 33° in those with upper-lumbar neurosegmental levels.

Muscle imbalance cannot be solely responsible as those with thoracic neurosegmental levels, who have no muscles acting across the hip, have the greatest deformities. Stillwell and Menelaus[57] felt that their data suggested that sitting, rather than muscle imbalance, was the most important causative factor. Indeed, a direct relationship between the time spent sitting and the severity of the deformity has been suggested.

Fixed flexion of up to 30° can be accommodated in orthoses. Beyond that it cannot. Correction should be offered to children with the capacity to ambulate. Coexisting hip dislocations can be ignored. The iliopsoas is excised through an anterior approach. The apophysis is split and the rectus femoris, sartorius, and anterior hip capsule, as well as any other tight structures, are divided until full extension is possible.

Extension femoral osteotomy is indicated in more severe deformities (more than 50°) or in the older child.

Arthrogryposis multiplex congenita

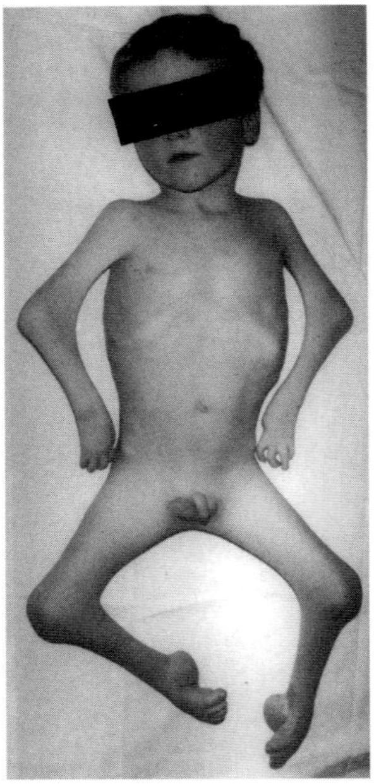

Fig. 4.3
Amyoplasia.

Motion is a prerequisite for normal joint development. In arthrogryposis there would appear to be some intra-uterine event, perhaps at 8–12 weeks of gestation, which damages the spinal cord. This may be a virus or teratogen. As a consequence there is altered joint and muscle development. Amyoplasia is a specific arthrogrypotic syndrome characterized by multiple congenital contractures, symmetrical posturing of the limbs, and decreased muscle bulk. The muscles are atrophic and, to a large extent, replaced by fibrofatty tissue. The skin is shiny and tense, and lacks subcutaneous fat (Fig. 4.3). Despite their neonatal appearance, most of these children have a good prognosis in that they should be able to ambulate and function independently.

Hip problems are common, affecting 80 per cent of children with arthrogryposis.[61,62] Friedlander *et al.*[63] found that 82 per cent had hip contractures and 58 per cent had dislocations. The aim of hip management is a painfree joint in a functional position.

Fixed flexion deformity

This is the most common deformity.There is little disagreement that, once it reaches a severity that affects function, it should be corrected. Up to about 35° it can be compensated by increasing the lumbar lordosis.[62] Anything greater than than 35° needs correction. Drennan[64] pointed out that when there is fixed flexion at the hip, there is almost invariably the same deformity at the knee and that this should be corrected first as it may limit or prevent walking. Surgical correction should not be undertaken until it is certain that the child will walk.

The technique is also generally agreed. The tight anterior structures, including the anterior hip capsule, are released through an anterolateral approach. The legs should be draped free so that releases can continue until it can be seen that the fixed flexion, as evidenced by the Thomas test, has been obliterated. Post-operatively, children should be managed in a hip spica with the hips in extension. This can be maintained for about 2 weeks after which it may be bivalved and used only as a night splint for a further 6 weeks.

Dislocation

Dislocation is common, affecting between 15 and 30 per cent of children with arthrogryposis.[65] It is teratological. The anatomy is more distorted than is usually found in a dislocated hip; the head is flattened, the ligamentum teres is thickened, and the soft-tissue planes are poorly developed. It is likely to be stiff and irreducible.[66]

Perceived wisdom is that unilateral dislocated hips should be reduced. The rationale of this view is that unilateral dislocations lead inexorably to the development of pelvic obliquity and scoliosis.[67] Once this has happened, reduction of the hip will not improve the curve.[62]

Bilateral dislocations are usually left alone. St Clair and Zimbler[67] felt that there was little likelihood of independent ambulation in the stiff patient with bilateral dislocations. Where there is a satisfactory range of motion, walking is possible but is likely to be limited (Sarwar and McEwan 1990).[68] Huurman and Jacobsen[62] found that attempted reduction almost invariably caused some loss of movement. In their experience of six such cases, all ended up with stiff hips. Gibson and Urs[69] were of the same opinion, feeling that there was a significant risk of producing either stiff painful hips or high bilateral dislocation surrounded by scar tissue. Pain is uncommon in untreated hips. Untreated bilateral dislocations do not seem to affect the ambulatory potential of the child.

The traditional approach to these hips is anterolateral and usually involves femoral shortening, perhaps preceded by traction.[62] Using this approach, Gruel et al.[66] reported fairly typical results with a redislocation rate of 19 per cent; 22 per cent of the others were subluxed, 48 per cent had avascular necrosis, and 15 per cent were infected. Overall, 70 per cent had complications, of which 37 per cent were serious.

This contrasts with the results of Szoke et al.[65] who used a medial approach in the first year of life. In this technique the dissection is between pectineus and adductor longus. The psoas is divided at the lesser trochanter. The capsule is exposed and the joint opened. The ligamentum teres and transverse ligament are divided. The pulvinar is excised. Once reduced, the hip is immobilized in a spica for 6 weeks. These authors believe that acetabular dysplasia corrects without the need for intervention. Twenty-five hips in 16 patients were managed with this method. The average age at operation was 8.9 months. There was one redislocation. Avascular necrosis, invariably mild, occurred in 11 per cent. Overall the results were reported as 80 per cent good, 12 per cent fair, and 8 per cent poor. They recommend performing reduction in both unilateral and bilateral dislocations at between 3 and 6 months, combining the procedure with other soft-tissue corrections at the knee and foot as indicated. These results are so much better than traditional methods that it would be hard to defend the previously held nihilistic management.

References

1 Watts H: Gait laboratory analysis for preoperative decision making in spastic cerebral palsy. Is it all it's cracked up to be? *Journal of Pediatric Orthopaedics* **14**: 703–4, 1994.
2 Ziv I, Blackburn N, Rang M, Koreska J: Muscle growth in normal and spastic mice. *Developmental Medicine and Child Neurology* **26**: 94–9, 1984.

3 Samilson RL, Tsou P, Aamoth G, Green W: (1972) Dislocation and subluxation of the hip in cerebral palsy *Journal of Bone and Joint Surgery* [Am] **54**: 863–73, 1972.

4 Howard DB, McKibben B, Williams LA, Mackie I: Factors affecting the incidence of hip dislocation in cerebral palsy. *Journal of Bone and Joint Surgery* [Br] **67**: 530–2, 1985.

5 Letts M, Shapiro L, Mulder K, Klasen O: The windblown hip syndrome in total body cerebral palsy. *Journal of Pediatric Orthopaedics* **4**: 55–62, 1984.

6 Cooperman D, Bartucci E, Dietrick E, Miller F: Hip dislocation in spastic cerebral palsy: long term consequences. *Journal of Pediatric Orthopaedics* **7**: 268–76, 1987.

7 Lonstein J, Beck K: Hip dislocation in cerebral palsy. *Journal of Pediatric Orthopaedics* **6**: 521–6, 1986.

8 Nwaobi O, Sussman M: Electromyographic and force patterns of cerebral palsy patients with windblown hip deformities. *Journal of Pediatric Orthopaedics* **10**: 382–8, 1990.

9 Robb J: Orthopaedic management of cerebral palsy. In *Children's orthopaedics and fractures* (ed. MKD Benson, JA Fixsen, MF McNicol). Churchill Livingstone, Edinburgh, 1994.

10 Selva G, Miller F, Dabney K: Anterior hip dislocation in cerebral palsy. *Journal of Pediatric Orthopaedics* **18**: 54–61, 1998.

11 Cooke P, Cole W, Carey R: Dislocation of the hip in cerebral palsy: natural history and predictability. *Journal of Bone and Joint Surgery* [Br] **71**: 441–6, 1989.

12 Hoffer M: The hip in cerebral palsy. *Journal of Bone and Joint Surgery* [Am] **68**: 629–31, 1986.

13 Pritchett JW: The untreated unstable hip in severe cerebral palsy. *Clinical Orthopaedics and Related Research* **173**: 169–72, 1983.

14 Gamble J, Rinsky L, Beck EE: Established hip dislocation in children with cerebral palsy. *Clinical Orthopaedics and Related Research* **253**: 90–9, 1990.

15 Banks HH, Green WT: Adductor myotomy and obturator neurectomy for correction of adduction of the hip in cerebral palsy. *Journal of Bone and Joint Surgery* [Am] **42**: 11–126, 1960.

16 Renshaw T: Cerebral palsy. In *Lovell and Winter's Pediatric orthopaedics* (ed. R Morrisey, S Weinstein). JB Lippincott, Philadelphia, PA, 1996.

17 Brunner R, Baumann J: Clinical benefits of reconstruction of dislocated or subluxed hip joints in patients with spastic cerebral palsy. *Journal of Pediatric Orthopaedics* **14**: 290–4, 1994.

18 Castle M, Schneider C: Proximal femoral resection interposition arthroplasty. *Journal of Bone and Joint Surgery* [Am] **60**: 1051–4, 1978.

19 McCarthy R, Douglas B, Reese N: Proximal femoral resection to allow adults who have cerebral palsy to sit. *Journal of Bone and Joint Surgery* [Am] **70**: 1011–16, 1988.

20 McHale K, Bagg M, Nason S: Treatment of chronically dislocated hip in adolescents with cerebral palsy with femoral head resection and subtrochanteric valgus osteotomy. *Journal of Pediatric Orthopaedics* **10**: 504–9, 1990.

21 Root L, Mendes J: The treatment of the painful hip in cerebral palsy by total hip replacement or hip arthrodesis. *Journal of Bone and Joint Surgery* [Am] **68**: 590–8, 1986.

22 Cabanala M, Weber M: Total hip arthroplasty in patients with neuromuscular disease. *Journal of Bone and Joint Surgery* [Am] **82**: 426–32, 2000.

23 Scrutton D: The early management of the hip in cerebral palsy. *Developmental Medicine and Child Neurology* **31**: 108–16, 1989.

24 Eilert R: Hip subluxation in cerebral palsy: what should be done for the spastic child with hip subluxation. *Journal of Pediatric Orthopaedics* **17**: 561–2, 1997.

25 Reimers J: The stability of the hip in children. A radiological study of the results of muscle surgery in cerebral palsy *Acta Orthopaedica Scandinavica Supplementum* **184**: 1–97, 1980.

26 Miller F, Cardosa, Dias R, Dabney K, Lipton G, Triana M: Soft tissue release for spastic hip subluxation in cerebral palsy. *Journal of Pediatric Orthopaedics* **17**: 571–84, 1997.

27 Miller F, Bagg M: Age and migration percentage as risk factors for progression in spastic hip disease. *Developmental Medicine and Child Neurology* **37**: 449–55, 1995.

28 Bagg M, Farber J, Miller F: Long term follow up of hip subluxation in cerebral play patients. *Journal of Pediatric Orthopaedics* **13**: 32–6, 1993.

29 Hoffer M, Stein G, Koffmann M, Prietto M: Femoral varus derotation osteotomy in spastic cerebral palsy. *Journal of Bone and Joint Surgery* [Am] **67**: 1229–35, 1985.

30 Houkim J, Roach J, Wenger D, Speck G, Herring J, Norris E: Treatment of acquired hip subluxation in cerebral palsy. *Journal of Pediatric Orthopaedics* **6**: 285–90, 1986.

31 Buckley SL, Sponseller PD, Magid D: The acetabulum in congenital and neuromuscular hip instability. *Journal of Pediatric Orthopaedics* **11**: 498–501, 1991.

32 Abel M, Wenger D, Mubarak S, Sutherland D: Quantitative analysis of hip dysplasia in cerebral palsy: a study of radiographs and 3D reformatted images. *Journal of Pediatric Orthopaedics* **14**: 283–9, 1994.

33 Zimmermann S, Sturm P: Computed tomographic assessment of shelf acetabuloplasty. *Journal of Pediatric Orthopaedics* **12**: 581–5, 1992.

34 Pope D, Bueff U, deLuca P: Pelvic osteotomies for subluxation of the hip in cerebral palsy. *Journal of Pediatric Orthopaedics* **14**: 724–30, 1994.

35 Kalen A, Bleck EE: Prevention of paralytic dislocation of the hip. *Developmental Medicine and Child Neurology* **27**: 17–24, 1985.

36 Turker R, Lee R: Adductor tenotomies in children with quadriplegic cerebral palsy. a longer term follow up. *Journal of Pediatric Orthopaedics* **20**: 370–4, 2000.

37 Cornell M: The hip in cerebral palsy. *Developmental Medicine and Child Neurology* **37**: 3–18, 1995.

38 Onimus M, Allamel G, Manzone P, Laurins J: Prevention of hip dislocation in cerebral palsy by early psoas and adductor tenotomies. *Journal of Pediatric Orthopaedics* **11**: 432–5, 1991.

39 Bleck EE: *Orthopaedic management of cerebral palsy*. Blackwell Scientific, Oxford, 1987.

40 Deitz F, Knutson L: Chiari pelvic osteotomy in cerebral palsy. *Journal of Pediatric Orthopaedics* **15**: 372–80, 1995.

41 Song H, Carroll N: Femoral varus osteotomy with or without acetabuloplasty for unstable hips in cerebral palsy. *Journal of Pediatric Orthopaedics* **18**: 62–8, 1998.

42 Song K: Myelomeningocele. In *Orthopaedic knowledge update: pediatrics*, pp. 65–76. AAOS, Rosemont, IL, 1996.

43 Menelaus M: The hip in myelomeningocele. *Journal of Bone and Joint Surgery* [Br] **51**: 448–52, 1976.

44 Beatty J, Canale T: Orthopedic aspects of myelomeningocele. *Journal of Bone and Joint Surgery* [Am] **72**: 626–30, 1990.

45 Lee E, Carroll N: Hip stability and ambulatory status in myelomeningocele. *Journal of Pediatric Orthopaedics* **15**: 522–7, 1985.

46 Shurtleff D, Menelaus M, Staheli L *et al.*: Natural history of flexion deformity of the hip in myelodysplasia. *Journal of Pediatric Orthopaedics* **6**: 666–73, 1986.

47 Wright J, Menelaus M, Broughton N, Shurtleff D: Natural history of knee contractures in myelomeningocele. *Journal of Pediatric Orthopaedics* **11**: 725–30, 1991.

48 Mazur J, Shurtleff D, Menelaus M, Colliver J: Orthopaedic management of high level spina bifida. *Journal of Bone and Joint Surgery* [Am] **71**: 56–61, 1989.

49 Sharrard WJW: Posterior iliopsoas transplantation in the treatment of paralytic hip dislocation. *Journal of Bone and Joint Surgery* [Br] **46**: 426–44, 1964.

50 Fiewell E: Surgery of the hip in myelomeningocele as related to adult goals. *Clinical Orthopaedics and Related Research* **148**: 87–93, 1980.

51 Fiewell E, Sakai D, Blatt T: The effect of hip reduction on function in patients with myelomeningocele. *Journal of Bone and Joint Surgery* [Am] **60**: 169–73, 1978.

52 Fraser R, Hoffmann E, Sparks L, Buccimazza S: The unstable hip in midlumbar myelomeningocele. *Journal of Bone and Joint Surgery* [Br] **74**: 143–6, 1992.

53 Broughton N, Menelaus M: *Orthopedic management of spina bifida cystica*. WB Saunders, London, 1998.

54 Broughton N, Menelaus M, Cole W, Shurtleff D: The natural history of hip deformity in myelomeningocele. *Journal of Bone and Joint Surgery* [Br] **75**: 750–63, 1993.

55 Alman B, Handari M, Wright J: Function of dislocated hips in children with lower level spina bifida. *Journal of Bone and Joint Surgery* [Br] **78**: 294–8, 1996.

56 Fraser R, Bourke H, Broughton N, Menelaus M: Unilateral dislocation of the hip in spina bifida. *Journal of Bone and Joint Surgery* [Br] **77**: 615–19, 1995.

57 Stillwell A, Menelaus M: Walking ability in mature patients with spina bifida. *Journal of Pediatric Orthopaedics* **3**: 184–90, 1983.

58 Heeg M, Broughton N, Menelaus M: Bilateral dislocation of the hip in spina bifida. *Journal of Pediatric Orthopaedics* **18**: 434–6, 1998.

59 Tachdjian M: *Clinical pediatric orthopedics*. Appleton and Lange, Stamford, CT, 1996.

60 Lindseth R: In *Lovell and Winter's Pediatric orthopaedics*. Lippincott–Raven, Philadelphia, PA, 1996.

61 Tachdjian M: *Pediatric orthopedics*. WB Saunders, Philadelphia, PA, 1990.

62 Huurman W, Jacobsen S: The hip in arthrogryposis multiplex congenita. *Clinical Orthopaedics and Related Research* **194**: 81–6, 1985.

63 Friedlander HL, Westin W, Wood WL: Arthrogryposis multiplex congenita. A review of 45 cases. *Journal of Bone and Joint Surgery* [Am] **50**: 89–112, 1968.

64 Drennan J: *Orthopaedic management of neuromuscular disorders*. JB Lippincott, Philadelphia, PA, 1983.

65 Szoke G, Staheli L, Jaffe K, Hall J: Medial approach open reduction of hip dislocation in amyoplasia type arthrogryposis. *Journal of Pediatric Orthopaedics* **16**: 127–30, 1996.

66 Gruel C, Birch J, Roach J, Herring J: Teratologic dislocation of the hip. *Journal of Pediatric Orthopaedics* **6**: 693–702, 1986.

67 St Clair S, Zimbler S: A plan of management and treatment results in the arthrogrypotic hip. *Clinical Orthopaedics and Related Research* **194**, 74–80, 1985.

68 Sarwar J, McEwan D: Amyoplasia. *Journal of Bone and Joint Surgery* [Am] **72**: 465–9, 1990.

69 Gibson DA, Urs NDK: Arthrogrypoisis multiplex congenita. *Journal of Bone and Joint Surgery* [Br] **52**: 483, 1970.

5

Controversies in acetabular fracture surgery

M.D. MacLeod

Treatment of fractures of the acetabulum has changed dramatically in the last five decades. Surgical treatment has evolved rapidly as surgeons have recognized the need to intervene and have developed techniques to improve outcomes associated with these injuries. Orthopaedic surgeons of today stand on the shoulders of Emile Letournel and Robert Judet and their pioneering work in the field of acetabular fracture surgery, and their commitment to reporting on their work and instructing others. Subspecialty training in acetabular fracture surgery is now readily available and, in many larger trauma referral centres, surgeons with interest in this area can tailor practices around acetabular and pelvic surgery. However, despite the advances in understanding and surgical treatment of acetabular fractures, it is evident that not all fractures of the acetabulum will do well. Poor results can and do occur despite the best intentions of the surgeon and despite his or her skill and attention to detail. Perhaps the greatest controversy in acetabular fracture surgery is, in fact, to determine the role of the surgeon in the ultimate outcome of the patient with an acetabular fracture.

The ultimate treatment objective for a patient with an acetabular fracture must be to restore function, minimize pain and disability, eliminate or minimize post-traumatic degenerative change, and minimize the incidence of complications. Anatomical reconstruction of the acetabulum optimizes the biomechanical characteristics and minimizes post-traumatic arthrosis. In the younger patient, anatomical reconstruction remains the gold standard. The role of the orthopaedic surgeon in a patient with an 'unreconstructible' acetabular fracture or in an older patient population with acetabular fractures is perhaps not so clear.

The purpose of this chapter is to discuss controversial areas in acetabular fracture treatment. I have specifically chosen the term 'fracture care' instead of 'fracture surgery' as there are a small number of acetabular fractures that can be successfully managed non-operatively. This is in and of itself controversial. Although many areas of the management of acetabular fractures could be discussed, I have chosen to restrict this discussion to topics of current concern, in particular those topics where answers are more elusive rather than matters simply of personal preference. I shall discuss classification schemes as a starting point for the discussion. Despite the known benefits of surgery, surgical indications bear reviewing, particularly where surgery has the potential to have a deleterious effect on outcome. Recently, reports of minimally invasive surgical techniques and percutaneous internal fixation have been made, and the role of these techniques versus traditional open surgery is unclear. In an attempt to improve patient outcomes, all interventions should minimize the risk of unnecessary complications, and I will examine the role of neurological monitoring and the prophylaxis of heterotopic ossification. For those patients who develop post-traumatic arthrosis of the hip after acetabular fracture, salvage becomes the next question. I shall discuss the various options for salvage including arthrodesis and total hip arthroplasty, both acute and delayed.

Ultimately, many of these questions will not have absolute answers. I hope that this chapter will serve to spark some thought and some evaluation of the way that we manage these difficult fractures.

Classification

The most widely used classification system is that proposed originally by Judet et al.[1] Although subsequently modified,[2] the classification remains an anatomical descriptive one (Fig. 5.1). The ten fracture types are divided into two groups of simple and associated fracture types. The five simple fracture patterns are fractures of the posterior column, the posterior wall, the anterior column, the anterior wall, and the transverse type. The associated fractures are those of the posterior column and posterior wall, the T-type fracture, the transverse fracture with posterior wall fracture, the anterior column with posterior hemitransverse fracture, and the both-column fracture. Because this classification system is anatomical and descriptive, it remains useful for purposes of discussion and communication between surgeons. However, this classification scheme does not have mechanisms to capture and, for the purposes of research, record other aspects of the injuries to the acetabulum and hip joint that are potentially important determinants of outcome. These important associated injuries include chondral and osteochondral injuries of the femoral head, marginal impaction of the acetabulum, and other chondral lesions of the acetabulum.

A more recent classification scheme has been developed in an attempt to aid in establishing a precise diagnosis. Developed in accordance with the general principles of the AO classification scheme for articular fractures, this scheme separates acetabular fractures into three main types: partial articular fractures of one column, partial articular fractures of transverse orientation, and

Fig. 5.1

Letournel classification.
(a) Simple forms: 1, posterior
wall fracture; 2, posterior
column fracture; 3, anterior
wall fracture; 4, anterior
column fracture; 5, transverse
fracture. (b) Associated forms:
1, posterior column posterior
wall fracture; 2, transverse
posterior wall fracture;
3, T-type fracture;
4, anterior column posterior
hemi-transverse fracture;
5, both-column fracture.
(Reproduced from
Jupiter *et al.* (2nd edn),
pp. 1184, 1185.)

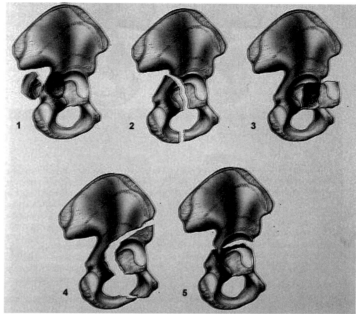

a

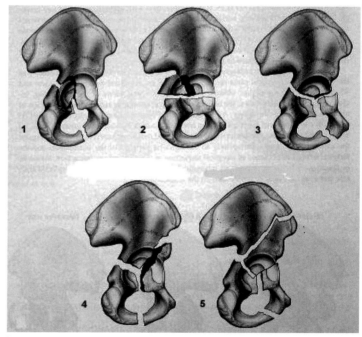

b

complete articular fractures of both columns[3] (Fig. 5.2). It was
proposed for the identification and accurate description of the
anatomical location and the morphological characteristics of the

81

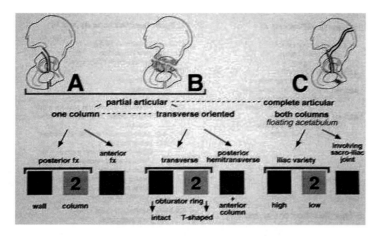

Fig. 5.2
AO classification of acetabular fractures. Type A, partial articular, one column: A1, posterior wall; A2, posterior column; A3, anterior. Type B, partial articular, transverse oriented: B1, transverse; B2, T type; B3, anterior column/wall, posterior hemi-transverse. Type C, complete articular, both columns: C1, high variety; C2, low variety; C3, involving the sacro-iliac joint. (Reproduced from *The comprehensive classification of fractures of the pelvis and acetabulum*, pp. 16–23.)

fracture. It includes qualifiers including femoral head subluxation and dislocation, chondral lesions of both the acetabulum and the femoral head, and retained intra-articular fragments. While Letournel's descriptive classification remains the common language of communication, the comprehensive classification will allow a more rigorous characterization of injury patterns and a clearer determination of prognosis and the influence of various interventions on ultimate outcome.

The natural history of surgically treated acetabular fractures

The outcome of an acetabular fracture is intrinsically tied to congruity of the joint surfaces, both femoral and acetabular, and to the stability of the joint surface. The two most general indications for surgical treatment of acetabular fractures are joint incongruity and joint instability. Several reports confirm the association of improved outcomes with the increased congruity of the acetabulum.[4-10] Matta et al.[6] supported the work of Letournel and Judet[2] showing a difference in clinical outcome if the residual displacement after intervention was less than 3 mm. Further longitudinal follow-up of this group of patients allowed Matta[4] to refine further the correlation between reduction and outcome. He was able to demonstrate a difference in outcome between fractures with 1 mm or less of residual radiographic displacement and fractures with more than 1 mm of residual displacement. This study has set the gold standard for acceptable displacement after fractures of the weight-bearing portion of the acetabulum.

From this clinical evidence, it is clear that small displacements of the acetabulum are important in long-term outcome after acetabular fractures. Normal low-level loading of the intact hip joint results in perimeter contact or rim loading of the acetabulum; full contact between the femoral head and the acetabulum does not occur until higher loading levels.[11,12] This has been likened to a ball or sphere articulating with a Gothic arch.[13] Presumably, small displacements of the weight-bearing joint surface result in significant biomechanical alterations as the joint is loaded. Finkenberg et al.[14] evaluated the effect of malreduction in the dog acetabulum. Residual step displacements of 1 mm or more uniformly resulted in arthrosis. Gap displacements of up to 3 mm resulted in minimal arthrosis. Olsen et al.[15,16] have shown the biomechanical consequences after posterior wall fractures both before and after fixation. Posterior wall fractures are perhaps the most simple acetabular fractures; however, Olsen et al.[16] demonstrated that fractures involving even small amounts of the posterior wall dramatically changed the loading pattern and decreased the total absolute contact area of the acetabulum. In the intact acetabulum, 48 per cent of the total articular contact was in the superior acetabulum. When a posterior wall defect of only one-third was created, this increased to 64 per cent. At the same time the absolute contact area significantly decreased. There are obvious implications for the survival of articular cartilage when the load per unit area is altered in this fashion. In a second cadaveric study, Olsen et al.[15] demonstrated that the loading patterns were not restored after open reduction and internal fixation. It should be noted that this study, given the inherent limitations, could not evaluate the biomechanical characteristics of the hip joint after healing of a posterior wall fracture subsequent to successful open reduction and internal fixation.

Previously, the anterior column was thought to be of lesser importance in the function of the acetabulum. This view was perhaps a natural consequence of the early work that identified the posterior and superior aspects to be the prime weight-bearing portions of the acetabulum. Fractures of the anterior aspect of the acetabulum were not thought to be as significant and the threshold for surgical intervention was higher. Recent work by Konrath et al.[17] suggests that the anterior column is an important contributor to the load-bearing characteristics and contact area of the acetabulum. This study demonstrated that small gap and step deformities of the superior aspect of the acetabulum resulted in similar alterations in the load-bearing pattern and total contact area as was shown with defects of the posterior wall. Presumably, any alteration in the peripheral zone of the acetabulum decreases peripheral loading and allows the femoral head to 'settle in' to the acetabulum during all contact rather than only under increased loads.

The goal of open reduction and internal fixation of the acetabulum is to restore the anatomy and improve or restore the biomechanical function of the hip joint. However, the role of internal fixation in changing the stiffness of subchondral bone is also of some concern. It has been speculated that altered stiffness of the subchondral bone may be significant in the development of articular cartilage damage.[18]

The role of changes in acetabular volume on loading characteristics of the hip joint is unclear. Given the nature of the known loading characteristics of the hip joint, changes in acetabular volume may conceivably decrease peripheral or rim loading of the acetabulum and increase the central and superior loading of the joint. Great attention has been given to fractures of the superior aspect of the acetabulum and the necessity for anatomical restoration of these fractures. The alterations in biomechanics caused by other fractures of the acetabulum, in particular those involving the more inferior aspects of the hip joint, is unknown. Conceptually, fractures that involve the margins of the hip joint may decrease peripheral loading and increase central loading of the hip joint.

Matta[4] has hypothesized that some degree of residual displacement exists even when an open reduction is thought to be anatomical and therefore the acetabulum must have some capacity to tolerate some changes in biomechanics. Clinical experience supports this contention, as an imperfect reduction, although associated with poorer long-term outcome, is not always associated with a poor outcome. This observation does not substantively alter the goal of the acetabular surgeon—to restore an anatomically reduced and congruent hip joint in fractures that are amenable to reconstruction.

Indications for fracture reduction and fixation

Not all acetabular fractures and not all displaced acetabular fractures require operative intervention. Careful patient selection, in addition to meticulous surgical technique, will result in improved results in patients managed both non-operatively and operatively.

The decision-making process begins with characterization and understanding of the injury. Plain radiographs of high quality, including an anteroposterior pelvis and obturator oblique and iliac oblique views should be obtained (Fig. 5.3). Additionally, a fine-cut CT scan is necessary for further determination of the bony anatomy (Figs 5.4(a)–(d)). Understanding imaging is one of the major struggles in the development of the acetabular and pelvic surgeon. Determining the nature of the injury is not as straightforward as it is in the case of an injury to a long bone. The pelvis is a curvilinear three-dimensional structure; developing an accurate three-dimensional image of the injury pattern is a challenge when working from plain radiographs and transverse CT images that are two-dimensional. The plain radiographs are used to determine the principle fracture lines and the CT scan is used to determine, in greater detail, the bony patho-anatomy. In the light of the importance of associated injuries such as marginal impaction, chondral injury, and femoral head fractures on ultimate outcome, careful evaluation of the CT scan is vital. A complete understanding of the injury pattern is necessary before the surgeon can make prudent decisions regarding treatment, plan appropriate surgical approaches, and plan an orderly progression to any proposed surgical intervention.

Fig. 5.3
Standard radiographs for
acetabular fractures.
(a) Anteroposterior pelvic
radiograph. (b) Judet view of
the pelvis: right acetabulum,
obturator oblique view; left
acetabulum, iliac oblique view.
(c) Judet view of the pelvis
(alternate to (b)): right
acetabulum, iliac oblique
view; left acetabulum,
obturator view.

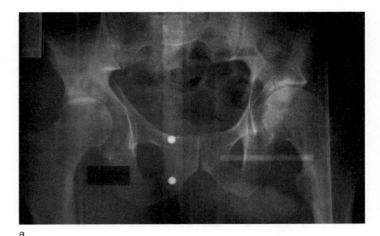

a

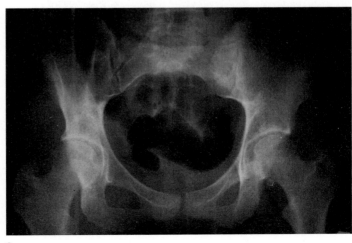

b

c

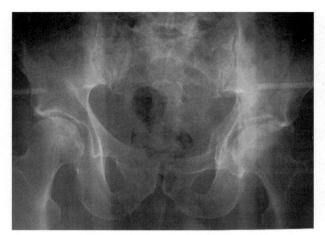

a

Fig. 5.4

(a), (b) Anteroposterior and obturator oblique views of the right acetabulum demonstrating a transverse posterior wall acetabular fracture. (c) Two-dimensional CT image. (d), (e), (f) Three-dimensional CT reconstructions.

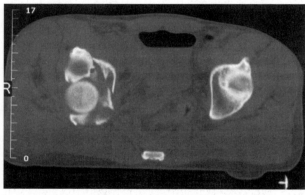

b

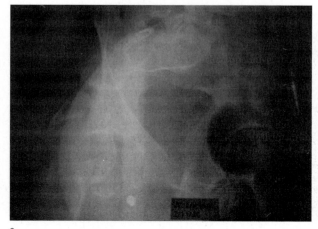

c

Fig. 5.4 *(continued)*

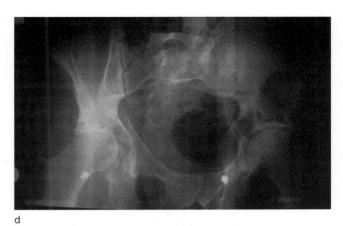

d

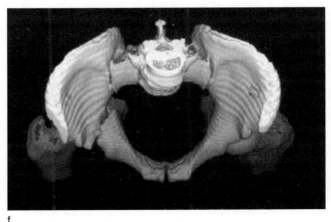

e

f

Two-dimensional CT scans should be used in conjunction with the plain radiographs. As the scan images are linear and transverse and the fracture lines are not usually linear and may be in any orientation to the transverse plain, CT images may be confusing if not correlated with the plain radiographs. For instance, a curvilinear fracture line may be imaged twice by a single CT cut and then could be interpreted as two individual fracture lines.

Computer-generated three-dimensional reconstructions of the two-dimensional CT scans can be useful but must be of good quality (Figs 5.4(e)–(g)). If the slices are not fine enough and the reconstruction is not of high quality, the true nature of the injury may be over- or underestimated. Cuts that are not sufficiently fine may result in obliterated fracture lines in the case of small displacements. Over-averaging during the computer reconstruction may obliterate fracture lines. I find the three-dimensional reconstructions to be particularly helpful if the fracture pattern is very complicated; in this instance the addition of three-dimensional images may be invaluable in determining surgical strategies. The reconstructed three-dimensional images can be rotated in any plane to allow the surgeon to evaluate the fracture pattern from different perspectives. The femoral head can be extracted from the images to allow visualization of the articular surface from the interior of the joint. Although not always indispensable, reconstructed three-dimensional images may be invaluable during preoperative planning and increase the efficiency of the surgeon in the operating room.

Once the surgeon has a thorough understanding of the fracture pattern and pertinent patient factors have been appreciated, a decision can be made as to whether to manage the patient's fracture operatively or non-operatively. Non-operative intervention may be selected for patient reasons. Severe concomitant medical illnesses, infection, either local or systemic, and severe osteopenia may all preclude successful open reduction and internal fixation of the acetabulum. Non-operative intervention may also be chosen for fracture reasons. Undisplaced fractures are usually treated non-operatively. Certain highly comminuted fractures may be determined not to be reconstructible. In these fractures, the opinion of another experienced acetabular fracture surgeon may be helpful before a final decision is made.

The decision to intervene surgically, given acceptable patient factors, is made on the basis of incongruity and instability of the hip joint after acetabular fracture. Incongruity of the acetabulum may be seen as actual articular surface displacement, subluxation of the femoral head within the acetabulum, or subluxation resulting from retained intra-articular fragments. Fractures with displacements of 2 mm or less can be managed non-operatively.[19,20] However, in view of Matta's recent results,[4] the previously accepted threshold for open reduction may be too generous. These results demonstrated a difference in outcome between fractures with 1 mm or less of residual displacement after open reduction and fractures with 2 mm or more of displacement. The indications regarding displacement for surgical intervention may change with continued long-term follow-up of larger series of patients.

Articular displacement is not the only issue when determining whether or not a particular fracture should be treated surgically. The location of the fracture is very important. Roof arc measurements, as described by Matta and coworkers[5,21] and Olsen et al.[19,22] are useful for quantifying the amount of the acetabulum that remains intact and in congruent contact with the femoral head. Roof arc measurements can be determined from either plain radiographs[5,21] or CT scans.[19,22] The three roof arc angles are generated on the three standard acetabular radiographic views. Each angle is generated by drawing a vertical line from the geometric centre of the acetabulum and a second line from the displaced fracture line to the geometric centre. The angle subtended by these two lines is the roof arc. If any of the three roof arc measurements on the three plain radiographic views is less than 45°, surgical intervention is indicated. A CT scan of the acetabulum can be used in similar fashion for the predictable identification of significant fractures of the superior aspect of the acetabulum. The superior 10 mm of the acetabulum is equivalent to the area described by the roof arc margins on the plain radiographs.[19,23] If displaced fracture lines involve the superior 10 mm of the acetabulum, surgery should be undertaken. It is important to note that roof arc measurements are of limited usefulness in posterior wall fractures.[19]

Instability of the hip joint is the second important indicator for surgery. Instability can be determined from imaging studies or may require dynamic evaluation of the patient. Any evidence of a change in relationship of the femoral head to the dome of the acetabulum on plain radiographs is an indication for surgery. Narrowing of the joint space or lateral displacement of the femoral head underneath the dome of the acetabulum is evidence of instability. Posterior wall fractures are common causes of instability. Previous studies have evaluated posterior wall fracture fragment size and attempted to correlate the size of the fracture with joint instability.[24-26] Although it is generally accepted that fractures involving less than 50 per cent of the posterior wall will not result in instability, one should be very careful when making this assumption. Examination under anaesthesia should be undertaken if there is any question of instability, particularly for fractures of the posterior superior wall. Under general anaesthesia, the hip joint is flexed and a posterior force is applied to the hip joint. Fluoroscopic examination is an important adjunct as the stress is applied. Any instability is an indication for surgery.

In summary, articular surface displacement is an indication for surgery if any roof arc measurement is less than 45°, if a displaced fracture line involves the superior 10 mm of the acetabular vertex, and if the femoral head is not congruous with the femoral head out of traction.

Finally, important consideration should be given to the concept of secondary congruence as described by Letournel and Judet.[2] This is a unique situation found in both-column fractures. The both-column fracture is unique in that the entirety of the acetabulum is detached from the ilium and the opportunity exists for all the individual fracture fragments to move into new positions around the femoral head. The fracture fragments may then assume a new but congruent relationship to the femoral head with gaps present between the fracture fragments but no step deformity.[5,19,20] It is important to note that, in addition to secondary congruence, there is no increase in cross-sectional diameter of the acetabulum. Although alterations in the loading characteristics of the acetabulum after both-column fractures are not known, the observations of good long-term outcome suggest that joint function remains acceptable given that the above secondary congruent relationship exists.[20] The standard plain radiographs of the acetabulum and the two-dimensional CT scan should be carefully evaluated to exclude a step deformity, any loss of the normal relationship between the femoral head and the dome segment of the acetabulum, and any increase in acetabular volume. If these conditions are not met, surgery is indicated. The surgical correction of these fractures is difficult, and if the patient is not selected carefully, the potential exists to convert a secondarily congruent fracture pattern to one of iatrogenic incongruity with potentially disastrous outcome.

Surgical management: open versus minimally invasive techniques

Surgical intervention for fractures of the acetabulum is challenging and requires training, devotion to the techniques, and meticulous attention to detail. The pelvis is a complicated curvilinear structure at the junctional level between the axial and appendicular skeleton. Important neurological and vascular structures lie in close proximity to the posterior and anterior margins of the acetabulum and intimately along the inner margin or quadrilateral plate. Initial surgical techniques were developed to expose large areas of the acetabulum to allow the surgeon to visualize both the extra-articular anatomy and, with incision of the hip capsule and dislocation of the femoral head, the articular surface of the acetabulum. However, experience has shown that the incidence of significant complications is increased with extensile lateral approaches to the acetabulum. Complications associated with surgery of the acetabulum are well recognized and can have devastating implications for the patient. Potential surgical complications include neurological injury, vascular injury, heterotopic ossification, avascular necrosis of the femoral head or fracture fragments, infection, soft-tissue devitalization and loss, abductor muscle weakness, and intra-articular hardware penetration.

The ultimate objective of the acetabular surgeon is to restore the articular anatomy and achieve stable fixation. Thus the surgical approach and surgical technique must allow these objectives to be met. As acetabular surgical techniques were developed, the initial exposures were designed to allow maximal visualization. The Kocher–Langenbach approach, the extended iliofemoral exposure, and the ilio-inguinal approach were the principle early surgical exposures. The triradiate exposure was developed as a modification of the Kocher–Langenbach approach to extend the exposure of the lateral wall of the acetabulum to include the anterior column to the medial eminence.

Although extensile approaches, such as the extended iliofemoral approach and the triradiate approach, allow maximum visualization of the lateral aspect of the acetabulum, there are problems associated with their use. Heterotopic ossification is a complication frequently seen with these extensile approaches to the lateral aspect of the ilium and acetabulum as well as with the Kocher–Langenbach approach. Heterotopic ossification does not always have significant clinical implications but can be highly problematic; pain, limitation of range of motion of the hip joint, and complete loss of motion of the hip joint can result. The use of an extensile approach to the acetabulum where an injury to the superior gluteal vessels has not been recognized can result in devitalization of the abductor muscle group and the gluteus maximus. Muscle death may occur and the soft-tissue envelope can be massively compromised with slough of the involved muscles. Infection, although uncommon, may be a difficult problem to manage after an extensile approach to the acetabulum. It is worth noting that simultaneous dissection on the medial and lateral walls of the ischium should be avoided if at all possible. If this is done and, unfortunately, postoperative infection ensues, such stripping may render the entirety of the ischium avascular and it may become a large sequestrum even though in continuity with the remainder of the pelvis. Radical bony debridement to eradicate such an infection may require removal of a large portion of the iliac wing.

The recognition of complications associated with the surgical approaches and the advent of new technologies has led to changes in surgical techniques, with the development of the modified iliofemoral approach and the modified triradiate approach. These modifications have been designed to reduce the surgical dissection around the hip joint capsule and the reflected head of rectus in an effort to reduce the incidence of heterotopic ossification. Simultaneous combined non-extensile surgical approaches are now commonly used for fractures of the acetabulum involving both the anterior and posterior column where the reduction of both columns cannot be effected through a single non-extensile approach.[27] When using a single non-extensile approach to treat complicated acetabular fractures, the surgeon often relies on indirect reduction techniques and percutaneous fixation techniques to reduce and stabilize the fracture.

Indirect reduction techniques allow fracture reduction without direct visualization of the fracture fragments. Reducing the extent of surgical dissection may reduce the incidence of surgical complications associated with larger exposures but is often challenging. There are two important factors that must be accounted for when a surgeon is considering relying on indirect reduction techniques to treat a fracture. Firstly, indirect reduction techniques rely on continuity between the articular surface and the associated fracture fragments. If the articular surface must be dealt with directly, as in the case of dissociated articular fragments and marginal impaction, or if there are retained intra-articular fragments, direct visualization of the acetabular joint surface is necessary. Indirect reduction techniques are not applicable when direct intervention at the articular surface must be undertaken. Occasionally, free fragments can be reduced by indirect or percutaneous techniques as demonstrated in Fig. 5.5. Secondly, the surgeon must be able to determine that the articular surface is reduced. The articular reduction is confirmed by the reduction of the extra-articular component of the fracture and by visualization intra-operatively. Large-field high-quality fluoroscopy, with or without digital subtraction techniques, is indispensable for the visualization of the quality of the articular reduction as well as the insertion of percutaneous fixation, particularly of the anterior and posterior column. Plain radiographs can determine small displacements; however, it is difficult to ensure that the radiographs are taken in the optimal plane. Multiplanar fluoroscopy can be used by the surgeon for optimal visualization of the reduction during the manoeuvre and after fixation. It is also worth noting that circumstances in the operating theatre are not always ideal, and the quality of the reduction on plain radiographs may appear better than it actually is in a significant number of cases.[28]

Internal fixation can also be inserted with minimally invasive techniques, avoiding the complications associated with large surgical dissections.[29] Internal fixation can be inserted in the anterior column in either an anterograde or retrograde[30] fashion and similar techniques can be used in the posterior column, although insertion of an anterograde screw in the posterior column requires a certain amount of dissection to allow access to the pelvic brim without injury to the adjacent femoral nerve and vessels.

As surgical techniques and technology improve, temptation will probably arise to attempt more difficult and complicated surgery with less invasive techniques. A balance between the potential reduction of risk factors and optimal articular surface reduction must be achieved. Ultimately, the quality of the reduction will determine the ultimate outcome in the absence of complications. Undertaking surgery must be based on a careful evaluation of all factors involved, developing and executing a surgical plan, being prepared for the unexpected, and taking steps to minimize potential complications.

Fig. 5.5

Clinical example: this 67-year-old man sustained a both-column fracture in a fall from a height of approximately 18 feet. In addition to the principal fracture lines, there was significant comminution of the dome of the acetabulum.

(a), (b), (c) Anteroposterior and Judet views of the pelvis. These images demonstrate a both-column fracture of the left acetabulum with impaction of the dome of the acetabulum. (d), (e) and (f) Two-dimensional CT images of the left acetabulum demonstrating the splitting of the anterior from the posterior column and extending into the iliac wing. (g), (h) Postoperative anteroposterior and Judet views of the pelvis. An ilio-inguinal approach was used to reduce and stabilize the anterior column fracture component. The dome component was reduced indirectly through the fracture lines and the posterior column was reduced with retractors and manipulating instruments placed through the interior of the pelvis. Fixation was placed in the supra-acetabular region from the lateral ilium using a percutaneous technique.

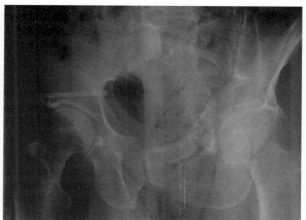

a

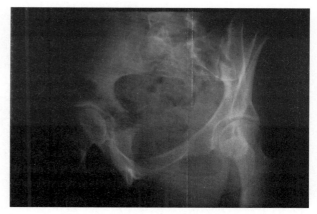

b

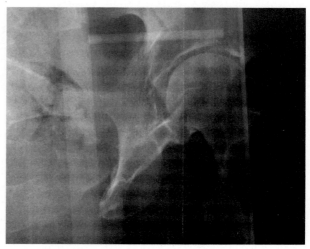

c

Fig. 5.5 (continued)

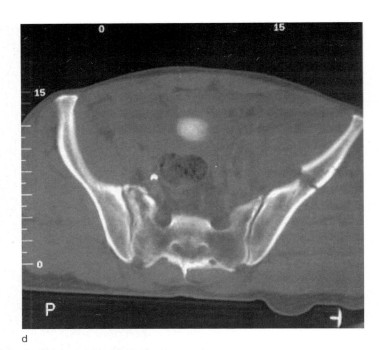

d

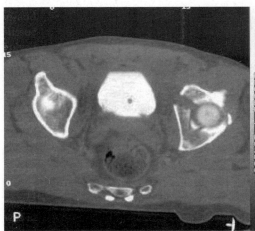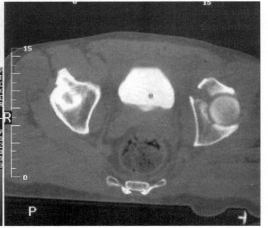

e

Neurological monitoring in acetabular fracture surgery

Post-traumatic neurological injury following acetabular fractures has been reported in 29–38 per cent of cases.[31-34]. The incidence of neurological injury after surgery of the acetabulum has been reported to be as high as 18 per cent.[2,5,6,31,35-40] The most common injury is to the sciatic nerve, and results from prolonged or over-vigorous retraction of the nerve in surgery during approaches to the posterior aspect of the acetabulum. Injuries to the sciatic nerve are associated with the Kocher–Langenbach, triradiate, and extended iliofemoral approaches.

Fig. 5.5 *(continued)*

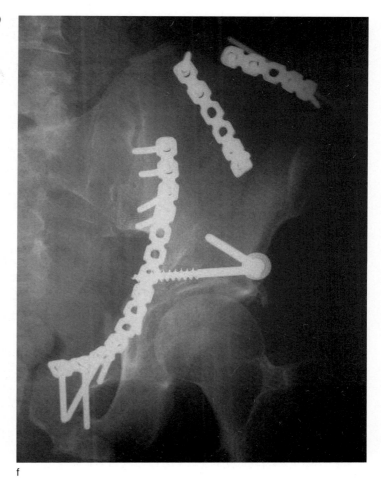

f

These approaches all have in common the exposure of the posterior column. The sciatic nerve is relatively fixed as it exits the pelvis and then again in the popliteal fossa. Retraction of the sciatic nerve against these two points of fixation can result in neurological injury which may be a result of local ischaemia from occlusion of local microcirculation or from direct axonal injury.[41] Injuries to the femoral nerve during an ilio-inguinal approach may also occur as a result of similar prolonged and/or excessive retraction of the nerve to facilitate exposure and the placement of instruments. Less commonly, neurological injury can arise as a result of direct trauma from sharp instruments, direct or indirect manipulation of sharp-margined adjacent bone fragments, or entrapment of the neurological structure within a fracture line during attempted reduction. Sharp injury can occur to the sciatic and femoral nerves, as well to the superior gluteal nerve. Injury to any of these neurological structures may have devastating functional implications for the patient despite successful acetabular reconstruction.

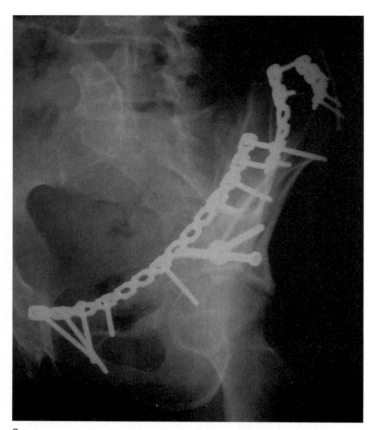

Fig. 5.5 *(continued)*

g

Direct precautions may be taken during surgery to minimize the potential for injury to neurological structures. The surgeon should exercise maximum caution to avoid injury to neurological structures by sharp instruments, bone fragments, and reduction manoeuvres. Additionally, attention to positioning and retraction techniques can reduce the potential for injury to the sciatic and femoral nerves during posterior and anterior approaches respectively.

When approaching the posterior aspect of the acetabulum, care should be taken to avoid injury to the sciatic nerve. Careful identification of the nerve and its relationship to the piriformis muscle is the first step. Retractors, which should be blunt tipped with a broad retracting surface, are placed in the greater and lesser sciatic notches. Retraction of the nerve should only be done with the hip in the extended position and the knee flexed to allow maximum relaxation of the nerve. Borelli[42] confirmed that positioning of the hip and knee influenced intraneural sciatic nerve pressures. Retraction should be relaxed as frequently as possible to avoid prolonged pressure on the nerve.

Fig. 5.5 *(continued)*

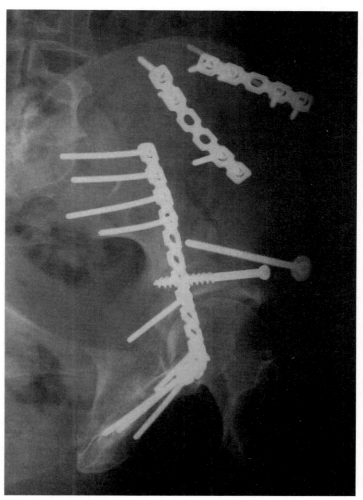

h

Similarly, during an ilio-inguinal approach, the femoral nerve is at risk and appropriate precautions should be undertaken. The femoral nerve lies on the anteromedial aspect of the iliopsoas muscle, immediately lateral to the iliopectineal fascia. Typically, the femoral nerve is most at risk when the muscle is retracted medially to expose the lateral window of the ilio-inguinal approach. At this point, the hip should be flexed to allow maximal relaxation of both the iliopsoas and the nerve. Similar frequent relaxation will reduce prolonged maximum pressure on the nerve.

Intra-operative neurological monitoring has been proposed as a method to reduce the incidence of iatrogenic neurological injury.[31,32,34,43,44] These studies have used somatosensory evoked potentials (SSEPs) to detect increasing dysfunction of the sciatic and femoral nerve during acetabular surgery. During exposure of the posterior column and manipulation of fracture fragments in this region, the peroneal division of the sciatic nerve is more sensitive to injury than the tibial division, and monitoring of the peroneal division is critical if SSEP monitoring is to be useful. Monitoring of the posterior tibial division alone will not detect critical levels of threatened injury to the peroneal division.[31,45] SSEP monitoring can detect changes in the function of the sciatic nerve intra-operatively. Unfortunately, there may be a significant delay from the time of application of significant and injurious pressure to the neurological structure and a change in the signal monitored by the SSEP. Consequently, after detection of a change in the SSEP signal, appropriate actions on the part of the surgeon, such as repositioning the limb and removing retractors, may not result in avoidance of postoperative nerve palsy. Unfortunately, false-negative and false-positive results have been reported.[34,46,47] Additionally, SSEP monitoring is not widely available and requires a high level of training for the technical staff. Despite these limitations, Helfet and Schmeling[31] felt that SSEP monitoring was a cost-effective method for the potential prevention of intra-operative neurological injury. Where SSEP monitoring is available and the surgeon and technical staff are trained in its use, this technique can be a useful adjunct in the prevention of iatrogenic nerve injury.

There are recent reports of motor evoked potential (MEP) monitoring[48,49] and electromyographic monitoring[50,51] during surgical treatment of pelvic and acetabular fractures. These newer monitoring techniques may provide more immediate feedback of impending neurological injury. A combination of MEP, electromyography, and SSEP has been promising in a preliminary study.[50] Further evaluations of MEP and electromyographic monitoring and large series comparison of MEP with SSEP are necessary to determine efficacy and cost effectiveness. Where available, experienced intra-operative neurological monitoring coupled with careful surgical technique is a useful adjunctive tool in the prevention of neurological injuries.

Prevention of heterotopic ossification after acetabular fracture surgery

Heterotopic ossification can result in significant limitation of motion, pain, and disability for patients after acetabular fracture surgery. It is uncommon in non-operative management of acetabular fractures, being reported as 1.8 per cent in a series of 90 patients.[52] The reported incidence of heterotopic ossification after acetabular fracture surgery without prophylaxis ranges from 18 to 70 per cent.[2,4,40,53-57] Routt and Swiontkowski[27] reported an incidence of heterotopic ossification of 100 per cent after surgical intervention, but significant limitation of hip motion was seen in only 8 per cent of the cases in the same series.

The mechanism for the development of heterotopic ossification is unclear. Chalmers et al.[58] proposed that an inducing agent, an osteogenic precursor cell line, and an environment conductive to osteogenesis are necessary for its development. Because of the significant difference in incidence of heterotopic ossification with and without surgery in acetabular fractures, it is evident that the act of surgery plays a role. The mechanism by which this occurs is unknown, although pleuripotential mesenchymal cells may be involved.[59,60] Regardless of the origin of the heterotopic ossification, the difference that exists in incidence rates between operative and non-operative groups indicates that the trauma associated with surgery is a potent stimulus for new bone formation.

Attempts have been made to identify risk factors for the development of heterotopic ossification associated with acetabular fracture surgery. Heterotopic ossification is commonly associated with the choice of surgical approach for acetabular fracture repair, being most frequent with extensile approaches to the lateral wall of the ilium including the Kocher–Langenbach, extended iliofemoral, and triradiate approaches.[2,4,6,45,60–63] It is less commonly associated with the ilio-inguinal approach.[4,61,63] However, it can occur even in cases where limited dissection is carried out to allow placement of reduction clamps on the lateral aspect of the posterior column of the acetabulum in conjunction with an ilio-inguinal approach. It is strongly associated with dissection around the hip joint capsule and the reflected head of the rectus femoris muscle. Other factors that have been associated with the development of heterotopic ossification include head injury,[2] male sex,[55] the severity of associated injuries,[60] the use of a trochanteric osteotomy,[64] and a prolonged interval to surgery.[65]

Heterotopic ossification is commonly graded according to the Brooker classification:[66] Brooker grades I and II are usually not symptomatic, while Brooker grades III and IV are strongly associated with joint dysfunction and patient disability.[64] The Brooker classification is limited because it is based on an anteroposterior radiograph alone and does not precisely determine the position of the new bone with respect to the joint in the anterior to posterior plane.[60,67] The position of the heterotopic ossification and the size of the deposits can be determined more accurately by two-dimensional CT scanning as described by Ritchie and Alonso[68] and Moed and Smith.[69]

Prophylaxis of heterotopic ossification after acetabular fracture surgery aims to prevent the formation of new bone in the soft tissues adjacent to the hip joint. Two principle prophylactic treatments have been developed: indomethacin treatment and controlled field radiation therapy.

Indomethacin is thought to act by inhibiting the cyclo-oxygenase pathway.[63,70] Although the end mechanism is unclear,

changes in cell function[71] or cell proliferation[72] reduce the formation of bone. Generally, indomethacin is given in a daily dose of
75 mg, started within the first 24 hours after surgery and continued for 6 weeks. There are no reports of impaired bone healing of
acetabular fractures associated with indomethacin administration.
However, the clinical efficacy of indomethacin is in question.
McLaren[63] reported that a 6-week course of indomethacin was
effective. Johnson et al.[62] found that 4 weeks of indomethacin was
effective only in cases treated by an extended iliofemoral
approach. Moed and Maxey[55] found that indomethacin was effective in reducing the occurrence of severe heterotopic ossification
but did not reduce the overall occurrence rate. Moore et al.[73]
found no difference between radiation therapy and indomethacin.
In a randomized prospective trial, Matta and Siebenrock[67] found
that indomethacin was not effective in preventing heterotopic
bone formation; however, the study power was found to be insufficient to allow conclusive determination. Indomethacin may not be
a treatment alternative for many some patients. Gastrointestinal
intolerance, allergy to non-steroidal anti-inflammatory drugs, and
concurrent anticoagulation with coumadin may preclude its use.
Patient compliance may be an issue, particularly in the patient
with a significant head injury.

Radiotherapy is a recognized alternative treatment modality for
the prophylaxis of heterotopic bone. It has been suggested that it
acts by preventing the proliferation of multipotential mesenchymal
cells.[58,73,74] The reported effective dose of radiation has fallen
to a current range of 700–800 cGy[73] administered as a single
dose[75–77] which should be administered as soon as possible in the
postoperative period. Childs et al.[76] found no difference in incidence
if radiation was delayed until the fourth postoperative day. Other
studies have shown a reduction in effectiveness if the radiation is
administered after the fourth postoperative day.[73,78–80] A combination of radiotherapy and indomethacin has been shown to be very
effective.[81] Theoretical concerns regarding the use of indomethacin
include carcinogenesis and sterility, but the risk is thought to
be low.[82,83] Radiotherapy has the advantage of full treatment in a
single dose; compliance issues are not a concern. However, radiotherapy is significantly more expensive than indomethacin[73], and
some patients, because of the extent of their injuries, cannot be
transported for radiotherapy.

My current protocol is to administer indomethacin 75–100
mg/day; the first dose is given in suppository form immediately after
surgery. If possible, 600cGy of radiation is administered within the
first 72 hours after surgery and then indomethacin is discontinued.
Indomethacin is reserved for those unable to be transported for
radiotherapy. Cytoprotective agents are also given for the 6 weeks of
indomethacin therapy in patients who cannot have radiotherapy
initiated within the first 72 hours postoperatively.

The role of total hip arthroplasty in acetabular fractures

Unfortunately, not all acetabular fractures will have a successful outcome, regardless of the intentions or skill of the surgeon. Extensive comminution, marginal impaction, articular cartilage injury, and avascular necrosis are factors associated with acetabular fractures which may preclude successful primary reconstruction or a successful outcome after what was believed to be an excellent primary open reduction and internal fixation. An instructive case is shown in Fig. 5.6. In this particular case, operative intervention could not be undertaken for this fracture with small displacements because of serious associated injuries. The decision to treat this patient non-operatively was not the treatment of choice. Four months after the injury, the patient had developed severe and unrelenting pain and progressive restriction of hip joint motion because of whole-head avascular necrosis and collapse; this patient had not had surgical intervention and did not have associated risk factors for avascular necrosis. This occurrence of a serious complication without surgical intervention illustrates that the ultimate outcome of an acetabular fracture may be independent of the primary surgical intervention. It is also interesting to note that, in this case, avascular necrosis had occurred without surgical intervention; in the past avascular necrosis after acetabular fractures was often attributed to iatrogenic causes.

The reported incidence of arthrosis after non-operative management of displaced acetabular fractures ranges from 12 to 57 per cent.[84–86] The incidence of arthrosis is significantly affected by open reduction and internal fixation techniques. The incidence of arthrosis after open reduction and internal fixation ranges from 12 to 14 per cent.[2,4,35,87] The development of post-traumatic arthrosis is a result of primary irreversible chondral injury or residual unacceptable incongruity of the hip joint leading to an unacceptable loading pattern.

Salvage options for post-traumatic arthrosis of the hip are principally arthrodesis and total hip arthroplasty. In the past, arthrodesis has been recommended as the treatment of choice for young patients with symptomatic arthrosis of the hip. This procedure has been recommended for monoarticular arthrosis that is non-inflammatory in nature, particularly in male patients who are involved in labouring professions. Arthrodesis is relatively contraindicated in patients with bilateral hip joint disease, particularly in women of childbearing years, and in patients with avascular necrosis, particularly if the disease process is bilateral.[88] The procedure is also relatively contraindicated in the patient with low back pain, contralateral hip arthrosis, and arthrosis or instability of either knee.[89]

Hip arthrodesis has been recommended after failed acetabular fracture; however, the procedure results in slowed gait and increased oxygen consumption[90] and therefore is confined to younger patients with greater functional reserves. The procedure can be very technically challenging in the patient who has had

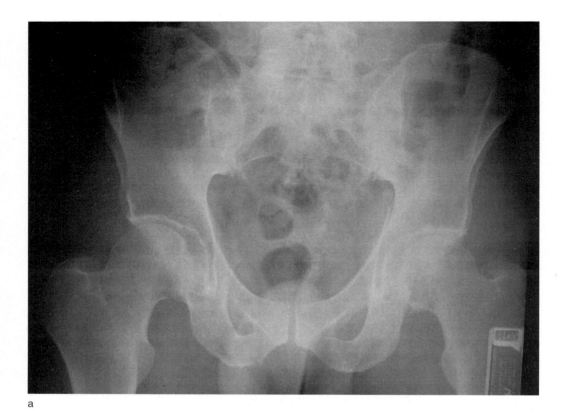

a

Fig. 5.6

Clinical example. This 45-year-old man sustained an acetabular fracture in a motor vehicle accident. He had no risk factors for avascular necrosis of the femoral head. Surgical intervention for the acetabular fracture could not be performed because of associated injuries. (a), (b), (c) Initial anteroposterior Pelvis and Judet views of the initial acetabular fracture. (d), (e) Anteroposterior pelvis and anteroposterior projection of the left hip 4 months after the initial fracture. The patient experienced increasing left hip pain, inability to weight-bear, and marked decrease in range of motion. Incongruity of the hip joint, irregularity of the femoral head articular surface,

failure of acetabular fracture surgery because of avascular necrosis of the femoral head. In this scenario, arthrodesis can be difficult to achieve and significant leg-length inequality may be difficult to avoid. After successful arthrodesis, patients will often develop symptoms in adjacent joints. Low back pain, contralateral hip pain, and knee pain commonly occur after arthrodesis.[88,91-94] Symptoms in these adjacent mobile joints occur in a delayed fashion, with onset usually between 20 and 25 years after arthrodesis.[91,93] Patients may also experience difficulty on a daily basis with activities that are reliant on hip flexion, including bending at the waist, climbing stairs, and sitting.

Largely because of the disability associated with the procedure, arthrodesis is rapidly becoming less acceptable to patients in favour of total hip arthroplasty. This is particularly true as the lay population becomes increasingly aware of the success of total hip replacement in the management of degenerative arthrosis. However, total hip arthroplasty is not a panacea for the problem of failed acetabular fracture surgery and post-traumatic arthrosis. Total hip replacement, while not having the associated functional disability associated with hip arthrodesis, is associated with a series of possible significant difficulties and problems.

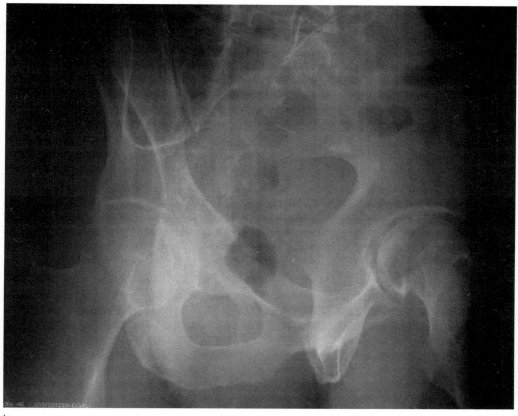

b

Fig. 5.6 *(continued)*
and hip joint-space loss are
noted. (f), (g) MRI of the left
hip demonstrates unilateral
avascular necrosis of the
femoral head with whole-head
involvement.

Total hip replacement for post-traumatic arthrosis is not a recent technique. Westerborn[95] and Kelly and Lipscomb[96] gave early reports of mould arthroplasty used to treat acetabular fracture failures. Boardman and Charnley[97] reported the use of low-friction arthroplasty in patients who had previous acetabular fractures and established post-traumatic arthrosis. More recent reports have been made of contemporary arthroplasty techniques for the treatment of post-traumatic arthrosis.[98–106] Failure rates as high as 58 per cent have been reported in these series with relatively short-term follow-up.[105]

Romness and Lewallen[98] reported 55 total hip replacements for post-traumatic arthrosis. The average age at implantation was 56 years and patients were followed for a mean of 7.5 years. The incidence of loosening of the acetabular components was 52.9 per cent, which was four to five times higher than the rate of acetabular loosening in a similar group of patients who had undergone arthroplasty for routine degenerative arthrosis.[107] The authors speculated that the high rate of acetabular component failure was attributable to deficiencies of acetabular bone stock.

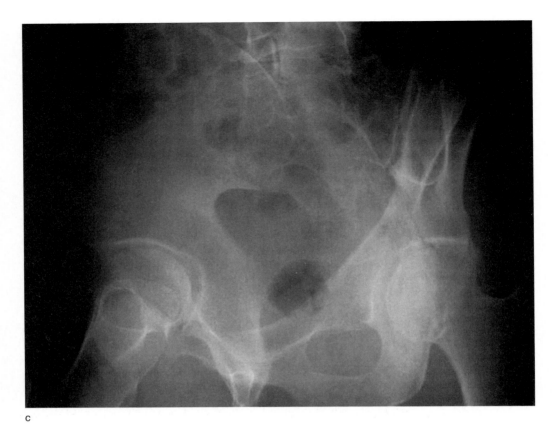

c

Fig. 5.6 *(continued)*

Karpos and Christie[103] reviewed 15 hip arthroplasty procedures with mean follow-up of 68 months. Significant numbers of the acetabular reconstructions required bone grafting: 40 per cent required structural grafting, presumably to re-establish rim support for the acetabular component, and 47 per cent required morsellized grafting to fill cavitary defects. The components were porous or mesh coated, and supplemental screws were used to improve acetabular fixation. At follow-up, although 27 per cent had one or more lucent zones, no symptomatic loosening had occurred.

Huo *et al.*[100] reported similar results in a series of 21 hip arthroplasties with a mean follow up of 65 months. Radiographic loosening was observed in 19 per cent; four of the five loose components were smooth and not porous coated. Acetabular component failures seemed predominantly related to component design, and the authors recommended that porous-coated components should be used in the scenario of post-traumatic arthrosis.

Weber *et al.*[99] reported one of the largest contemporary series of post-traumatic hip reconstructive procedures. The mean follow-up was 9.6 years and a combination of cemented and uncemented acetabular components were used; the mean duration was 14.9 years

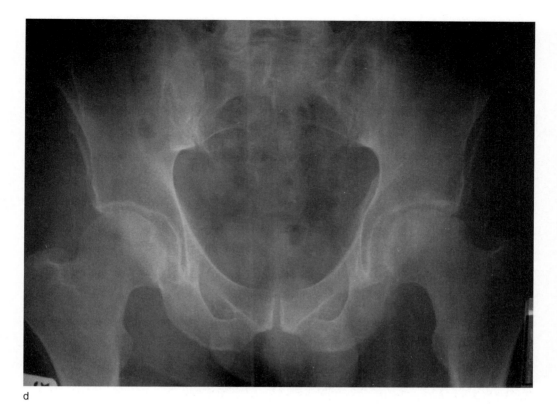

d

Fig. 5.6 *(continued)*

for the cemented components and 3.9 years for the uncemented components. None of the uncemented acetabular components were loose at follow-up, but 37 per cent of the cemented acetabular components were loose or had been revised because of aseptic loosening. Bone grafting had been performed in approximately a quarter of the reconstructions, but most of these were morselized grafts and not structural. These authors found that soft-tissue scarring, implants from previous open reduction and internal fixation, heterotopic bone, and bony deficiencies, including avascular necrosis of acetabular segments and non-union of acetabular fractures, complicated the surgical reconstructions. Analysis of the data showed that failure of the acetabular components was associated with patients less than 50 years of age, patients weighing more than 80 kg, and combined cavitary and segmental defects.

Total hip arthroplasty has also been reported as an immediate form of treatment for certain acetabular fractures.[108] However, the use of this procedure remains controversial. Joly and Mears[108] gave cautious relative recommendation of the technique in limited specific circumstances including patients of advanced age, obesity, osteopenia, high-risk fracture types, including those with associated severe femoral head chondral or osteochondral injury, and a delay

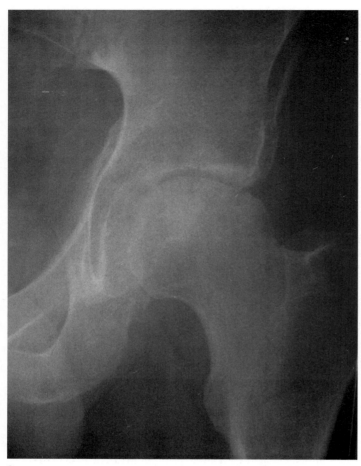

Fig. 5.6 *(continued)*

e

of more than 1 month in the initial management of the original acetabular fracture. It is important to note that these authors stress that this technique is not broadly recommended and has been applied in only a limited number of cases. It is also important to note that open reduction techniques have been used successfully in some of these circumstances.[109] Potentially the greatest obstacle facing successful outcome in acute total hip arthroplasty for acetabular fracture is achieving a stable acetabular bone construct in which to implant the acetabular component. In an effort to avoid the complications associated with an extensile lateral approach or simultaneous anterior and posterior approaches, Mears and Shirahama[110] have used braided cables passed around the acetabulum to stabilize the fracture fragments prior to insertion of the acetabular component (Fig. 5.7). This technique is technically difficult; it requires the surgeon to have a precise understanding of the fracture pattern and the technique for cable insertion to avoid injury to

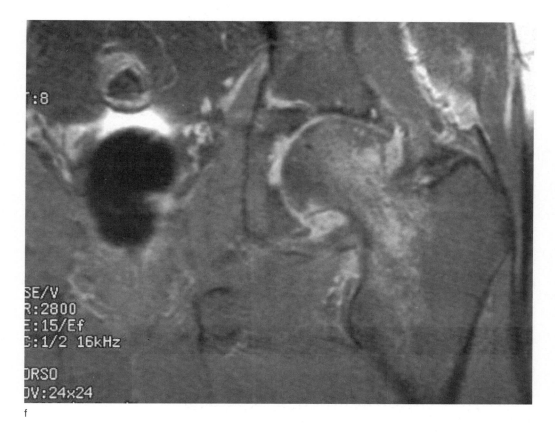

Fig. 5.6 *(continued)*

neurovascular structures and to obtain a stable construct. Additionally, the technique may be ineffective in highly comminuted fractures or severely osteopenic bone as these factors may by their very nature prohibit a stable construct. If in these circumstances fracture reconstruction is deemed impossible, delayed total hip arthroplasty after the fracture has united may be a preferable alternative. Although acute total hip arthroplasty has been used in the scenario of a pathological fracture of the acetabulum, it is important to recognize the critical distinction between that group of patients and patients with post-traumatic arthrosis of the hip. In patients with pathological fractures of the acetabulum, the objective is to decrease pain and improve quality of life; unfortunately, long-term survival is infrequent and the longevity of the hip joint is usually not the predominant concern. Acute total hip arthroplasty after acetabular fracture offers the potential advantages of one-stage treatment and minimization of the problems noted above with delayed total hip arthroplasty. Clearly, however, the technical challenges are significant given the objective of obtaining long-term implant function and survival.

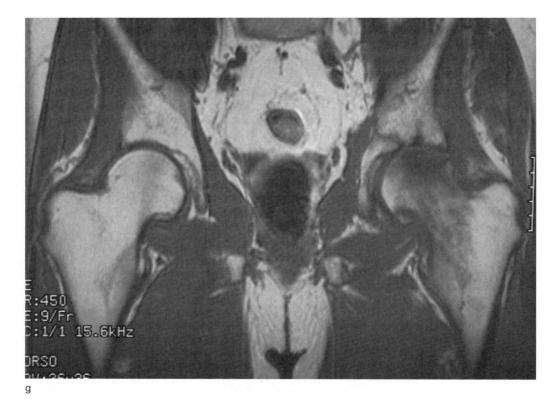

g

Fig. 5.6 *(continued)*

If a fracture of the acetabulum is determined not to be reconstructible and it is thought that the patient is eventually going
to come to total hip replacement as definitive management of
the fracture, controversy exists as to the role of acute surgery in
the ultimate management of the fracture. Up to the present, non-
operative management has been the mainstay of treatment in this
patient group. However, fractures that are left widely displaced
may result in non-union or severe malunion.[111] These problems
may significantly complicate eventual reconstruction arthroplasty.
Unfortunately, open surgical techniques predispose the patients
to the risks associated with surgery as discussed previously.
Additionally, the surgical exposure and disturbance of vascular
supply to the fracture fragments may result in avascular necrosis
of segments of the acetabulum, leading to non-union. It has been
shown by biopsy that segmental avascular necrosis may be
present in healed acetabular fractures.[111,112] The arterial supply
to the acetabulum is extensive, including branches of the obturator artery, the superior gluteal artery, and the inferior gluteal
artery as shown by the corrosion casting technique.[113] Although
the arterial supply is diverse, the predominant supply to the
acetabulum was shown in the same study to be the acetabular
branch of the obturator artery. This risk of injury can be minimized

Fig. 5.7

Clinical example of acute total hip arthroplasty for acetabular fracture. (a), (b) Posterior wall fracture-dislocation in an elderly patient. The CT images the extensive marginal impaction and total posterior wall involvement with subluxation of the femoral head. (c) The fracture treated with acute total hip replacement. The posterior wall was reconstructed with bulk allograft and posterior wall plating. The uncemented acetabulum was fixed with supplemental screws. (d), (e), (f) Acute acetabular fracture fixed with two cables and a cable-grip system. To prevent the cables from slipping into the acetabulum, they are passed through drill holes in the superior margin of the acetabulum. One cable is passed over the anterior column and the second is passed through the obturator foramen in this example. The cables are passed along the quadrilateral plate and through the greater sciatic notch to connectors in the supra-acetabular region.

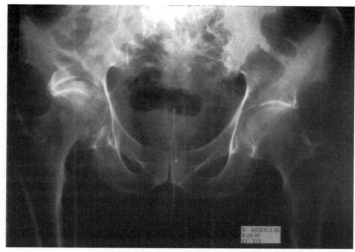

a

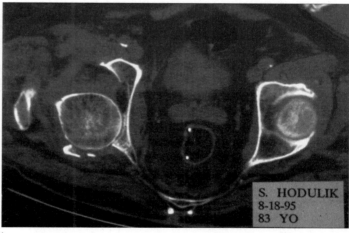

b

by reducing soft-tissue stripping on the surface of the quadrilateral plate, particularly in the inferior half. It is preferable to avoid injury to this arterial supply if any intervention is to be undertaken as a preliminary step to salvage with a total hip arthroplasty. Limited open reduction techniques and percutaneous fixation techniques[29] may result in decreased non-union and significant malunion rates. However, the benefits of these techniques may not be as great when accurate reconstruction of the acetabulum is not the primary goal, as limited internal fixation such as anterior and posterior column screws rely, to a large degree, on the intrinsic stability gained by accurate reconstruction and bony interdigitation. If bony stability is not achieved, limited internal fixation may not be as beneficial. Furthermore,

Fig. 5.7 *(continued)*

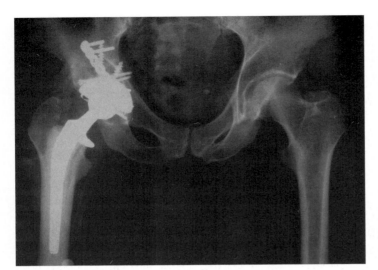

c

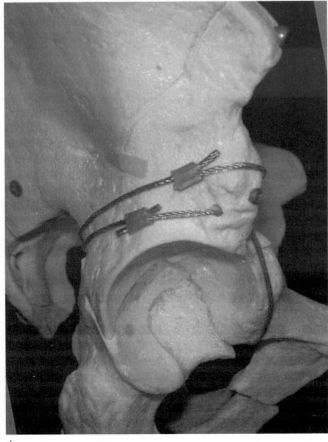

d

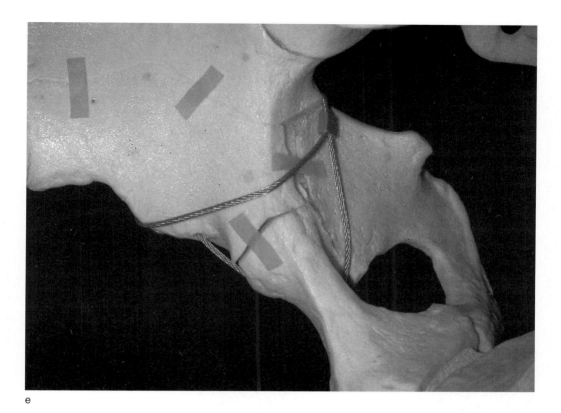

e

Fig. 5.7 *(continued)*

the internal fixation may still pose problems at the time of total hip arthroplasty. These techniques are very technically demanding, requiring specialized instruments and implants, high-quality intra-operative imaging and guidance systems, and an experienced surgical team.

In general it would seem that delayed total hip arthroplasty is favoured over acute total hip arthroplasty when it can be determined that the hip joint cannot be successfully reconstructed by standard means. Generally, the hip joint should be salvaged wherever possible, particularly if the patient is younger. This is particularly true in cases of malunions and non-unions.[114,115] There is no conclusive evidence that open reduction and internal fixation improves the outcome of total hip arthroplasty over initial non-operative management. In fact, the initial surgery may complicate the eventual arthroplasty by promoting soft-tissue scarring, avascular necrosis of the acetabulum, heterotopic ossification, infection, and neurological injury. If an arthroplasty is to be undertaken, the surgical challenges are typically those associated with revision total hip arthroplasty rather than with primary hip arthroplasty. The principle challenge is to obtain a satisfactory bony bed for implantation of the acetabular component. The surgeon must recognize non-unions and malunions

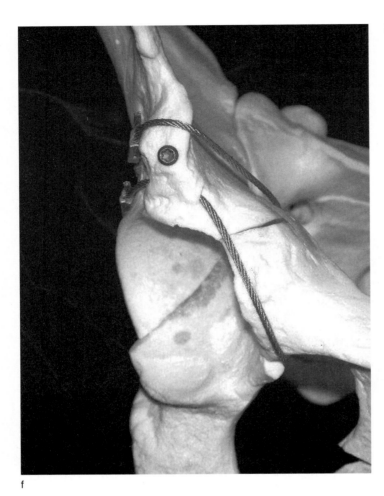

Fig. 5.7 *(continued)*

f

and be prepared to deal with significant bony defects. It appears that non-cemented acetabular components have met with greater success. Nonetheless, it would appear that the longevity of total hip arthroplasty is not comparable to that seen with total hip arthroplasty for routine degenerative arthrosis.

Summary

Acetabular fracture care is a demanding field of orthopaedic surgery. Many areas in the care of acetabular fractures have not yet been fully studied. These controversies do not mean that our understanding and ability to treat acetabular fractures have not improved. On the contrary, imaging techniques, surgical techniques and techniques to prevent or treat complications have improved dramatically. Unfortunately, these fractures remain complicated entities. Perhaps the principal challenge for the future will be to determine those fractures that will not be helped by open reduction and internal fixation as new techniques for long-term salvage and function become available.

References

1 Judet R, Judet J, Letournel E: Fractures of the acetabulum: classification and surgical approaches for open reduction. *Journal of Bone and Joint Surgery* [Am] **46**: 161538, 1964.

2 Letournel E, Judet R: In *Fractures of the acetabulum* (ed. RA Elson). pp 63–6. Springer-Verlag, New York, 1993.

3 Helfet DL, Nazarrian S: The comprehensive classification of fractures of long bones, spine, and pelvis, second edition. Springer-Verlag, New York, 1996.

4 Matta JM: Fractures of the acetabulum: accuracy of reduction and clinical results in patients managed operatively within three weeks after the injury. *Journal of Bone and Joint Surgery* [A] **78**: 1632–45, 1996.

5 Matta JM, Merritt PO: Displaced acetabular fractures. *Clinical Orthopaedics and Related Research* **230**: 83–97, 1988.

6 Matta JM, Mehne DK, Roofi R: Fractures of the acetabulum: early results of a prospective study. *Clinical Orthopaedics and Related Research* **205**: 241–50, 1986.

7 Rowe CR, Lowell JD: Prognosis of fractures of the acetabulum. *Journal of Bone and Joint Surgery* [Am] **43**: 30, 1961.

8 Pantazopoulos T, Mousafiris C: Surgical treatment of central acetabular fractures. *Clinical Orthopaedics and Related Research* **246**: 57–64, 1989.

9 Kebaish A, Roy A, Rennie W: Displaced acetabular fractures: long term follow up. *Journal of Trauma* **31**: 1539–42, 1991.

10 Knight RA, Smith H: Central fractures of the acetabulum. *Journal of Bone and Joint Surgery* [Am] **40**: 1–16, 1958.

11 Greenwald AS, O'Connor JJ: The transmissions of load through the human hip joint. *Journal of Biomechanics* **4**: 507–28, 1971.

12 Bay BK, Hamel A, Olson SA: Statically equivalent load and support conditions produce different hip joint contact pressures and periacetabular strains. *Journal of Biomechanics* **30**: 193–6, 1997.

13 Bullough P, Goodfellow J, O'Connor J: The relationship between degenerative changes and the loading bearing in the human hip. *Journal of Bone and Joint Surgery* [Br] **55**: 746–58, 1973.

14 Finkenberg JG, Kim WC, Wolgin WA, Dickman P: Acetabular fractures role of joint incongruity in the development of osteoarthritis. *Orthopaedic Transactions* **12**: 526, 1988.

15 Olson SA, Bay BK, Chapman MW, Sharkey NA: Biomechanical consequences of fracture and repair of the posterior wall of the acetabulum. *Journal of Bone and Joint Surgery* [Am] **77**: 1184–92, 1995.

16 Olson SA, Bay BK, Polak AN, Sharkey NA, Lee T: The effect of variable size posterior wall acetabular fractures on contact characteristics of the hip joint. *Journal of Orthopaedic Trauma.* **10**: 395–482, 1996.

17 Konrath GA, Hamel AJ, Sharkey NA, Bay BK, Olson SA: Biomechanical consequences of anterior column fracture of the acetabulum. *Journal of Orthopaedic Trauma* **12**: 547–52, 1998.

18 Radin EL, Rose RM: Role of subchondral bone in the initiation and progression of cartilage damage. *Clinical Orthopaedics and Related Research* **213**: 34–40, 1986.

19 Olson SA, Matta JM: Surgical treatment of acetabular fractures. In *Skeletal trauma* (2nd edn) (ed. B. Browner). WB Saunders, Philadelphia, PA, 1998.

20 Tile M: In *Fractures of the pelvis and acetabulum* (2nd edn) (ed. M Tile), p. 327. Williams and Wilkins, Philadelphia, PA, 1995.

21 Matta J: Operative indications and choice of surgical approach for fractures of the acetabulum. Techniques Orthopédiques 1:13–22, 1986.

22 Olson SA, Maurizi MG, Hassien J, Pearl AJ: A review of computerized tomography evaluation of acetabular fractures. *Contemporary Orthopaedics* 23: 436–47, 1991.

23 Olson SA, Matta JM: The computerized tomography subchondral arc: a new method of assessing acetabular articular continuity after fracture: a preliminary report. *Journal of Orthopaedic Trauma* 7: 402–13, 1993.

24 Keith JE, Brashear HR, Guilford WB. Stability of posterior fracture-dislocations of the hip: quantitative assessment using computed tomography. *Journal of Bone and Joint Surgery* [Am] 70: 711–14, 1988.

25 Vailas JC , Hurwitz S, Wiesel SE: Posterior acetabular fracture-dislocations: fragment size, joint capsule, and stability. *Journal of Trauma* 29: 1494–6, 1989.

26 Calkins MS, Zych G, Latta L *et al.*: Computerized tomography evaluation of stability in posterior facture dislocations of the hip. *Clinical Orthopaedics and Related Research* 227: 152–63, 1988.

27 Routt ML Jr, Swiontkowski MF: Operative treatment of complex acetabular fractures: combined anterior and posterior exposures during the same procedure. *Journal of Bone and Joint Surgery* [Am] 72: 897–904, 1990.

28 Moed BR, Willson Carr SE, Watson JT: Open reduction and internal fixation of posterior wall fractures of the acetabulum. Presented at the Orthopaedic Trauma Association, San Antonio, TX, 12–14, October 2000.

29 Starr AJ, Borer DS, Reinert CM, Jones AL: Early results and complications following limited open reduction and percutaneous screw fixation of displaced fractures of the acetabulum. Presented at the Orthopaedic Trauma Association, San Antonio, TX, 12–14, October 2000.

30 Routt ML Jr, Simonian, PT, Grujic L: The retrograde medullary superior pubic ramus screw for the treatment of anterior pelvic ring disruptions: a new technique. *Journal of Orthopaedic Trauma* 9: 33–44, 1995.

31 Helfet DL, Schmeling GJ: Somatosensory evoked potential monitoring in the surgical treatment of acute, displace acetabular fractures: results of a prospective study. *Clinical Orthopaedics and Related Research* 301: 213–20, 1994.

32 Helfet DL, Hissa EA, Sergay S, Mast JW: Somatosensory evoked potential monitoring in the surgical management of acute acetabular fractures. *Journal of Orthopaedic Trauma* 2: 161–6, 1991.

33 Helfet DL, Schmeling GJ: Management of acute, displaced acetabular fractures using indirect reduction techniques and limited approaches. *Orthopaedic Transactions* 15: 833, 1991.

34 Vrahas M, Bordon RG, Mears DC, Krieger D, Sclabassi RJ: Intraoperative somatosensory evoked potential monitoring of pelvic and acetabular fractures. *Journal of Orthopaedic Trauma* 6: 50–8, 1992.

35 Letournel E: Acetabular fractures: classification and management. *Clinical Orthopaedics and Related Research* 151: 81–106, 1980.

36 Matta JM: Acetabulum fractures: results of a combined operative and nonoperative protocol. Presented at the 58th Annual Meeting of the American Academy of Orthopaedic Surgeons, 1991.

37 Matta J, Merritt P: Displaced acetabular fractures. *Clinical Orthopaedics and Related Research* **230**: 83–97, 1989.

38 Mears D, Rubash H: *Pelvic and acetabular fractures* Slack, Thorofare, NJ, 1986.

39 Matta JM, Anderson LM, Epstein HC, Hendricks P: Fractures of the acetabulum. A retrospective analysis. *Clinical Orthopaedics and Related Research* **205**: 230–40, 1986.

40 Goulet JA, Bray TJ: Complex acetabular fractures. *Clinical Orthopaedics and Related Research* **240**: 9–20, 1989.

41 Fassler PR, Swiontkowski MF, Kilroy AW, Routt ML Jr: Injury of the sciatic nerve associated with acetabular fracture. *Journal of Bone and Joint Surgery* [Am] **75**: 1157–66, 1993.

42 Borelli J Jr: Intraneural sciatic nerve pressures relative to the position of the hip and knee: a human cadaveric study. *Journal of Orthopaedic Trauma* **14**: 255–8, 2000.

43 Calder HB, Mast J, Johnstone CA: Intraoperative evoked potential monitoring in acetabular surgery. *Clinical Orthopaedics and Related Research* **305**: 160–7, 1994.

44 Baumgaertner MR, Wegner D, Booke J: SSEP monitoring during pelvic and acetabular fracture surgery. *Journal of Orthopaedic Trauma* **2**: 127–33, 1994.

45 Moed BR, Maxey JW, Minster GJ: Intraoperative somatosensory evoked potential monitoring of peripheral nerves in an animal model. *Journal of Orthopaedic Trauma* **6**: 59–65, 1992.

46 Templeman DC, Olson S, Moed BR, Duwelius P, Matta JM: Surgical treatment of acetabular fractures. *Instructional Course Lectures* **48**: 481–96, 1999.

47 Middlebrooks ES, Sims SH, Kellam JF, Bosse MJ: Incidence of sciatic nerve injury in operatively treated acetabular fractures without somatosensory evoked potential monitoring. *Journal of Orthopaedic Trauma* **11**: 327–9, 1997.

48 Arrington ED, Hochschild DP, Steinagle TJ, Mongan PD, Martin SL: Monitoring of somatosensory and motor evoked potentials during open reduction and internal fixation of pelvic and acetabular fractures. *Orthopedics* **23**: 1081–3, 2000.

49 Kawaraguchi Y, Kakimoto M, Inoue S *et al.*: Monitoring of motor evoked potentials during insertions of iliosacral screws for reconstruction of pelvic fracture in two patients. *Masue* **49**: 514–18, 2000.

50 Helfet DL, Anand N, Malkani AL *et al.*: Intraoperative monitoring of motor pathways during operative fixation of acute acetabular fractures. *Journal of Orthopaedic Trauma* **11**: 2–6, 1997.

51 Moed BR, Ahmad BK, Craig JG, Jacobson GP, Anders MJ: Intraoperative monitoring with stimulus-evoked electromyography during placement of iliosacral screws: an initial clinical study. *Journal of Bone and Joint Surgery* [Am] **80**: 537–46, 1998.

52 Stewart MJ, Milford LW: Fracture-dislocation of the hip: an end result study. *Journal of Bone and Joint Surgery* **36A**: 315–342, 1954.

53 Bray TJ, Esser M, Fulkerson L: Osteotomy of the trochanter in open reduction and internal fixation of acetabular fractures. *Journal of Bone and Joint Surgery* [Am] **69**: 711–17, 1987.

54 Mears DC, Rubash HE: Extensive exposure of the pelvis. *Contemporary Orthopaedics* **6**: 21, 1983.

55 Moed BR, Maxey JW: The effect of indomethacin on heterotopic ossification following acetabular fracture surgery. *Journal of Orthopaedic Trauma* **7**: 33–8, 1993.

56 Bosse M, Poka A, Reinert C, Ellwanger F, Slawson R, McDevitt E: Heterotopic ossification as a complication of acetabular fracture. *Journal of Bone and Joint Surgery* [Am] **70**: 1231–7, 1988.

57 Burd TA, Anglen JO: Indomethacin vs. localized irradiation for the prevention of heterotopic ossification following acetabulum fractures: a 7-year prospective randomized trial of 182 patients. Presented at the Orthopaedic Trauma Association, San Antonio, TX, 12–14, October 2000.

58 Chalmers J, Gray DH, Rush J: Observations on the induction of bone and soft tissue. *Journal of Bone and Joint Surgery* [Br] **57**: 36–44, 1975.

59 Hall BK: Histiogenesis and morphogenesis of bone. *Clinical Orthopaedics and Related Research* **263**: 94–101, 1991.

60 Ghalambor N, Matta JM, Bernstein L: Heterotopic ossification following operative treatment of acetabular fracture: an analysis of risk factors. *Clinical Orthopaedics and Related Research* **305**: 96–105, 1994.

61 Matta JM, Anderson LM, Epstein HC, Hendricks P: Fractures of the acetabulum: a retrospective analysis. *Clinical Orthopaedics and Related Research* **205**: 230, 1986.

62 Johnson EE, Kay RM, Dorey FJ: Heterotopic ossification prophylaxis following operative treatment of acetabular fracture. *Clinical Orthopaedics and Related Research* **305**: 88–95, 1994.

63 McLaren AC: Prophylaxis with indomethacin for heterotopic bone after open reduction of fractures of the acetabulum. *Journal of Bone and Joint Surgery* [Am] **72**: 245–7, 1990.

64 Kaempffe FA, Bone LB, Border JR: Open reduction and internal fixation of acetabular fractures: Heterotopic ossification and other complications of treatment. *Journal of Orthopaedic Trauma* **5**: 439–45, 1991.

65 Daum WJ, Scarborough MT, Gordon W Jr, Uchida T: Heterotopic ossification and other perioperative complications of acetabular fractures. *Journal of Orthopaedic Trauma* **6**: 427–32, 1992.

66 Brooker LF, Bowerman JW, Robinson RA, Riley LH: Ectopic Ossification following total hip replacement: incidence and a method of classification. *Journal of Bone and Joint Surgery* [Am] **55**: 1629–32, 1973.

67 Matta JM, Siebenrock KA: Does indomethacin reduce heterotopic bone formation after operations for acetabular fractures? A prospective randomized study. *Journal of Bone and Joint Surgery* [Br] **79**: 959–63, 1997.

68 Ritchie W, Alonso JE: CT classification of heterotopic ossification after reconstruction of acetabular fractures. *Proceedings of the 1st International Pelvic and Acetabular Surgery Symposium, Pittsburgh, PA, 1992.*

69 Moed BR, Smith S: Radiographic assessment of heterotopic ossification following acetabular fracture surgery. Presented at the 62nd Annual Meeting of the American Academy of Orthopaedic Surgeons, Orlando, FL, February 1995.

70 Bruno LP, Stern PJ, Wyrick JD: Skeletal changes after burn injuries in an animal model. *Journal of Burn Care and Rehabilitation* **9**: 148–51, 1988.

71 Bhalla AK, Simon LS: A clinical evaluation of the antiarthritic agents. *Comprehensive Therapy* **10**: 40–50, 1984.

72 Nilsson OS, Bauer CF, Brosjo O, Tornkvist H: Influence of indomethacin on induced heterotopic bone formation in rats. *Clinical Orthopaedics and Related Research* **207**: 239–45.

73 Moore KD, Gosss K, Anglen JO: Indomethacin versus radiation therapy for prophylaxis against heterotopic ossification in acetabular fractures: a randomized, prospective study. *Journal of Bone and Joint Surgery* [Br] **80**: 259–63, 1998.

74 Pellegrini VD, Gregoritch SH: Preoperative irradiation for prevention of heterotopic ossification following total hip arthroplasty. *Journal of Bone and Joint Surgery* [Am] **78**: 870–81, 1996.

75 Lo TCM, Healy WL, Covall DJ *et al.*: Heterotopic bone formation after hip surgery: prevention with single-dose postoperative hip irradiation. *Radiology* **168**: 851–4, 1988.

76 Childs HA 3rd, Cole T, Falkenberg E *et al.*: *International Journal of Radiation, Oncology, Biology, Physics* **47**: 1347–52, 2000.

77 Anglen JO, Moore KD: Prevention of heterotopic bone formation after acetabular fracture fixation by single-dose radiation therapy: a preliminary report. *Journal of Orthopaedic Trauma* **10**: 258–63, 1996.

78 Ayers DC, Pellegrini VD, Evars CM: Prevention of heterotopic ossification in high-risk patients by radiation therapy. *Clinical Orthopaedics and Related Research* **263**: 87–9, 1991.

79 Gregoritch SJ, Chadha M, Pellegrini VD, Rubin P, Kantorowitz DA: Randomized trial comparing preoperative versus postoperative irradiation for prevention of heterotopic ossification following prosthetic total hip replacement: preliminary results. *International Journal of Radiation, Oncology, Biology, Physics* **30**: 55–62, 1994.

80 Seegenschmiedt MH, Martus P, Goldman AR *et al.*: Preoperative versus postoperative radiotherapy for prevention of heterotopic ossification(HO): first results of a randomized trial in high-risk patients. *International Journal of Radiation, Oncology, Biology, Physics* **30**: 63–73, 1994.

81 Moed BR, Letournel E: Low-dose irradiation and indomethacin prevent heterotopic ossification after acetabular fracture surgery. *Journal of Bone and Joint Surgery* [Br] **76**: 895–900, 1994.

82 Brady LW: Radiation induced sarcomas of bone. *Skeletal Radiology* **4**: 72–8, 1979.

83 Kim JH, Chu FC, Woodard HQ *et al.*: Radiation induced soft tissue and bone sarcoma. *Radiology* **129**: 501–8, 1978.

84 Rowe CR, Lowell JD: Prognosis of fractures of the acetabulum. *Journal of Bone and Joint Surgery* [Am] **43**: 30–59, 1961.

85 Pennal GF, Davidson J, Garside H, Plewes J: Results of treatment of acetabular fractures. *Clinical Orthopaedics and Related Research* **151**: 115–23, 1980.

86 Carnesale PJ, Stewart MJ, Barnes SN: Acetabular disruption and central fracture dislocation of the hip. *Journal of Bone and Joint Surgery* [Am] **57**: 1054–9, 1975.

87 Mayo KA: Open reduction and internal fixation of fractures of the acetabulum: results in 163 fractures. *Clinical Orthopaedics and Related Research* **305**: 31–7, 1994.

88 Pellegrini VD Jr: Arthrodesis of the hip. In *Surgery of the musculoskeletal system* (ed. CM McAllistair). Churchill Livingston, New York, 1990.

89 Callaghan JJ, McBeath AA: Arthrodesis. In *The adult hip* (ed. JJ Callaghan, AG Rosenberg, HE Rubash). Lippincott–Raven, PA, 1998.

90 Waters RL, Barnes G, Husserl T, Liss R: Comparable energy expenditure after arthrodesis of the hip and ankle. *Journal of Bone and Joint Surgery* [Am] **70**: 1032–7, 1988.

91 Callaghan J, Brand RA, Pedersen DR: Hip arthrodesis: a long-term follow-up. *Journal of Bone and Joint Surgery* [Am] **67**: 1328–35, 1985.

92 Carnesale PG: Arthrodesis of the hip: a long-term study. *Orthopaedic Digest* **4**: 12, 1976.

93 Sponseller P, McBeath A, Perpich M: Hip arthrodesis in young patients: a long-term follow-up study. *Journal of Bone and Joint Surgery* [Am] **66**: 853–9, 1984.

94 Stewart MJ, Coker TP: Arthrodesis of the hip: a review of 109 patients. *Clinical Orthopaedics and Related Research* **62**: 136–50, 1969.

95 Westerborn A: Central dislocation of the femoral head treated with mold arthroplasty. *Journal of Bone and Joint Surgery* [Am] **36**: 307–14, 1954.

96 Kelly PJ, Lipscomb PR: Primary vitallium-mold arthroplasty for posterior dislocation of the hip with fracture of the femoral head. *Journal of Bone and Joint Surgery* [Am] **40**: 675–80, 1958.

97 Boardman KP, Charnley J: Low-friction arthroplasty after fracture-dislocation of the hip. *Journal of Bone and Joint Surgery* [Br] **60**: 495–7, 1972.

98 Romness DW, Lewallen DG: Total hip arthroplasty after fracture of the acetabulum: long-term results. *Journal of Bone and Joint Surgery* [Br] **72**: 761–4.

99 Weber M, Berry DJ, Harmsen WS: Total hip arthroplasty after operative treatment of an acetabular fracture. *Journal of Bone and Joint Surgery* [Am] **80**: 1295–1305.

100 Huo MH, Solberg BD, Zatorski LE, Keggi KJ: Total hip replacements done without cement after acetabular fractures: a 4 to 8 year follow-up study. *Journal of Arthroplasty* **14**: 827–831, 1999.

101 Pritchett JW, Bortel DT: Total hip replacement after central fracture dislocation of the acetabulum. *Orthopaedic Review* **20**: 607–10, 1991.

102 Waddell JP, Morton J: Total hip arthroplasty following acetabular fracture. Presented at the Annual Meeting of the Orthopaedic Trauma Association, Los Angeles, CA, September 1994.

103 Karpos PAG, Christie MJ: THR following acetabular fracture using cementless acetabular components: 4 to 8 years results. Presented at the Annual Meeting of the American Association of Hip and Knee Surgeons, Dallas, TX, October 1995.

104 Karpos PAG, Chrisitie MJ, Chenger JD: Total hip arthroplasty following acetabular fracture: the effect of prior open reduction, internal fixation. *Orthopaedic Transactions* **17**: 598, 1993.

105 Mears DC, Ward AJ: Late results of total hip arthroplasty to manage post-traumatic arthritis of acetabular fractures. Presented at Fractures of the Pelvis and Acetabulum: The 3rd International Consensus, Pittsburgh, PA, October 1996.

106 Mont MA, Marr DC, Krackow KA, Jacobs JA, Jones LC, Hungerford DS: Total hip replacement without cement for non-inflammatory osteoarthrosis in patients who are less than forty-five years old. *Journal of Bone and Joint Surgery* [Am] **75**: 740–51, 1993.

107 Stauffer RN: Ten year follow-up study of total hip replacement: with particular reference to roentgengraphic loosening of the components. *Journal of Bone and Joint Surgery* [Am] **64**: 983–90, 1982.

108 Joly JM, Mears DC: The role of total hip arthroplasty in acetabular fracture management. *Operative Techniques in Orthopaedics* **3**: 80–102, 1993.

109 Helfet DL, Borelli J Jr, Dipasquale DO, Sanders R: Stabilization of acetabular fractures in elderly patients. *Journal of Bone and Joint Surgery* [Am] **74**: 753–65, 1992.

110 Mears DC, Shirahama M: Stabilization of an acetabular fracture with cables for acute total hip arthroplasty. *Journal of Arthroplasty* **13**: 104–7, 1998.

111 Mears DC, Velyvis JH: Primary total hip arthroplasty after acetabular fracture. *Journal of Bone and Joint Surgery* [Am] **82**: 1328–53, 2000.

112 Mears DC: Avascular necrosis of the acetabulum. *Operative Techniques in Orthopaedics* **7**: 241–9, 1997.

113 Itokazu M, Takahashi K, Matsunaga T *et al.*: A study of the arterial supply of the human acetabulum using a corrosion casting method. *Clinical Anatomy* **2**: 77–81, 1997.

114 Johnson EE, Matta JM, Mast JW, Letournel E: Delayed reconstruction of acetabular fractures 21–120 days following injury. *Clinical Orthopaedics and Related Research* **305**: 20–30, 1994.

115 Mayo KA, Letournel E, Matta JM, Mast JW, Johnson EE, Martimbeau CL: Surgical revision of malreduced acetabular fractures. *Clinical Orthopaedics and Related Research* **305**: 47–52, 1994.

6

Femoral neck fractures: epidemiology and results and controversies in treatment

Harry Tsigaras and Steven J. MacDonald

Introduction

Hip fractures are a major public health issue globally. The morbidity and mortality associated with these injuries exacts a significant economic and social cost to the patient, the health care provider, and the community.[1] Hip fracture is a universal problem with an escalating incidence.[2] As longevity continues to increase, the proportion of the population at greatest risk, the elderly, grows. The most rapidly growing segment of the population is, in fact, the over-85 age group.[3] If current incidence trends continue, a doubling or tripling of the number of hip fractures can be expected in the next 25–50 years.[4-6] This has far-reaching implications for health care systems worldwide. As we begin this new century there will be a tremendous challenge and opportunity in the management of the hip fracture patient.

This chapter will review the epidemiology of femoral neck fractures and results and controversies in treatment. It is only through a thorough understanding of our current knowledge of this condition that we can help to produce changes in the future.

Epidemiology

Incidence

The actual number of hip fractures that occur worldwide is not accurately known. It has been estimated that in 1990 there were 1.26 million fractures.[7] Generally, there is a significant underestimation in the incidence secondary to many factors including a decreasing mortality rate in the elderly in all regions of the world. Lifetime risks of hip fracture at the age of 50 are 4.6 per cent for men and 13.9 per cent for women based on current mortality; however, based on predicted mortality these numbers increase to 11.1 per cent and 22.7 per cent respectively.[8] Many studies have relied on hospital discharge data, but it has been demonstrated[9] that actual incidences can range from 15 per cent lower to 89 per cent higher than these records indicate, depending on the country of origin.

There is a well-documented enormous geographic variation in the incidence of hip fracture (Table 6.1). The highest rates are demonstrated in Scandinavia and North America, with intermediate rates in western Europe and the lowest rates in Asia. Even within each country there are significant regional differences in hip fracture incidence despite controlling for independent variables such as age and race (Bacon *et al.* 1989; Jacobsen *et al.* 1990; Stroup *et al.* 1990 and Hinton *et al.* 1995).[23-26] The reasons for these variabilities are still incompletely understood, however, will be discussed at greater length later in the text.

Unquestionably, the incidence of hip fractures is rising worldwide. Over a 23-year period (1970–1993) in Scotland there was an overall increase of 101 per cent in the number of patients admitted with hip fractures, and an increase of 158 per cent in the cohort of patients aged 75 years and over.[27] In a Danish study[28] there was an annual increase of 9–10 per cent in a 16-year interval (1970–1986), with an increase in the age-specific incidence observed for both males and females. In Australia there was a 45 per cent increase in the total number of fractures between 1979 and 1990.[29] In a study covering a 65-year period (1928–1992) in Rochester, Minnesota, a fivefold increase in the prevalence of hip fractures was thought to be mainly determined by change in incidence.[30] Recently, however, several authors have noted either smaller increases in the incidence or a plateauing of these rates. Rogmark *et al.*[11] reported a significant break in previous trends in

Table 6.1 Country-specific hip fracture incidence (in order of decreasing frequency)

	Current incidence per 100 000		Reference
	Female	Male	
Norway	1293	551	Finsen and Benum[10]
Sweden	850	360	Rogmark *et al.*[11]
New Zealand	540–790	185–360	Norton *et al.*[12]
Argentina	513	122	Bagur *et al.*[13]
United States	510	174	Gallagher *et al.*[14]
Canada	479	187	Papadimitropoulos *et al.*[15]
Finland	467	233	Kannus *et al.*[16]
Kuwait	295	200	Memon *et al.*[17]
Iceland	274	141	Schwartz *et al.*[9]
France	269	122	Baudoin *et al.*[18]
United Kingdom	257	72	Lau *et al.*[19]
Italy	228	81	Mazzuoli *et al.*[20]
China	87	97	Xu *et al.*[21]
Taiwan	45	36	Huang *et al.*[22]

that the incidence in Sweden was no longer increasing. Possible explanations included prevention of osteoporosis, increasing immigration of those with a lower genetic predisposition to fracture, and a healthier cohort of elderly patients. A report from Finland[31] demonstrated that, although there was an 11 per cent increase in the number of hip fractures over a 10 year period, there was no change in the age-standardized incidence of fractures and that the increase reflected a change in the age distribution of the population. Conversely, a second Finnish report,[32] studying a 27-year period, demonstrated an increase in the specific age-adjusted incidence of hip fractures. Wildner *et al.*[33] reported an annual increase of 2 per cent in East Germany over an 18-year period. Therefore trends are still emerging and careful evaluation will be required in this new millennium.

Predicting the future incidence of hip fractures is obviously difficult with the many variables involved. A conservative estimate would assume no change in the age-specific incidences. Gullberg[7] have done just that, estimating current worldwide totals at 1.26 million, doubling to 2.6 million by 2025, and reaching 4.5 million by 2050. A similar report from Australia,[34] again assuming no changes in the age- and gender-specific incidences, predicts that the number of fractures in South Australia will increase by 66 per cent by 2021 and by 190 per cent by 2051. In the United States the rate is also expected to more than double over the next 50 years, with a current rate of 238 000 rising to 512 000 by 2040.[6]

The economic impact of hip fractures is staggering. The costs include not only the initial medical care but also aftercare, reduction in quality of life, loss of work years, and costs to the family and the community.[1] It is estimated that the annual cost to the health care system in the United Kingdom is just under £1 billion.[35] The annual cost in the United States is approximately $7 billion.[6] Worldwide, it is estimated that, by 2050, $131.5 billion will be spent on managing hip fractures.[36] If we hope to effect a change in the incidence and costs associated with these fractures, an understanding of the risk factors involved is critical to future research.

The risk factors associated with hip fractures are multifactorial with significant overlap. Obviously some of these risk factors can be altered while others cannot. They can be broadly classified as follows:

- demographic factors
- gender
- age
- race
- genetics
- lifestyle factors
- body mass
- diet

- smoking
- alcohol
- activity level
- medical history/medication
- geographic factors
- climate
- location of residence
- biomechanical factors
- femoral anatomy
- bone density.

Demographic factors

Gender

Gender plays a significant role in the risk of sustaining a hip fracture. Women account for 72–73 per cent of all fractures worldwide.[7,37] The lifetime risk of a hip fracture is 16–18 per cent in white women and 5–6 per cent in white men.[32] In most reviews, women are at least twice as likely to suffer a hip fracture compared with their male counterparts. The exception to this has been in Asia where the risk has been equal or slightly higher in males.[21] The doubling of the incidence of hip fractures is only true in the over-65 age group, and the rates are almost identical in those aged 50–54 years (Table 6.2). Other factors, particularly the incidence of osteoporosis, influence the fracture rate in elderly women. Documented significant risk factors include the age of menarche and menopause,[38] with a long reproductive period being protective for hip fracture mortality and the use of postmenopausal hormone therapy[39] reducing its incidence.

Age

A patient's age is clearly an independent risk factor for hip fracture. Gullberg et al.[7] summarized the incidence of hip fracture by age for men and women by region of the world (Table 6.2). The incidence of hip fracture in women in their early eighties is over a 50 times that in women in their early fifties. In a large review it was noted that the incidence of hip fracture doubled every 7 years, and that age-associated factors common to both sexes provided the main risk factors.[40] A similar review demonstrated comparable results, with annual age-specific incidences increasing exponentially with age, doubling every 6 years, and equalling 4 per cent in women aged over 90 years.[41] This has significant implications with the global ageing of the population. In the United States, 13 per cent of the population are over 65 years of age at present, but by 2040 over 20 per cent will be in this category. Currently, this group accounts for 25 per cent of all prescription drugs, 33 per cent of all health care dollars spent, and over 50 per cent of all hospital bed utilization.[42] Clearly, as one ages, many other factors are involved in increasing the incidence of hip fracture.

Table 6.2 Incidence of hip fracture in 1990 by age, sex, and region

Region	Incidence per 100 000 Men							Women						
	50–54	55–59	60–64	65–69	70–75	75–79	80+	50–54	55–59	60–64	65–69	70–74	75–79	80+
W. Europe	28	33	67	103	203	331	880	33	54	115	184	362	657	1808
S. Europe	10	16	34	55	81	190	534	11	21	47	100	170	380	1075
E. Europe	38	38	88	88	194	194	475	58	58	155	155	426	426	1251
N. Europe	58	66	97	198	382	682	1864	74	78	190	327	612	1294	2997
N. America	33	33	81	123	119	338	1230	60	60	117	252	437	850	2296
Oceania	20	34	63	92	180	445	1157	31	63	112	204	358	899	2476
Asia	19.5	19.5	36.5	46.5	102	150	364	14	14	38	74.5	155.5	252	562.5
Africa	6	10	14	27	8	0	116	4.0	12	17	12	16	50	80
Latin America	25	40	40	106	106	327	327	19.5	50	50	162.5	162.5	622	622
World	22.5	24.5	47.3	68.7	119.1	219.4	630.2	23.9	28.4	69.1	121.6	239.8	457.7	1289.3

Race

Clearly, there are differences in hip fracture incidence that are related to race. Many reviews from the United States have documented a much lower incidence of hip fractures in the black population than in the white population. Fracture rates for white females have been reported to be 1.5 to 4 times higher than those for black females after the age of 40. [43] Hinton and Smith [44] demonstrated that the rate of hip fracture was highest in white women with a successively decreasing rate in white men, black women, and black men. Lauderdale *et al.*[45] found that the age-adjusted hip fracture incidence for three Asian-American groups (Chinese, Japanese, and Korean Americans) was lower than for white Americans. The natural question arises as to whether the effect is due to race or culture. Ross *et al.*[46] studied native Japanese, Japanese Americans, and American Caucasians and demonstrated the age-specific hip fracture rates of those of Japanese ancestry were half those of Caucasians for both sexes. The Japanese Americans were presumed to have much more westernized diet and other cultural influences than native Japanese but their fracture rates were similar. One possible explanation for these differences in bone density variability. However, this could not explain all the differences as Japanese have significantly lower bone mineral content, as measured by dual X-ray absorptiometry, than Caucasians.[47] A potential explanation lies in the differences in the actual femoral anatomy between the races. Women of African origin have thicker cortical bone, a shorter hip axis length (the distance from below the lateral aspect of the greater trochanteric to the inner pelvic brim), and smaller intertrochanteric widths than Caucasians. It was felt that these differences could contribute to a 25 per cent decreased risk of hip fracture among black women.[48] Similarly, Japanese women have lower risks of hip fracture, possibly due to a shorter femoral neck and a smaller femoral neck angle.[47]

Genetics

Tremendous advances have been made in molecular biology and genetics research. If patients at risk for fracture could be identified with simple screening then prevention protocols could potentially be initiated. The apolipoprotein E (apoE) allele has been associated with Alzheimer's disease and osteoporosis in patients on hemodialysis. Cauley *et al.*[49] performed a prospective evaluation and found that women with the apoE polymorphism were at an increased risk of hip fracture which could not be explained by bone density, mental impairment, or frequency of falls, but could perhaps be due to an effect of apoE on vitamin K, bone turnover, or weight loss. Also, the vitamin D receptor genotype has been associated with a twofold increase risk of hip fracture in the BB genotype.[50] Family history has also been shown to be a risk factor for hip fracture even when adjusted for bone density.[51]

Lifestyle factors

Body mass

The body mass index (BMI) is calculated by dividing the patient's weight (kg) by height (m²). As the BMI increases so does the patient's risk of hypertension, hypercholesterolaemia, type 2 diabetes, coronary heart disease, and stroke.[52] Conversely, a low BMI has been shown to increase the risk of hip fracture.[53-55] It has been postulated that the adipose tissue may offer a degree of protection during a fall. The association between body size and hip fracture risk was assessed in an analysis of over 8000 women followed prospectively.[56] Looking at multiple factors including total body weight, percentage weight change since age 25, hip girth, lean mass, fat mass, percentage body fat, BMI, and modified BMI, the authors demonstrated that women with a smaller body size had a higher risk of subsequent hip fracture than all others. After careful analysis it was concluded that the effect was probably due to a lower hip bone mineral density in women with a smaller body size. Not only are patients who maintain a low BMI at increased risk, but so are those who loose weight later in life. Weight loss (>10 per cent) in both men and women after the age of 50 increases the risk for hip fracture, and weight gain (>10 per cent) appears to offer some protection.[57,58] Height has been implicated as an independent risk factor for hip fracture. Hemenway *et al.*[59] reported on a prospective study of 50 000 men and noted that patients who were 1.8 m (6 feet) or taller were more than twice as likely to sustain hip fracture as those under 1.75 m (5 feet 9 inches). The same group reported on a prospective cohort of over 92 000 women and demonstrated that women who were 1.73 m (5 feet 8 inches) or taller were more than twice as likely to sustain a hip fracture than those under 1.57 m (5 feet 2 inches).[60] Height was seen to be an important independent risk factor for hip fracture in both these studies.

Diet

As explained above, malnutrition with weight loss is a significant risk factor for hip fracture for both men and women. Therefore diet in the elderly is a very important issue. Postmenopausal women admitted with hip fractures have been shown to have vitamin D deficiency and elevated levels of parathyroid hormone.[61] Vitamin D deficiency is both treatable and preventable, and if treated should reduce future fracture risk. In a prospective randomized trial, women received either vitamin D and calcium or placebo for 18 months.[62] Among the women treated with vitamin D and calcium, the number of hip fractures was 43 per cent lower than among those taking placebo and the total number of non-vertebral fractures was 32 per cent lower. In a cohort of patients followed prospectively, dietary calcium was the only nutrient that was consistently associated with hip fracture when deficient.[63]

Other dietary influences have been evaluated with respect to their influence on hip fracture rates. Osteoblast activity is stimulated by higher concentrations of fluoride which can lead to an increase in cancellous bone mass. Water fluoridation has proven advantages for dental health; however, it has been suggested that there is an increased rate of hip fractures in areas of high fluoride concentrations in drinking water. Evaluating this is obviously very difficult because of the presence of multiple covariables. In an extensive analysis, Hillier et al.[64] were unable to find a correlation between fluoride consumption and risk of hip fracture. However, Kurttio et al.[65] felt that fluoride consumption increased the risk of hip fracture in women aged 50–64 years. This question may never be answered as it has been estimated that more than 400 000 patients would need to be entered into an appropriately designed study to solve the issue.[66] Vitamin K insufficiency may also play a role in osteoporosis in hip fracture risk; however, this is unclear at the present. Both decreased circulating levels of vitamin K_1 and equivocal levels have been shown in patients presenting with hip fractures.[67,68]

Smoking

Tobacco smoking exacts an enormous toll on our society. It has been estimated that as many as 20 per cent of all deaths in developed countries are caused by smoking.[69] Law and Hackshaw[70] reported a meta-analysis of published studies correlating smoking and hip fractures. Smoking increased the lifetime risk of hip fracture by about 50 per cent and, among all women, one hip fracture in eight was attributable to smoking. Forsen et al.[71] reported on almost 35 000 adults and again demonstrated that smoking increased the chance of hip fractures in women by 50 per cent. The correlation was much stronger among thinner women with a relative risk of 3.0, which was equivalent to adding 10 years to their age in terms of hip fracture risk. The effects of smoking are not quickly reversible. Five years after cessation of smoking there is still an increased risk of hip fracture,[72] and only by 10 years did former smokers have a reduced risk of hip fracture compared with current smokers.[73] In a prospective study[74] it was shown that smoking was positively and significantly associated with decreased hip bone mineral density in old age. However, there are other reports[58,59,75] have failed to show a correlation. Therefore further evaluation is required to confirm that smoking is an independent risk factor.

Alcohol

Alcohol has been evaluated as a potential risk factor for hip fracture. A quantitative association between alcohol consumption and hip fracture was demonstrated in an evaluation of over 30 000 patients.[76] A low to moderate alcohol intake (less than 27 drinks for men and less than 13 drinks for women weekly) was not associated with hip fracture incidence. As alcohol consumption increased, particularly in men, so did risk of fracture. Alcohol was seen as an independent risk factor[77] after multivariate analysis, and results obtained with a retrospective cohort design[78] concluded that alcohol consumption, particularly if it was heavy and long term did indeed increase the risk of hip fracture. However, many other authors[58,59,75] have been unable to show a correlation between alcohol consumption and hip fracture. Alcohol intake is yet another variable that warrants further evaluation in its relationship to hip fracture incidence.

Activity level

There have been many reports evaluating the importance of maintaining physical activity in elderly men and women. Gregg et al.[79] followed 9700 women and assessed physical activity and risk of hip fracture. After controlling for other factors, very active women had a statistically significant 36 per cent reduction in hip fractures compared with the least active women. Kujala et al.[80] followed over 3000 men and noted a statistically significant reduction in hip fractures in those who participated in vigorous physical activity. Coupland et al.[81] noted that patients who were inactive were more than twice as likely to sustain a hip fracture. In a large review of potential risk factors for hip fractures it was concluded that lifestyle factors were associated with hip fracture risk and that a low degree of physical exercise and a low BMI accounted for a large component of total risk.[77]

Medical history/medications

Many medical conditions have been associated with an increased risk for hip fracture (Table 6.3). Any comorbidity that makes the likelihood of a fall higher could potentially elevate the hip fracture risk. A variety of conditions have this association. In addition, disorders that lead either directly or indirectly to osteopenia could increase the risk for fracture.

Different medications have been associated with hip fracture risk. Psychotropic medications in the elderly increase the propensity for falls. Cumming and Klineberg[92] studied the effect of a short-acting benzodiazepine and found an odds ratio of 3.5 in patients with hip fractures over controls after adjusting for multiple confounders by logistic regression. Other authors[93] have also shown an increased risk for fracture in the elderly receiving opioid analgesics. The long-term use of corticosteroids has been associated with an increased risk of hip fracture,[94] which is expected from the osteopenia that results from their use. The prolonged use of anti-epileptic drugs can lead to osteomalacia. A correlation with hip fracture risk has been demonstrated in one investigation of patients taking these medications[94] but not shown in another,[95] and further study is required. Decreased endogenous oestrogen levels lead to bone resorption[96] and the absence of oestradiol results in

Table 6.3 Medical comorbidities and increased risk for hip fracture

Medical comorbidity	Risk increase	Etiology	Reference
Diabetes	1.5–6.9×	Possibly due to to decreased bone mass	Forsen et al. (1999)[82]
Parkinson's disease	4–5×	Multiple falls (due to gait abnormality, reflexes) Osteoporosis	Johnell et al. (1992)[83]
Stroke	2–4×	Paresis Falls	Ramnemark et al. (1998)[84]
Epilepsy	5× (femoral neck) 10× (intertrochanteric)	Multifactorial (falls, osteomalacia due to anticonvulsant drugs, seizure frequency)	Desai et al. (1996)[85]
Cardiac arrhythmia		Falls due to dizziness and syncope	Abdon et al. (1980)[86]
Carotid sinus hypersensitivity		Falls	Ward et al. (1999)[87]
Alzheimer's disease	2.7×	Falls	Melton et al. (1994)[88]
Decreased visual activity	2.2×	Falls (especially. if stereoscopic vision)	Felson et al. (1989)[89]
Graves' disease (thyrotoxicosis)	2.3×	Bone mass	Gallagher et al. (1980)[14]
Rheumatoid arthritis	2×	Functional impairment in activities of daily living	Cooper et al. (1995)[90]
Bilateral oophorectomy	1.8×	Oestrogen Type I osteoporosis	Kreiger et al. (1982)[91]

osteocyte death.[97] There is now a clear body of literature[39,98–100] supporting the hypothesis that postmenopausal use of oestrogens protects against hip fractures in women.

Geographic factors

Climate

Many authors have published analyses of regional and seasonal variation in the incidence of hip fracture. Stroup et al.[25] reporting on regional variations in the United States, demonstrated that the rate of hip fracture was highest in the South and lowest in the Northeast. These patterns were seen after adjusting for age and race, and were especially marked in woman. In a large series of almost 700 000 patients with hip fractures in the United States, an increased incidence of hip fractures was found for males and females of all ages in the South.[26] Interestingly, the higher rates of fractures in the South depended on the level of the fracture, with the incidence of cervical fracture being disproportionately elevated in the South. The authors were unsure of the exact reasons for this regional variation but felt that the cervical area of the femur may be more sensitive to environmental, nutritional, or socio-economic factors. The causes of geographical variations in hip fracture rates remain unknown. Lauderdale *et al.* (1998)[45] felt that it was the region of residence early in life, and not the current region, that was associated with substantial variation in hip fracture rates.

Seasonal variations in hip fracture incidence have also been noted. The question remains as to why the incidence of hip fracture increases in the winter. Logically, one would assume that it would be secondary to weather conditions such as snow and ice. Levy *et al.*[101] in a Canadian study, showed a increases of 5 per cent and 12 per cent in hip fracture incidence in women and men respectively in the winter, and thought that it was probably due to slips, slower reaction times, or winter bone loss. Chiu *et al.*[102] reported a 36 per cent increase in hip fracture incidence in the winter months in Hong Kong. However, other authors believe that factors other than weather must be playing an important role. Jacobsen *et al.*[103] felt that ice and snow were not strongly associated with fracture occurrence and that the winter-related increase in risk was essentially unchanged after controlling for weather. In a recent study, Douglas *et al.*[104] compared hip fracture incidence at three different latitudes (Scotland, Hong Kong, and New Zealand) and noted a significant seasonal variation in all three countries. They point out that there is no snow or ice in Hong Kong and therefore other factors must be exerting an influence. The distinct seasonal variation could be due to variation in sunlight, with decreased vision and a higher potential for falls.[105] Vitamin D synthesis and serum parathyroid hormone levels also have seasonal variations[106] which could affect fracture rates.

Location of residence

We have already discussed the variation in hip fracture incidence between countries and between climates within a single country. Many authors have also shown that, even within smaller regions, there are variations between urban and rural places of residence. Kaastad *et al.*[107] demonstrated in Oslo, Norway, that the incidence of hip fractures in the rural county was only two-thirds of that in the city. Other reports from Scandinavia[108,109] have also shown lower incidences of hip fracture in the rural setting than in urban centres. This trend is also seen in other countries. Madhok *et al.*[110] demonstrated that urban residents of Rochester, Minnesota, had a 35 per cent greater age- and sex-adjusted incidence of proximal femur fractures than those from the surrounding rural area. However, Luthje *et al.*[111] however, found no difference between hip fracture incidences in urban and rural populations in a Finnish study.

Even within a confined urban versus rural setting, there is a further subdivision of location that is important, namely the residential status. There are many reports comparing individuals living in institutions with those in private residences. Norton *et al.*[112] demonstrated that patients in institutions were almost four times more likely to sustain a hip fracture than those living in private homes. In another study, Butler et al.[113] showed the risk of hip fractures for those living in institutions to be 10.5 times higher than for those living in private homes when unadjusted for age and sex. They concluded that strategies to minimize hip fracture incidence should focus on those in institutions. Many explanations for these findings have been suggested, such as poor vision, overall poorer general health, and the higher use of drugs that may lead to falls. However, in an interesting review, Cumming,[114] after adjusting for multiple confounders, demonstrated that living in a nursing home was not an independent risk factor for hip fracture. Instead, he suggested that those living in nursing homes represented a cohort of patients with multiple risk factors compared with those in private homes and it was not the place of residence that was significant.

Biomechanical factors

Femoral anatomy

As was discussed previously, a proposed etiology for the differences in hip fracture incidence between races has been geometry of the proximal femur. Various anatomical measures have been evaluated. Hip axis length was first discussed by Faulkner et al.[115] who concluded that a longer hip axis was associated with an increased risk of both femoral neck and trochanteric fractures. They were unable to find an association between the neck width or the neck–shaft angle and hip fracture risk. The hip axis has been shown to be longer in white women than in black and Asian women,[116,117] and this longer bending moment could be a factor in hip fracture incidence. Hip axis length has been shown to predict hip fracture incidence independently of bone mineral density.[118] Other anatomical variables seen in women of African origin that are protective against hip fracture include thicker cortical bone and smaller bone widths.[48] Neither femoral neck diameter[119] nor neck–shaft angle[116] are predictors of hip fracture.

Bone density

Bone mineral density (BMD) is clearly related to hip fracture risk. Each standard deviation decrease in BMD has been shown to increase the risk of femoral neck fracture by 1.9 and of intertrochanteric fracture by 2.6.[120] The challenge is to identify those at risk early and initiate effective treatment. There is much ongoing research in osteoporosis.

Results and controversies of treatment

The magnitude of the epidemic in femoral neck (or 'hip') fractures can be appreciated from the results reported in the previous section. In training and in practice, the orthopaedic surgeon will be faced with the management of this common, but often complex, condition. Hip fracture patients are often burdened with pre-existing medical conditions, and so there will always be an inherent morbidity and mortality related to the management of this patient population.

A review of current practice reveals that our personal approaches are not always based on what may be advocated in the scientific literature. An example of this is the management of intracapsular hip fractures (Fig. 6.1). There is good evidence to suggest that a patient who is successfully managed with internal fixation will have superior function to a similar patient who is successfully managed with a hemi-arthroplasty, and there is also evidence that at least 65 per cent of patients with an intracapsular fracture treated with internal fixation will go on to uneventful union.[121] However, in direct contrast to this point, medical record and reimbursement analysis[122] reveals that 70 per cent of intracapsular fractures in North America (including non-displaced and impacted fractures) are managed with an arthroplasty. Obviously, many factors, both patient and surgeon related, influence and contribute to this finding.

It is not possible to do justice to all the philosophies, results, and controversies regarding the management of hip fractures in a single chapter. The purpose of this section is to provide an overview of the clinical, radiographic, and surgical factors which are commonly encountered in the management of hip fracture patients. Also, the results of treatments, as well as the virtues and shortcomings of the more common treatment modalities, will be discussed.

Clinical assessment

A complete history (including a previous fracture history) and physical examination, with good-quality radiographs, will aid the clinician in deciding a specific treatment protocol. In addition, the treating doctor must also adopt the role of a 'clinical detective', as often the patient cannot volunteer all information needed, because of dementia, disorientation, advanced age, dehydration, or other factors.

The age of the fracture itself should be determined, and one may be suspicious of this if the patient reveals established bruising or pressure areas. An examination for advanced osteoporosis (e.g. a kyphotic spine, heavily nicotine-stained fingers, fragile skin secondary to steroid therapy) should also be undertaken. This should be considered highly, as there is now evidence showing that underlying bone quality is a significant factor contributing to the failure of internal fixation devices.[123–125]

As well as the more obvious patient characteristics, such as age, infirmity, and pre-existing medical conditions, one should be alert for more subtle conditions such as impaired vision, a history of poor balance, early dementia, or parkinsonism—all features that may not

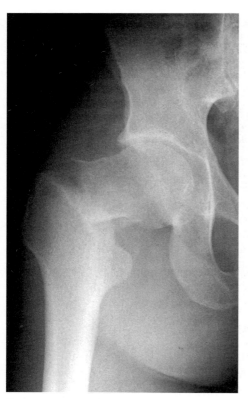

a

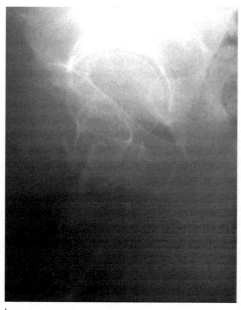

b

Fig. 6.1

An example of two displaced intracapsular femoral neck fractures. The preoperative radiographs ((a), (b) patient A; (c), (d) patient B) show the significant displacement induced at the time of injury. The treating physician elected to fix the fracture internally in the active younger patient A (e), whereas the same fracture pattern was managed with a bipolar arthroplasty in the more elderly and less active patient B who had extensive medical comorbidities (f). Patient A went on to uneventful union and has excellent function; patient B has also regained independent mobility and, equally importantly, has required no further surgery.

Fig. 6.1 *(continued)*

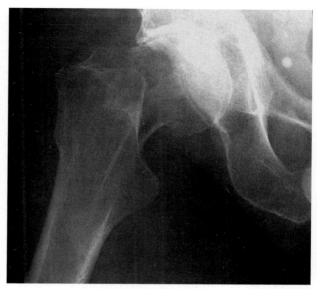

c

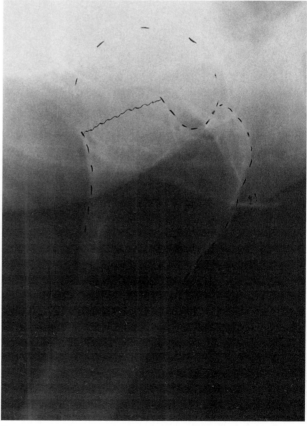

d

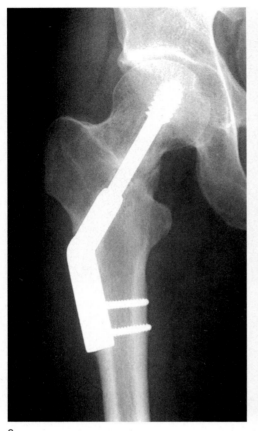
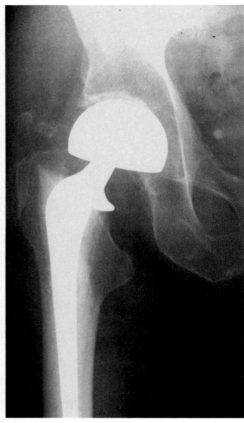

e   f

Fig. 6.1 *(continued)*

be readily identifiable. In fact, it is well established that dementia can present in the form of falls and fractures.[123] This may or may not contribute to the final surgical result, but may adversely affect the functional outcome.[126] Also, routine interview of family and caregivers will often prove to be an invaluable tool. For further aid in this area, both pre- and postoperatively, many hospitals have now set up specific teams of medical, nursing, and allied health members.

Today's orthopaedic surgeon is often part of these multidisciplinary teams which specifically address the acute and longer-term needs of these patients. Recently, through the use of clinical pathways, these specialized 'hip fracture service' teams have been shown to reduce in-patient hospital days significantly, whilst also influencing a dramatic reduction in short-term mortality and morbidity.[127,128] In one review, 30-day mortality decreased from 22 to 7 per cent; in the other, the incidence of major complications fell from 12.5 to 5 per cent.

It has also become apparent that the chronological age of the patient is now less influential in decision-making. This is justifiable with data extrapolated from present day life-tables demonstrating that modern populations in developed countries are living to an older age (see above). Many clinicians now prefer to view the activity and the lifestyle of the patient (or 'physiological' age) as the major factor in deciding whether to recommend a particular surgical treatment. In a similar vein, one group recently recommended that such treatment decisions be based on whether the patient is 'housebound or institutionalized'.[129]

Radiographs and classification

To date, treatment protocols have largely been determined by the patient's radiographs.[130] It is important that a systematic approach be taken with this investigation, so that the most important radiographic parameters are included in the decision-making process.

Firstly, the literature is abundant with inconsistent nomenclature in this area. Terms such as subcapital, basicervical, pertrochanteric and intertrochanteric should be avoided, in preference for the simpler terms intracapsular and extracapsular. We believe that this classification is easier to understand, has excellent repeatability, and carries distinct implications for treatment. Obviously, further qualification, such as the degree of displacement in an intracapsular fracture or noting whether an extracapsular fracture has an unstable pattern (such as a 'reverse obliquity' fracture, or if a fracture has significant posteromedial comminution), is required in practice.

At present there is no reliable preoperative investigation that will predict the ultimate viability of the femoral head.[131,132] Displacement of the fracture (including rotation) is still considered the most important predictive factor in the fate of intracapsular fractures, and should continue to be highly regarded in determining treatment.[130,133] A variety of classification systems have been proposed, but some of their limitations have been recently emphasized.

The Garden classification[134] has been questioned as a predictor of outcome,[135] and recently has been criticized because of poor inter- and intra-observer repeatability.[136] It had previously been criticized because it relied on the anteroposterior radiograph only, which masks the degree of posterior neck comminution.[137] Its main use now appears to be distinguishing 'undisplaced' fractures (Garden types 1 and 2) from 'displaced' fractures (Garden types 3 and 4).

The more modern AO classification has also been downgraded.[138] Again, the criticism is that it only reliably distinguishes displaced from non-displaced fractures. The Pauwel classification, which uses the inclination of the fracture 'line', is simple to apply and makes one consider the biomechanical characteristics of the fracture. Even though smaller reviews have suggested a relationship between fracture 'verticality' and non-union rates,[139] a recent meta-analysis[140] could not find any such predictive value. We have not completely dismissed the notion of 'fracture angle', using it mainly as an important intra-operative guide to facilitate what constitutes an acceptable reduction.

Further controversies in intracapsular fractures are the level of the neck fracture,[141] with the more proximal assumed to have a worse prognosis, and the degree of posterior neck comminution.[137] The latter feature must be strongly appreciated, as the normal hip undergoes rotary movements during gait, and the integrity of the posterior neck is essential in protecting internal fixation devices from excessive rotary and shear forces which may predispose to implant failure.

In our opinion radiographs should be examined specifically for each of the following.

- Classification of the fracture as intracapsular or extracapsular.
- The degree of displacement, including rotation (this requires good-quality anteroposterior and lateral radiographs).
- The degree of comminution, specifically in the posterior neck for intracapsular fractures and in the posteromedial and subtrochanteric regions for extracapsular fractures.
- Evidence of severe osteoporosis (remember that 'normal' bone mass must be reduced by approximately 30 per cent before osteopenia becomes evident on radiographs).
- Any unusual radiographic features, such as periosteal new bone formation, which may be suggestive of underlying pathological processes such as malignancy or infection. Callus formation may also provide a clue to the age of the fracture.

We also advocate routinely obtaining anteroposterior pelvic radiographs (as opposed to a similar view of the injured hip only) to allow preoperative templating of the contralateral hip. The use of other investigative modalities, including plain and computed tomography, nuclear medicine scans, and MRI, is reserved for selected patients such as those who pose a diagnostic dilemma, those with a known malignancy presenting with possible metastatic disease or fracture, and those who present with a potential primary tumour which requires proper staging and ultimately a biopsy.

Treatment protocols

Non-operative treatment

The literature has been cautious in advocating internal fixation in the treatment of minimally displaced intracapsular hip fractures. Even though the rates of non-union have been reported to be higher with non-operative management,[142] the rate of surgical complications can be significant, especially in the more elderly patient.[143] Primarily, *in situ* fixation of these fractures is advised to prevent displacement,[129] but there may be some caveats to this approach, including patients with non-acute fractures and patients with significant medical and anaesthetic risks. Others adopt a conservative approach to the valgus impacted intracapsular fracture[134,144] as this is one pattern, with its inherent stability, that has demonstrated acceptable results with non-surgical treatment.

With respect to the displaced intracapsular hip fracture, the frail elderly patient with a shortened life expectancy may be considered for conservative management. Non-union will be inevitable in this group, and the patient and/or the caregivers should be made aware that there is a distinct risk of delayed surgery to address this outcome. This will be indicated for pain and inability to bear or transfer weight, and also to provide comfort during nursing or to allow the patient to perform personal activities of daily living. The distinct advantage of a delayed total hip arthroplasty (THA) in this scenario is that the risk of prosthetic dislocation lessens with time, presumably secondary to capsular scarring.

Studies also favour internal fixation for the extracapsular hip fractures, based mainly on the potential for improved rehabilitation and the reduced incidence of deformity.[145] The surgical management of extracapsular fractures has been so successful, for both patients and health care providers, that conservative management is now rarely indicated.[137] If one decides to treat these fractures non-operatively (for whatever reason), the patient and others must be aware of the documented shortcomings of this approach.[145] These include a higher risk of malunion, malrotation and shortening, a prolonged period of immobilization (with the risks of recumbency increasing dramatically after 48 hours), a period of protective ambulation, prolonged patient discomfort, distortion of the proximal femoral anatomy (one may have to consider future hip surgery), and the theoretical, but devastating, risks of having an unstable long-bone fracture, such as fat embolism, acute respiratory distress syndrome, and deep venous thrombosis. Despite a recent review suggesting that functional outcomes were not significantly different between the two approaches, our belief is that surgical management is indicated almost universally for these fractures.

Operative treatment

INTRACAPSULAR FRACTURES

The debates and controversies regarding the management of intracapsular fractures have not altered appreciably over the last 25 years. The major questions that the treating surgeon has to ask include the following.

- For an undisplaced or minimally displaced intracapsular fracture, which provides superior results—multiple screws or a 'sliding' hip screw device?
- For a displaced fracture, when do I decide to try and 'save' the femoral head?

- If I choose an arthroplasty option, which is most appropriate for my patient?

Minimally displaced fractures

An undisplaced intracapsular fracture is simply defined, but one with 'minimal' displacement is more ambiguous. We define a minimally displaced fracture as one that has less than 10° of varus angulation on the anteroposterior view and/or 10° (apex anterior) angulation on the lateral radiograph. Deformity beyond these ranges implies that there is associated rotation of the fracture and/or significant posterior comminution,[137] and thus the fracture should be reclassified as 'displaced'.

The reported rates of avascular necrosis and non-union are significantly lower in this group than in displaced fractures,[134,146,147] and so procedures preserving the femoral head (internal fixation) are the almost universal surgical treatment. We reserve replacement procedures for patients with severe osteopenia and as salvage for the complications and/or poor outcomes of internal fixation. The central issue for most surgeons is deciding the optimal form of internal fixation.

At the forefront of this debate, especially in North America, has been the battle between the various 'sliding' hip screw devices and the use of multiple bone screws. Secondary arguments regarding the latter technique include the surgical approach (standard open versus limited/percutaneous), the number of screws employed, solid versus cannulated screws, the implant material (stainless steel versus titanium), and crossed versus parallel screws.[147]

In a recent review of over 450 intracapsular hip fractures[148] it was reported that the rates of failure for minimally displaced fractures were similar—14 per cent for the dynamic hip screw and 15 per cent for three parallel screws. The final functional outcomes were similar for the remaining patients, irrespective of the internal fixation device used. Similar findings have been observed by others,[142,149] and these authors agree that it is the inherent stability of this fracture pattern, not the virtues of one implant over another, that justify their results.

Essentially, there are very few questions that we should ask of these implants.

- Is the surgical technique simple and quick in its application?
- Does the implant have a proven track record of maintaining reduction until union?
- What are the common complications distinctive to these implants?

Like the authors cited above, our belief is that either method is effective for treating these minimally displaced intracapsular fractures. But whatever method is preferred, the surgeon should be familiar with the established technical 'pearls' for each approach, such as screw placement, number of screws, site of lateral cortical entry, and the use of anti-rotation wires/screws. These points will be discussed in more detail in subsequent sections. It is of paramount importance that the fracture position, or reduction, should not be compromised by the internal fixation device, both intra-operatively and until union has occurred.

DISPLACED FRACTURES—THE 'YOUNGER' PATIENT

As we have discussed, chronological age should have little bearing on dictating treatment. However, in this section we have divided patients into life 'phases' to highlight the controversies surrounding management issues with respect to the 'unsolved' fracture—the displaced intracapsular fracture.

Owing to well-documented long-term problems with arthroplasty procedures in 'younger' patients, current opinion is that all displaced intracapsular hip fractures in these patients (aged about 60 years) should be considered for reduction and internal fixation. This should be undertaken expeditiously, preferably within 6–8 hours of injury,[150] with an anatomical reduction and secure internal fixation. The patient should then be rehabilitated with protected postoperative weight-bearing and monitored for the risks of failure of fixation, non-union, and avascular necrosis. The last of these can surface many years later, with a recent review documenting that approximately one-third of cases developing avascular necrosis did so between 4 and 10 years after the injury.[151] The patient should not be assessed with MRI preoperatively because, as well as being time consuming, a recent study has shown that it is not predictive of the development of avascular necrosis.[133]

The surgeon should have no hesitation in performing an open reduction if an acceptable position is not achieved with closed methods. The bone quality in these patients is usually adequate, and so the main factor in optimizing results is the quality of the reduction. With an anatomical reduction, a stable mechanical environment is created for the implants, thus reducing the likelihood of failure.[124]

Performing a 'decompressive' capsulotomy in association with a closed reduction is controversial. The literature appears divided on this point, not so much because the contained fracture haematoma poses a threat to the intracapsular vessels through a 'tamponade' effect,[152] but rather because some believe that a displaced intracapsular fracture implies a torn capsule. Recently, Swiontkowski[122] has suggested that this is not necessarily the case.[122] The same author estimates that this procedure helps 15–20 per cent of patients. Thus, on the basis of the risk–benefit ratio, it appears that a capsulotomy/capsulectomy procedure can be justified.

Obviously, these principles will apply if one adopts a philosophy of internal fixation for those patients we shall describe as 'middle-aged' (60–80 years) presenting with a displaced intracapsular fracture. The dilemma here becomes one of careful patient selection, followed by implant choice.

DISPLACED FRACTURES—THE 'MIDDLE-AGED' PATIENT

This is the patient group that most management debate revolves around. Again, for the reasons cited above including the extensive literature documenting significant failure rates for these fractures with internal fixation (40 per cent in one large series[148]), many surgeons (especially in North America) have adopted an almost blanket approach to treating this 'arthroplasty' age range by replacing the femoral head.

However, this is not a universal approach, as much of the European literature has revealed.[153,154] Some groups will attempt to save most femoral heads, and only use THA as a salvage procedure to address avascular necrosis or secondary degenerative arthritis. Non-unions are addressed by osteotomy, refixation, and bone grafting.

Comparisons of studies have been difficult, primarily because of the heterogenous nature of hip fracture populations worldwide. Variables have included demographic factors (BMI, smoking rates, etc.), access to expeditious treatment, and attitudes towards rehabilitation and postoperative surveillance. As well as these factors, there are 'surgeon' factors to consider: the level of trauma experience, the appreciation of implant biomechanical principles, and the limitations of fixation in osteopenic bone.

If one does decide on internal fixation, adherence to certain key principles is paramount.[130,137] These pertain to both the reduction and the fixation of the fracture. The consensus for what constitutes an acceptable reduction (other than the ideal anatomical reduction) for these fractures includes no varus, up to 20° of valgus, and no more than 10°–20° of anterior–posterior angulation.[155] These guidelines become even more important in the presence of extremely osteopenic bone. A recent article[124] examining the biomechanical factors contributing to failure of fixation of intracapsular hip fractures using multiple parallel screws concluded that the most important factor was underlying bone quality. When these fractures are the result of low-energy force, as is usual in this group, clinical osteoporosis is implied.

Other investigators,[156,157] who acknowledge bone quality as a serious consideration, believe that screw placement is of equal importance. For a sliding hip screw device, the 'centre–centre' position is essential in preventing varus malunion and even lag screw 'cut-out.'[130] Others have employed mathematical calculations, from radiographic measurements, to quantify this point, and even provide a predictive threshold value for implant failure.[158]

Another approach with hip screw devices has been to advocate that an anti-rotation device (such as a parallel superiorly placed threaded wire or screw) be employed while the track for the lag screw is prepared. This prevents excessive rotation of the femoral head fragment, which may compromise the reduction, and even have a further effect on the (already) damaged microcirculation. What remains controversial is whether such a device should be left *in situ* in combination with the sliding hip screw implant. The proponents of this believe that this device plays a role in preventing rotary moments at the fracture site during gait, whereas others think that it may contribute to complications by not allowing the hip screw device to compress ('dynamize') the fracture—a key element in the stability and success of this implant.

Surgeons who favour the multiple-screw approach must also pay special attention to technique. Multiple screws have comparable union rates,[159] with their main advantage being that they are inserted through a percutaneous approach. Other advantages of this approach are that it can be performed with cannulated screws, and even titanium screws, which are useful if one has to perform an MRI (as in the assessment of non-union and avascular necrosis). A limitation of this technique was recently highlighted in a biomechanical report, where three parallel screws were compared with a sliding hip screw device in a vertical fracture pattern. One of the findings under cyclical axial loading (reproduced to mimic daily gait) was that the multiple screws were inferior in the parameters tested.[160] These included degree of femoral head displacement and load to failure.

Again, key to the success of these screws is that an anatomical reduction is achieved first—this implies an open reduction, if required. It has been established that three screws are biomechanically sufficient[149] and that they should be inserted in an 'inverted triangle' configuration. The spacing between the screws should be as wide as possible, as this increases fixation strength, with the screws skirting as close as possible to the cortex of the femoral neck, especially the inferior and the posterior screws. The inferior screw should be inserted first, but final compression should only occur once all screws are in place. The screw tips should rest 5 mm from the subchondral bone, and the screw threads should not rest across the fracture site (therefore both 16-mm and 32-mm partially threaded screws should be available). It is also important that the lateral cortical entry point of the lowest screw not be at a level distal to the level of the lesser trochanter, as this is associated with an increased risk of creating a femoral shaft fracture.[155] In most proximal femurs, this will result in the screws being inserted at an angle of 130°–135°.

DISPLACED FRACTURES—THE 'ELDERLY' PATIENT

The incidence of these fractures is more common in the later decades of life, and it is these patients who are also of greatest concern with respect to medical comorbidities and surgical risk.

For this reason, the treating surgeon has a responsibility to choose a procedure that will restore pain-free mobility quickly and allow the patient many months or years of good function. Just as important, the surgeon will have to decide if the patient can withstand secondary procedures, as these are often indicated to address the complications of the index treatment.

Because of these important considerations, surgeons have favoured arthroplasty options for this patient group, primarily because the incidence of complications requiring surgical management is less. This is supported by the results of two recent large randomized studies[161,162] which compared these replacement options (hemi-arthroplasty, bipolar replacement, and total hip replacement) with internal fixation. Both concluded that functional outcomes were similar for the two groups, and that the main differences lay in the rates of complication and reoperation. To help further in this decision-making process, an excellent summary of the advantages and disadvantages of the two approaches has recently been provided (Table 6.4).[129]

Because larger studies do not strongly favour one approach over the other, surgeons have resolved the issue on the grounds that they

Table 6.4 Differences between internal fixation and arthroplasty

Advantages	Disadvantages
INTERNAL FIXATION	
Patients retain their own femoral head	Risk of nonunion (10%–20% in the young; 20%–35% in the elderly)
Less surgical trauma in intial operation	Risk of avascular necrosis (10%–20%)
Mortality and morbidity may be slightly reduced	Risk of fracture around the implant (1%–2%)
Lower risk of wound sepsis (up –1%)	Increased rate of reoperation (20%–36%)
ARTHROPLASTY	
Lower rate of reoperation (6%–18%)	More extensive operation than internal fixation
	Higher risk of deep infection around the implant (3%)
	Higher risk of superficial wound infection (5%–15%)
	Risk of dislocation incurred (2%–5%)
	Risk of fracture around implant (1%–3%)
	Later risk of prosthetic loosening (2%–10%)
	Later risk of acetabular wear (4%–20%)

perceive to be most important.[163] The treating doctor may place more emphasis on eventual hip function, thus favouring internal fixation, or may want to avoid reoperation on his/her elderly patient, thus opting for an arthroplasty procedure. Other factors, which are less discussed, include the influence of surgical training and local 'bias' provided by peers in one's own hospital or even town.

Retrospective reviews which provide 'local' experience in treating these common fractures are of equal value to larger studies. One recent review,[164] with an 8-year follow-up of 367 patients, documented important guidelines, which included that there is a significantly higher revision rate associated with internal fixation for the treatment of displaced intracapsular hip fractures in patients aged over 80 years. This difference was not observed in the 65- to 80-year-old age group, but there was a significantly higher mortality rate in this age bracket for the group undergoing internal fixation.

We have adopted a parallel stance with the older patient (greater than 80 years) presenting with a displaced intracapsular fracture. Since an arthroplasty will most likely 'rob' the previously more vigorous patient of some natural hip function, we believe that a bipolar replacement will provide excellent pain relief, mobility, and stability, and carry a low rate of re-operation. Like others, we have observed satisfactory function with bipolar replacements.[165] We counsel the patient specifically regarding the slightly higher risk of infection and dislocation, and also that later conversion to a THA may be required. However, other proponents of arthroplasty favour the use of unipolar (hemi-arthroplasty) or total hip replacement.

Unipolar replacements (hemi-arthroplasties), such as the Austin Moore and Thompson prostheses, can provide an excellent solution for the elderly, frail, and/or housebound patient. However, it is our opinion that the advantages of low cost and speed of implantation do not make up for the many shortcomings that have been documented. Jadhav et al.[166] found that 75 per cent of patients complained of pain within 6 months of surgery and the majority exhibited acetabular wear, protrusion, and subsidence of the implant. In a more recent analysis[167] the group undergoing hemi-arthroplasty exhibited a reoperation rate of 24 per cent (compared with 7 per cent for the THA group), a significantly inferior average Harris hip score (55 versus 80), and a poor outcome with respect to pain and mobility. Finally, a review that specifically compared these two procedures in a mobile and socially independent group of patients[168] concluded that THA provided vastly superior functional outcomes compared with hemi-arthroplasty. In this series, 38 per cent of the hemi-arthroplasties required conversion to THA (mean review time less than 4 years).

We are also guarded about employing THA as the primary option for this group of patients. Despite the dislocation rate of 2–5 per cent reported in Table 6.4, there are many studies with smaller patient samples in the literature revealing alarming rates of dislocation—up to 32 per cent.[167-169] This is of relevance, as surgeons who do not perform many hip arthroplasties on an annual basis[170] are often faced with performing them on this particular patient population. The lax articular capsule, the surgical approach, improper implant placement, and patient mental dysfunction have all been cited as important factors contributing to this significant complication.[146,171] The current use of constrained acetabular components may reduce the incidence of dislocation, but they have distinct disadvantages of wear and even premature loosening.

Proponents of total hip replacement will often argue that this procedure provides the patient with optimal function and a low risk of reoperation, which is usually to address instability.[171] A recent prospective study[172] used six outcome measures to evaluate the 'theoretical' superiority of THA as a treatment for these fractures, and concluded that the procedure did not do better on any of them up to 1 year postoperatively. Another clinical review[173] has revealed an alarmingly high early loosening rate of these hip replacements compared with matched patients undergoing the procedure for osteoarthritis (up to 14 per cent at 5 years).

The use of total hip replacement, as an index procedure, in this group of patients should be reserved for the patient with pre-existing osteoarthritis of the hip.[146] Relative indications also include osteoarthitis of the contralateral hip, metabolic or inflammatory conditions (which may predispose other arthroplasty alternatives to acetabular protrusion), high activity demands or expectations, and a life expectancy of more than 5 years.

EXTRACAPSULAR FRACTURES

These fractures constitute approximately half of all hip fractures, and the potential complications of non-union and avascular necrosis are significantly lower than for intracapsular fractures. It is most important to determine whether the fracture is inherently unstable.[174] The key to this rests with the posteromedial wall or 'buttress'—whether this is intact, or not, is highly significant to fracture stability. As stability is compromised, there is a greater degree of collapse at the fracture site. The amount of this collapse can play havoc with fixation devices (Table 6.5).[174]

Sliding hip screw devices take advantage of the potential for collapse by 'controlled compression' of the fracture fragments and the establishment of bony support across the fracture site. These devices have been proven biomechanically to unload the proximal medial cortex.[175] The clinical results of these implants since their introduction have been extremely satisfying. They have allowed previously bed-bound patients to be mobilized without the documented disadvantages of previous implants, which included fixed nail-plate devices and the first-generation flexible intramedullary nails, such as the Ender and condylocephalic nails.[137,176,177]

Table 6.5 Kyle–Gustilo classification system for intertrochanteric fractures

Type	Features	Degree of collapse (mm)
I	Stable: nondisplaced fractures with comminution	6.4
II	Stable: displaced fracture with minimal comminution; can be reduced to a stable construct	9.9
III	Unstable fractures with a large area of posteromedial comminution	14.8
IV	Unstable intertrochanteric fracture with subtrochanteric extension	17.0
V	Unstable intertrochanteric fracture with femoral neck component	17.8

The most common mode of failure of a sliding hip screw device is 'cut out' of the lag screw.[158,178] The reasons for this are multifactorial, but obviously relate to fracture instability, bone quality, and improper technique.[137] Kyle *et al.*[137] also acknowledge that an appreciation of the biomechanics of sliding devices, and their interplay with forces around the hip, is imperative in understanding their limitations.

To counter this complication, modifications to treatment have been proposed, and others advocate the use of intramedullary implants to deal with unstable fracture patterns. Modifications have included performing adjuvant medializing and/or 'valgizing' displacement osteotomies,[179] theoretically increasing fracture stability and reducing excessive loads across the implant. The principles of these procedures were established in the era of 'rigid' nail-plate devices, such as the Jewett nail.[137] The modern consensus is that this practice provides no advantage over anatomical reduction in unstable extracapsular fractures,[180–182] and may even predispose to mechanical problems of the hip and knee by altering hip offset and the mechanical weight-bearing axis respectively. It also has the disadvantage of limb-length discrepancy. A recent meta-analysis[183] also highlighted that an osteotomy increased operative time, blood loss, and hospital stay compared with a group of patients who underwent anatomical reduction. This review recommended that osteotomy may have a role if a 'fixed' nail-plate device is used, but such implants are now rarely employed.

Intramedullary implants, with their ability to load share, were the obvious alternative to the problem of fracture instability.[176,184] Even though flexible nails had fallen out of favour earlier (because of migration, varus malunion, and knee pain related to their insertion points), there was a resurgence of interest in the 1980s with the second-generation rigid and interlocked devices. The implant that gained most attention was the Gamma nail (Howmedica, Rutherford, NJ).

It is not surprising that the most modern controversy surrounding unstable extracapsular fractures concerns the use of intramedullary or reconstruction nails. The Gamma nail gained widespread popularity in the late 1980s and early 1990s because it promised to combine the advantages of both the sliding hip screw devices and intramedullary fixation, thus providing stable fixation and permitting the patient early mobilization and full weight-bearing.

The first-generation nail was plagued with the burden of an unacceptable complication rate, which included migration of the proximal screw, implant breakage, and, most devastating, femoral shaft fracture.[185] The incidence of these femoral fractures was, in part, related to a mismatch of the nail design and the normal geometry of the proximal femur.[186] Various modifications of technique to reduce the incidence of this complication were reported.[187,188] Using a smaller diameter nail, over-reaming the canal (by 1–2 mm), manually passing the nail without the use of the hammer, and only drilling one hole for each of the distal locking screws were advocated as important factors in minimizing this disastrous scenario. This complication also led many surgeons to abandon the device or, at the very least, not to support its use for the more stable fracture patterns.[189] A second-generation implant was introduced with new design features which attempted to reduce these complications.

However, two recent large European randomized studies[190, 191] were unable to demonstrate distinct superiority of this newer design over a standard sliding hip screw device. In the first series,[190] the functional outcomes were similar at 1 year, although the rate of femoral shaft fracture and lag screw cut-out were still greater in the Gamma nail group. In the second series,[191] the incidence of femoral shaft fracture was significantly higher in the Gamma nail group. Both groups recommended that the Gamma nail should not be used as the 'routine' device for extracapsular (intertrochanteric) fractures. A meta-analysis of nearly 1800 patients comparing these two treatments[192] concurred with the above studies, stating that the Gamma nail had a significantly increased risk of femoral shaft fracture and need for reoperation.

In distinct contrast, there are also studies that document fewer complications with the Gamma nail than with screw–plate constructs,[193–195] and these studies also demonstrate reduced surgical time and blood loss. Another study[196] reported a significant reduction in 30-day mortality, from 17 to 6 per cent. The major explanation for this finding was that the Gamma nail allowed immediate weight-bearing. This is an important consideration in dealing with patients with significant comorbidities and those patients who are unable to restrict their weight-bearing voluntarily. Despite having to overcome a steep 'learning curve', the advantages of intramedullary fixation continue to be highly favoured by many authors who also claim that the complication rate reduces dramatically with increased use.[197–199]

New implants, or modifications of established implants, are continually being introduced to address these complications. An example of one such device is the Intramedullary Hip System (IMHS) (Smith & Nephew, Memphis, TN) which is gaining extensive use in North America. In limited reviews,[200,201] this system has been favourably compared with the Gamma nail in terms of incidence of complications, but the fact remains that similar devastating complications have been observed. Despite favourable finite-element and other biomechanical analyses, large randomized studies are lacking on these new devices, both comparing 'nail versus nail' and, more importantly, 'nail versus hip screw' designs.[202,203] Until such results are available, routine application of these devices cannot be advised.

Before concluding this section, we should also acknowledge that there is a distinct extracapsular fracture pattern, termed 'reverse obliquity', that has unique biomechanical characteristics. This uncommon, but relatively unstable, fracture pattern[204] behaves more like a subtrochanteric fracture, and warrants the use of either smaller-angle (90° or 95°) screw/blade-plate implants or intramedullary devices.[205] The routine use of 135° sliding hip screws in these fractures has not met with the same success as their application for other extracapsular fractures.

SUBTROCHANTERIC FRACTURES

This region of the femur has a distinct vascular watershed, and the medial subtrochanteric region also encounters the highest compressive stresses in the body.[137] Therefore it is not surprising that there is an established risk of non-union and implant failure in the operative management of these fractures. Extramedullary implants, such as blade plates and sliding hip screw devices, have not met with the same success in dealing with these fractures (compared with 'trochanteric' fracture patterns). This is especially true with markedly comminuted subtrochanteric fractures; it has been advocated that, for these implants to work effectively as tension-band devices, anatomical reduction should be employed, particularly of the medial fragments.[137] Anyone who deals with this fracture can appreciate that this is not a simple request—it is technically demanding and often requires extensive periosteal stripping.

Kyle[174] has shown that 'indirect' fracture techniques can provide superior results to open reduction and internal fixation (ORIF).

Table 6.6 Series of patients with subtrochanteric fractures

Group	Delayed non-union
I (24): ORIF	17 per cent
II (23): indirect reduction	0 per cent

Data from Kyle.[174]

The rate of delayed union was zero in the former group and 17 per cent in the latter (Table 6.6). This exemplifies the point that surgical technique and philosophy (not implant choice) are the key factors in successfully treating these fractures.

An intramedullary nail allows indirect techniques to be instituted. They are load-sharing devices which can be implanted distant from the fracture and thus do not disturb the fracture haematoma, and they have a low risk of disturbing soft tissue attachments to bone fragments. They allow alignment of the fracture and, provided that bone quality is adequate, they can prevent excessive collapse and malrotation.

These distinct advantages have led many to use intramedullary devices for both subtrochanteric fractures and in the treatment of metastatic deposits (prefracture). For these indications, the Gamma nail comes in a longer version, and good results have recently been reported.[196,206-208]

Clinical and laboratory studies support the use of intramedullary devices in dealing with comminuted and/or 'low' subtrochanteric fractures. In comparing the Gamma nail with a number of internal fixation devices, described collectively as 'angular type with lateral cortical support', such as the dynamic condylar screw and blade plates, one group[209] demonstrated superior results with the nail. There were significantly fewer complications in this group—7.5 per cent compared with 30 per cent in the ORIF group. The latter group also had a 10 per cent non-union rate, with none reported in the Gamma nail group. Also, there were distinct differences in the duration of surgery, blood transfusion requirements, and the delay to ambulation without aids. These results are supported by one bio-mechanical study[210] which demonstrated superior fixation strength with Gamma nails, compared with both 135° sliding hip screws and 95° dynamic condylar screws, in subtrochanteric fractures.

Overview

No algorithm can cater for the variety and complexity of hip fracture patients presenting to an orthopaedic surgeon. An assessment of the patient—physical and medical condition, cognitive limitations, and future activity demands—must be the primary concern of the treating physician. Enlisting the assistance of other health professionals will also be beneficial in optimizing functional outcome. Identification of patient age alone can no longer be the only clinical criterion on which to base management.

Likewise, the identification of fracture displacement should not produce 'reflex' surgical responses. Radiographic classification should strive not only to be anatomical, but also biomechanical. Attempts to categorize the fracture pattern, as stable versus unstable, will invoke more careful consideration in deciding which surgical procedure is most appropriate.

Once a management decision is made, the biomechanical and material limitations of the selected implant have to be appreciated and respected. Proper and disciplined surgical technique is imperative for the success of these procedures. Despite this, however, there will be factors outside the control of the management team, such as underlying bone quality and rehabilitation compliance.

Finally, the modern literature cannot be ignored. The busier a surgeon becomes, the more emphasis will be placed on evidence-based outcome studies to support, or change, current practice. Recent meta-analyses have strongly shown that more powerful studies are needed before the current controversies of hip fracture management can be concluded.

References

1 Youm T, Koval KJ, Zuckerman JD: The economic impact of geriatric hip fractures. *American Journal of Orthopedics* **28**: 423–8, 1999.

2 Dubey A, Koval KJ, Zuckerman JD: Hip fracture epidemiology—a review. *American Journal of Orthopedics* **28**: 497–506, 1999.

3 Fowles DG (ed.): *A profile of older Americans*. American Association of Retired Persons, Washington, DC, 1990.

4 Luthje P: Incidence of hip fracture in Finland. A forecast for 1990. *Acta Orthopaedica Scandinavica* **56**: 223–5, 1985.

5 Kelsey JL, Hoffman S: Risk factors for hip fracture. *New England Journal of Medicine* **316**: 404–6, 1987.

6 Cummings SR, Rubin SM, Black D: The future of hip fractures in the United States. Numbers, costs, and potential effects of postmenopausal estrogen. *Clinical Orthopaedics and Related Research* **252**: 163–6, 1990.

7 Gullberg B, Johnell O, Kanis JA: World-wide projections for hip fracture. *Osteoporosis International* **7**: 407–13, 1997.

8 Oden A, Dawson A, Dere W, Johnell O, Jonsson B, Kanis JA: Lifetime risk of hip fractures is underestimated. *Osteoporosis International* **8**: 599–603, 1998.

9 Schwartz AV, Kelsey JJ, Maggi S *et al.*: International variation in the incidence of hip fractures: cross-national project on osteoporosis for the World Health Organization. Program for Research on Aging. *Osteoporosis International* **9**: 242–53, 1999.

10 Finsen V, Benum P: Changing incidence of hip fractures in rural and urban areas of central Norway. *Clinical Orthopaedics and Related Research* **218**: 104–10, 1987.

11 Rogmark C, Sernbo I, Johnell O, Nilsson JA: Incidence of hip fractures in Malmo, Sweden, 1992–1995. A trend-break. *Acta Orthopaedica Scandinavica* **70**: 19–22, 1999.

12 Norton R, Yee T, Rodgers A, Gray H, MacMahon S: Regional variation in the incidence of hip fracture in New Zealand. *New Zealand Medical Journal* **110**: 78–80, 1997.

13 Bagur A, Mautalen C, Rubin Z: Epidemiology of hip fractures in an urban population of Central Argentina. *Osteoporosis International* **4**: 332–5, 1994.

14 Gallagher JC, Melton LJ, Riggs BL: Examination of prevalence rates of possible risk factors in a population with a fracture of the proximal femur. *Clinical Orthopaedics and Related Research* **153**: 158–65, 1980.

15 Papadimitropoulos EA, Coyte PC, Josse RG, Greenwood CE: Current and projected rates of hip fracture in Canada. *Canadian Medical Association Journal* **157**: 1357–63, 1997.

16 Kannus P, Niemi S, Parkkari J, Palvanen M, Vuori I, Jarvinen M: Hip fractures in Finland between 1970 and 1997 and predictions for the future. *Lancet* **353**: 802–5, 1999.

17 Memon A, Pospula WM, Tantawy AY, Abdul-Ghafar S, Suresh A, Al-Rowaih A: Incidence of hip fracture in Kuwait. *International Journal of Epidemiology* **27**: 860–5, 1998.

18 Baudoin C, Fardellone P, Potard V, Sebert JL: Fractures of the proximal femur in Picardy, France in 1987. *Osteoporosis International* **3**: 43–9, 1993.

19 Lau EMC, Cooper C, Wickham C, Donnan S, Barber DJP: Hip fracture in Hong Kong and Britain. *International Journal of Epidemiology* **19**: 1119–21, 1990.

20 Mazzuoli GF, Gennari C, Passeri M *et al.*: Incidence of hip fracture: an Italian survey. *Osteoporosis International* **3** (Supplement 1): 8–9, 1993.

21 Xu L, Lu A, Zhao X, Chen X, Cummings SR: Very low rates of hip fracture in Beijing, People's Republic of China. The Beijing Osteoporosis Project. *American Journal of Epidemiology* **144**: 901–7, 1996.

22 Huang KY, Chang JK, Ling SY, Endo N, Takahashi HE: Epidemiology of cervical and trochanteric fractures of the proximal femur in 1996 in Kaohsiung City, Taiwan. *Journal of Bone and Mineral Metabolism* **18**: 89–95, 2000.

23 Bacon WE, Smith GS, Baker SP: Geographic variation in the occurrence of hip fractures among the elderly white US population. *American Journal of Public Health* **79**: 1556–8, 1989.

24 Jacobsen SJ, Goldberg J, Miles TP, Brody JA, Stiers W, Rimm AA: Regional variation in the incidence of hip fracture. US white women aged 65 years and older. *Journal of the American Medical Association* **264**: 500–2, 1990.

25 Stroup NE, Freni-Titulaer LW, Schwartz JJ: Unexpected geographic variation in rates of hospitalization for patients who have fracture of the hip. Medicare enrollees in the United States. *Journal of Bone and Joint Surgery* [Am], 72(9): 1294–98, 1990.

26 Hinton RY, Lennox DW, Ebert FR, Jacobsen SJ, Smith GS:(1995). Relative rates of fracture of the hip in the United States. Geographic, sex and age variations. *Journal of Bone and Joint Surgery* [Am] **77**: 695–702.

27 French FH, Johnstone AJ, Dougall T: Coping with the epidemic. The impact of proximal femoral fractures upon the acute orthopaedic services in northeast Scotland. *Bulletin of the Hospital for Joint Diseases* **58**: 15–18, 1999.

28 Schroder HM, Andreassen MD, Villadsen I, Sorensen JG, Erlandsen M: Increasing age-specific incidence of hip fractures in a Danish municipality. *Danish Medical Bulletin* **42**: 109–11, 1995.

29 Lord SR: Hip fractures: changing patterns in hospital bed use in NSW between 1979 and 1990. *Australian and New Zealand Journal of Surgery* **63**: 352–5, 1993.

30 Melton LJ 3rd, Therneau TM, Larson DR: Long-term trends in hip fracture prevalence: the influence of hip fracture incidence and survival. *Osteoporosis International* **8**: 68–74, 1998.

31 Huusko TM, Karppi P, Avikainen V, Kautiainen H, Sulkava R: The changing picture of hip fractures: dramatic change in age distribution and no change in age-adjusted incidence within 10 years in Central Finland. *Bone* **24**: 257–59, 1999.

32 Kannus P, Parkkari J, Sievanen H, Heinonen A, Vuori I, Jarvinen M: Epidemiology of hip fractures. *Bone* **18** (Supplement 1): 57S–63S, 1996.

33 Wildner M, Casper W, Bergmann KE: A secular trend in hip fracture incidence in East Germany. *Osteoporosis International* **9**: 144–50, 1999.

34 Chipchase LS, McCaul K, Hearn TC: Hip fracture rates in South Australia: into the next century. *Australian and New Zealand Journal of Surgery* **70**: 117–19, 2000.

35 Dolan P, Torgerson DJ: The cost of treating osteoporotic fractures in the United Kingdon female population. *Osteoporosis International* **8**: 611–17, 1998.

36 Johnell O: The socioeconomic burden of fractures: today and in the 21st century. *American Journal of Medicine* **103**: 5–265, 1997.

37 Cooper C, Campion G, Melton LJ 3rd: Hip fractures in the elderly: a world-wide projection. *Osteoporosis International* **2**: 285–9, 1992.

38 Jacobsen BK, Nilssen S, Hevch I, Kvale G: Reproductive factors and fatal hip fractures. A Norwegian prospective study of 63 000 women. *Journal of Epidemiology and Community Health* **52**: 645–50, 1998.

39 Grodstein F, Stampfer MJ, Falkeborn M, Naessen T, Persson I: Postmenopausal hormone therapy and risk of cardiovascular disease and hip fracture in a cohort of Swedish women. *Epidemiology* **10**: 476–80, 1999.

40 Hedlund R, Lindgren U, Ahlbom A: Age and sex specific incidence of femoral neck and trochanteric fractures. An analysis based on 20 538 fractures in Stockholm County, Sweden, 1972–1981. *Clinical Orthopaedics and Related Research* **222**: 132–9, 1987.

41 Martin AD, Silverthorn KG, Houston CS, Bernhardson S, Wajda A, Roos LL: The incidence of fracture of the proximal femur in two million Canadians from 1972 to 1984. Projections for Canada in the year 2006. *Clinical Orthopaedics and Related Research* **266**: 111–18, 1991.

42 Brummel-Smith K: Geriatrics for orthopaedists. *Instructional Course Lectures* **46**: 409–16, 1997.

43 Farmer ME, White LR, Brody JA, Bailey KR: Race and sex differences in hip fracture incidence. *American Journal of Public Health* **74**: 1374–80, 1984.

44 Hinton RY, Smith GS: The association of age, race and sex with the location of proximal femoral fractures in the elderly. *Journal of Bone and Joint Surgery* [Am] **75**: 752–9, 1993.

45 Lauderdale DS, Jacobsen SJ, Furner SE, Levy PS, Brody JA, Goldberg J: Hip fracture incidence among elderly Asian-American populations. *American Journal of Epidemiology* **146**: 502–9, 1997.

46 Ross *et al.* 1991.

47 Nakamura T, Turner CH, Yoshikawa T *et al.*: Do variations in hip geometry explain differences in hip fracture risk between Japanese and White Americans. *Journal of Bone and Mineral Research* **9**: 1071–6, 1994.

48 Theobald TM, Cauley JA, Gluer CC, Bunker CH, Ukoli FA, Genant HK: Black–white differences in hip geometry. Study of Osteoporotic Fractures Research Group. *Osteoporosis International* **8**: 61–7, 1998.

49 Cauley JA, Zmuda JM, Yaffe K *et al.*: Apolipoprotein E polymorphism: a new genetic marker of hip fracture risk—The Study of Osteoporotic Fractures Research Group. *Journal of Bone and Mineral Research* **14**: 1175–81, 1999.

50 Feskanich D, Hunter DJ, Willett WC *et al.*: Vitamin D receptor genotype and the risk of bone fractures in women. *Epidemiology* **9**: 535–9, 1998.

51 Fox KM, Cummings SR, Powell-Threets K, Stone K: Family history and risk of osteoporotic fracture. Study of Osteoporotic Fractures Research Group. *Osteoporosis International* **8**: 557–62, 1998.

52 Thompson D, Edelsberg J, Colditz GA, Bird AP, Oster G: Lifetime health and economic consequences of obesity. *Archives of Internal Medicine* **159**: 2177–83, 1999.

53 Bernstein J, Grisso JA, Kaplan FS: Body mass and fracture risk. A study of 330 patients. *Clinical Orthopaedics and Related Research* **364**: 227–30, 1999.

54 Dretakis EK, Papakitsou E, Kontakis GM, Dretakis K, Psarakis S, Steriopoulos KA: Bone mineral density, body mass index, and hip axis length in postmenopausal Cretan women with cervical and trochanteric fractures. *Calcified Tissue International* **64**: 257–8, 1999.

55 Pruzansky ME, Turano M, Luckey M, Senie R: Low body weight as a risk factor for hip fracture in both black and white women. *Journal of Orthopaedic Research* **7**: 192–7, 1989.

56 Ensrud KE, Lipschutz RC, Cauley JA *et al.*: Body size and hip fracture risk in older women: a prospective study. Study of Osteoporotic Fractures Research Group. *American Journal of Medicine* **103**: 274–80, 1997.

57 Langlois JA, Harris T, Looker AC, Madans J: Weight change between age 50 years and old age is associated with risk of hip fracture in white women aged 67 years and older. *Archives of Internal Medicine* **156**: 989–94, 1996.

58 Mussolino ME, Looker AC, Madans JH, Langlois JA, Orwoll ES: Risk factors for hip fracture in white men: the NHANES Epidemiologic Follow-up Study. *Journal of Bone and Mineral Research* **13**: 918–24, 1998.

59 Hemenway D, Azrael DR, Rimm EB, Feskanich D, Willett WC: Risk factors for hip fracture in US men aged 40 through 75 years. *American Journal of Public Health* **84**: 1843–5, 1994.

60 Hemenway D, Feskanich D, Colditz GA: Body height and hip fracture: a cohort study of 90 000 women. *International Journal of Epidemiology* **24**: 783–6, 1995.

61 LeBoff MS, Kohlmeier L, Hurwitz S, Franklin J, Wright J, Glowacki J: Occult vitamin D deficiency in postmenopausal US women with acute hip fracture. *Journal of the American Medical Association* **281**: 1505–11, 1999.

62 Chapuy MC, Arlot ME, Duboeuf F *et al.*: Vitamin D_3 and calcium to prevent hip fractures in the elderly women. *New England Journal of Medicine* **327**: 1637–42, 1992.

63 Holbrook TL, Barrett-Connor E, Wingard DL: Dietary calcium and risk of hip fracture: 14-year prospective population study. *Lancet* **ii**: 1046–9, 1988.

64 Hillier S, Cooper C, Kellingray S, Russell G, Hughes H, Coggon D: Fluoride in drinking water and risk of hip fracture in the UK: a case–control study. *Lancet* **355**: 265–9, 2000.

65 Kurttio P, Gustavsson N, Vartiainen T, Pekkanen J: Exposure to natural fluoride in well water and hip fracture: a cohort analysis in Finland. *American Journal of Epidemiology* **150**: 817–24, 1999.

66 Allolio B, Lehmann R: Drinking water fluoridation and bone. *Experimental and Clinical Endocrinology and Diabetes* **107**: 12–20, 1999.

67 Hodges SJ, Akesson K, Vergnaud P, Obrant K, Delmar PD: Circulating levels of vitamins K_1 and K_2 decreased in elderly women with hip fracture. *Journal of Bone and Mineral Research* **8**: 1241–5, 1993.

68 Roberts NB, Holding JD, Walsh HP *et al.*: Serial changes in serum vitamin K_1, triglyceride, cholesterol, osteocalcin and 25-hydroxyvitamin

D_3 in patients after hip replacement for fractured neck of femur or osteoarthritis. *European Journal of Clinical Investigation* **26**: 24–9, 1996.

69 Wald NJ, Hackshaw AK: Cigarette smoking: an epidemiological overview. *British Medical Bulletin* **52**: 3–11, 1996.

70 Law MR, Hackshaw AK: A meta-analysis of cigarette smoking, bone mineral density and risk of hip fracture: recognition of a major effect. *British Medical Journal* **315**: 841–6, 1997.

71 Forsen L, Bjorndal A, Bjartveit K *et al.*: Interaction between current smoking, leanness, and physical inactivity in the prediction of hip fracture. *Journal of Bone and Mineral Research* **9**: 1671–8, 1994.

72 Forsen L, Bjartveit K, Bjorndal A, Edna TH, Meyer HE, Schei B: Ex-smokers and risk of hip fracture. *American Journal of Public Health* **88**: 1481–3, 1998.

73 Cornuz J, Feskanich D, Willett WC, Colditz GA: Smoking, smoking cessation, and risk of hip fracture in women. *American Journal of Medicine* **106**: 311–14, 1999.

74 Hollenbach KA, Barrett-Connor E, Edelstein SL, Holbrook T: Cigarette smoking and bone mineral density in older men and women. *American Journal of Public Health* **83**: 1265–70, 1993.

75 Johnell O, Gullberg B, Kanis JA *et al.*: Risk factors for hip fracture in European women: the MEDOS Study. Mediterranean Osteoporosis Study. *Journal of Bone and Mineral Research* **10**: 1802–15, 1995.

76 Hoidrup S, Gronbaek M, Gottschau A, Lauritzen JB, Schroll M: Alcohol intake, beverage preference, and risk of hip fracture in men and women. Copenhagen Centre for Prospective Population Studies. *American Journal of Epidemiology* **149**: 993–1001, 1999.

77 Kanis J, Johnell O, Gullberg B *et al.*: Risk factors for hip fracture in men from southern Europe: the MEDOS study. *Osteoporosis International* **9**: 45–54, 1999.

78 Felson DT, Kiel DP, Anderson JJ, Kannel WB: Alcohol consumption and hip fractures: the Framingham Study. *American Journal of Epidemiology* **128**: 1102–10, 1988.

79 Gregg EW, Cauley JA, Seeley DG, Ensrud KE, Bauer DC: Physical activity and osteoporotic fracture risk in older women. Study of Osteoporotic Fractures Research Group. *Annals of Internal Medicine* **129**: 81–8, 1998.

80 Kujala UM, Kaprio J, Kannus P, Sarna S, Koskenvuo M: Physical activity and osteoporotic hip fracture risk in men. *Archives of Internal Medicine* **160**: 705–8, 2000.

81 Coupland C, Wood D, Cooper C: Physical inactivity is an independent risk factor for hip fracture in the elderly. *Journal of Epidemiology and Community Health* **47**: 441–3, 1993.

82 Forsen L, Meyer HE, Midthjell K, Edna TH: Diabetes mellitus and the incidence of hip fracture: results from the Nord–Trondelag Health Survey. *Diabetologia* **42**: 920–5, 1999.

83 Johnell O, Melton LJ 3rd, Atkinson EJ, O'Fallon WM, Kurland LT: Fracture risk in patients with parkinsonism: a population-based study in Olmsted County, Minnesota. *Age and Ageing* **21**: 32–8, 1992.

84 Ramnemark A, Nyberg L, Borssen B, Olsson T, Gustafson Y: Fractures after stroke. *Osteoporosis International* **8**: 92–5, 1998.

85 Desai KB, Ribbans WJ, Taylor GJ: Incidence of five common fracture types in an institutional epileptic population. *Injury* **27**: 97–100, 1996.

86 Abdon NJ, Nilsson BE: Episodic cardiac arrythmia and femoral neck fracture. *Acta Medica Scandinavica* **208**: 73–6, 1980.

87 Ward CR, McIntosh S, Kenny RA: Carotid sinus hypersensitivity—a modifiable risk factor for fractured neck of femur. *Age and Ageing* **28**: 127–33, 1999.

88 Melton LJ 3rd, Beard CM, Kokmen E, Atkinson EJ, O'Fallon WM: Fracture risk in patients with Alzheimer's disease. *Journal of the American Geriatrics Society* **42**: 614–19, 1994.

89 Felson DT, Anderson JJ, Hannan MT, Milton RC, Wilson PW, Kiel DP: Impaired vision and hip fracture. The Framingham Study. *Journal of the American Geriatrics Society* **37**: 495–500, 1989.

90 Cooper C, Coupland C, Mitchell M: Rheumatoid arthritis, corticosteroid therapy and hip fracture. *Annals of Rheumatic Diseases* **54**: 49–52, 1995.

91 Kreiger N, Kelsey JL, Holford TR, O'Connor T: An epidemiologic study of hip fracture in postmenopausal women. *American Journal of Epidemiology* **116**: 141–8, 1982.

92 Cumming RG, Klineberg RJ: Psychotropics, thiazide diuretics and hip fractures in the elderly. *Medical Journal of Australia* **158**: 414–17, 1993.

93 Shorr RI, Griffin MR, Daugherty JR, Ray WA: Opioid analgesics and the risk of hip fracture in the elderly: codeine and propoxyphene. *Journal of Gerontology* **47**: M111–15, 1992.

94 Melton LJ 3rd, Crowson CS, Khosla S, O'Fallon WM: Fracture risk after surgery for peptic ulcer disease: a population-based cohort study. *Bone* **25**: 61–7, 1999.

95 Annegers JF, Melton LJ 3rd, Sun CA, Hauser WA: Risk of age-related fractures in patients with unprovoked seizures. *Epilepsia* **30**: 348–55, 1989.

96 Heshmati HM, Khosla S, Robins SP, Geller N, McAlister CA, Riggs BL: Endogenous residual estrogen levels determine bone resorption even in late postmenopausal women. *Journal of Bone and Mineral Research* **12** (Supplement 1): S121, 1997.

97 Tomkinson A, Reeve J, Shaw RW, Noble BS: The death of osteocytes via apoptosis accompanies estrogen withdrawal in human bone. *Journal of Clinical Endocrinology and Metabolism* **82**: 3128–35, 1997.

98 Kiel DP, Felson DT, Anderson JJ, Wilson PW, Moskowitz MA: Hip fracture and the use of estrogens in postmenopausal women. The Framingham Study. *New England Journal of Medicine* **317**: 1169–74, 1987.

99 Michaelsson K, Baron JA, Farahmand BY *et al.*: Hormone replacement therapy and risk of hip fracture: population based case-control study. The Swedish Hip Fracture Study Group. *British Medical Journal* **316**: 1858–63, 1998.

100 Hoidrup S, Gronbaek M, Pedersen AT, Lauritzen JB, Gottschau A, Schroll M: Hormone replacement therapy and hip fracture risk: effect modification by tobacco smoking, alcohol intake, physical activity, and body mass index. *American Journal of Epidemiology*, **150**: 1085–93, 1999.

101 Levy AR, Bensimon DR, Mayo NE, Leighton HG: Inclement weather and the risk of hip fracture. *Epidemiology* **9**: 172–7, 1998.

102 Chiu KY, Ng TP, Chow SP: Seasonal variation of fractures of the hip in elderly persons. *Injury* **27**: 333–6, 1996.

103 Jacobsen SJ, Sargent DJ, Atkinson EJ, O'Fallon WM, Melton LJ 3rd: Population-based study of the contribution of weather to hip fracture seasonality. *American Journal of Epidemiology* **141**: 79–83, 1995.

104 Douglas S, Bunyan A, Chiu KH, Twaddle B, Maffulli N: Seasonal variation of hip fracture at three latitudes. *Injury* **31**: 11–19, 2000.

105 Jacobsen SJ, Goldberg J, Miles TP, Brody JA, Stiers W, Rimm AA: Seasonal variation in the incidence of hip fracture among white persons aged 65 years and older in the United States, 1984–1987. *American Journal of Epidemiology* **133**: 996–1004, 1991.

106 Lips P, Hackeng WH, Jongen MJ, von Ginkel FC, Netelenbos JC: Seasonal variation in serum concentrations of parathyroid hormone in elderly people. *Journal of Clinical Endocrinology and Metabolism* **57**: 204–6, 1983.

107 Kaastad TS, Meyer HE, Falch JA: Incidence of hip fracture in Oslo, Norway: differences within the city. *Bone* **22**: 175–8, 1998.

108 Larsson S, Eliasson P, Hansson LI: Hip fractures in northern Sweden 1973–1984. A comparison of rural and urban populations. *Acta Orthopaedica Scandinavica* **60**: 567–71, 1989.

109 Mannius S, Mellstrom D, Oden A, Rundgren A, Zetterberg C: Incidence of hip fracture in western Sweden 1974–1982. Comparison of rural and urban populations. *Acta Orthopaedica Scandinavica* **58**: 38–42, 1987.

110 Madhok R, Melton LJ 3rd, Atkinson EJ, O'Fallon WM, Lewallen DG: Urban versus rural increase in hip fracture incidence. Age and sex of 901 cases 1980–89 in Olmsted County, USA. *Acta Orthopaedica Scandinavica* **64**: 543–8, 1993.

111 Luthje P, Peltonen A, Nurmi I, Kataja M, Santavirta S: No differences in the incidences of old people's hip fractures between urban and rural populations—a comparative study in two Finnish health care regions in 1989. *Gerontology* **41**: 39–44, 1995.

112 Norton R, Campbell AJ, Reid IR *et al.*: Residential status and risk of hip fracture. *Age and Ageing* **28**: 135–9, 1999.

113 Butler M, Norton R, Lee-Joe T, Cheng A, Campbell AJ: The risks of hip fracture in older people from private homes and institutions. *Age and Ageing* **25**: 381–5, 1996.

114 Cumming RG: Nursing home residence and risk of hip fracture. *American Journal of Epidemiology* **143**: 1191–4, 1996.

115 Faulkner KG, Cummings SR, Black D, Palmero L, Gluer CC, Genant HK: Simple measurement of femoral geometry predicts hip fracture:the study of osteoporotic fractures. *Journal of Bone and Mineral Research* **8**: 1211–17, 1993.

116 Mikhail MB, Vaswani AN, Aloia JF: Racial differences in femoral dimensions and their relation to hip fracture. *Osteoporosis International* **6**: 22–4, 1996.

117 Cummings SR, Cauley JA, Palermo L *et al.*: Racial differences in hip axis lengths might explain racial differences in rates of hip fracture. Study of Osteoporotic Fractures Research Group. *Osteoporosis International* **4**: 226–9, 1994.

118 Gnudi S, Ripamanti C, Gualtieri G, Malavolta N: Geometry of proximal femur in the prediction of hip fracture in osteoporotic women. *British Journal of Radiology* **72**: 729–33, 1999.

119 Duboeuf F, Hans D, Schott AM *et al.*: Different morphometric and densitometric parameters predict cervical and trochanteric hip fracture: the EPIDOS Study. **12**: 1895–1902, 1997.

120 Schott AM, Cormier C, Hans D *et al.*: How hip and whole-body bone mineral density predict hip fracture in elderly women: the EPIDOS Prospective Study. *Osteoporosis International* **8**: 247–54, 1998.

121 Johnson RM: Current techniques with use of hemiarthroplasty in femoral neck fractures. *Program and Abstracts of the 14th Annual Vail Orthopaedic Symposium: Trauma Update, Vail, CO, 20–23 January 2000.*

122 Swiontkowski MF: Current treatment of femoral neck fractures. *Program and Abstracts of the 14th Annual Vail Orthopaedic Symposium: Trauma Update, Vail, CO, 20–23 January 2000.*

123 Boonen S, Broos P, Haentjens P: Factors associated with hip fracture occurrence in old age. Implications in the postsurgical management. *Acta Chirurgica Belgica* **99**: 185–9, 1999.

124 Spangler L, Cummings P, Tencer AF, Mueller BA, Mock C: Biomechanical factors and failure of transcervical hip fracture repair. *Injury* **32**: 223–8, 2001.

125 Swiontkowski MF., Harrington RM, Keller TS, Van Patten PK: Torsion and bending analysis of internal fixation techniques for femoral neck fractures: the role of implant design and bone density. *Journal of Orthopaedic Research* **5**: 433–44, 1987.

126 Edlund A, Lundstrom M, Lundstrom G, Hedqvist B, Gustafson Y: Clinical profile of delirium in patients treated for femoral neck fractures. *Dementia and Geriatric Cognitive Disorders* **10**: 325–9, 1999.

127 Parker MJ, Pryor GA, Myles JW: The value of a special surgical team in preventing complications in the treatment of hip fractures. *International Orthopaedics* **18**: 184–8, 1994.

128 Parker MJ, Pryor GA, Myles JW: 11-year results in 2846 patients of the Peterborough Hip Fracture Project: reduced morbidity, mortality and hospital stay. *Acta Orthopaedica Scandinavica* **71**: 34–8, 2000.

129 Parker MJ: The management of intracapsular fractures of the proximal femur. *Journal of Bone and Joint Surgery* [Br] **82**: 937–41, 2000.

130 Parker MJ: Prediction of fracture union after internal fixation of intracapsular femoral neck fractures. *Injury* **25** (Supplement 2): B3–6, 1994.

131 Holmberg S, Thorngren KG: Pre-operative 99mTc-MDP scintimetry of femoral neck fractures. *Acta Orthopaedica Scandanavica* **55**: 430–5, 1984.

132 Ragnarsson JI, Ekelund L, Karrholm J, Hietala SO: Low field magnetic resonance imaging of femoral neck fractures. *Acta Radiologica* **30**: 247–52, 1989.

133 Asnis SE, Wanek-Sgaglione L: Intracapsular fractures of the femoral neck. Results of cannulated screw fixation. *Journal of Bone and Joint Surgery* [Am] **76**: 1793–1803, 1994.

134 Garden RS: Reduction and fixation of subcapital fractures of the femur. *Orthopaedic Clinics of North America* **5**: 683–712, 1974.

135 Parker MJ: Garden grading of intracapsular fractures: meaningful or misleading? *Injury* **24**: 241–2, 1993.

136 Thomsen NOB, Jensen CM, Skovgaard N et al.: Observer variation in the radiographic classification of fractures of the neck of the femur using Garden's system. *International Orthopaedics* **20**: 326–9, 1996.

137 Kyle RF, Cabanela ME, Russell TA et al.: Fractures of the proximal part of the femur. *Instructional Course Lectures* **44**: 227–53, 1995.

138 Blundell CM, Parker MJ, Pryor GA, Hopkinson-Woolley J, Bhonsle SS: Assessment of the AO classification of intracapsular fractures of the proximal femur. *Journal of Bone and Joint Surgery* [Br] **80**: 679–83, 1998.

139 Hammer AJ: Nonunion of subcapital femoral neck fractures. *Journal of Orthopaedic Trauma* **6**: 73–7, 1992.

140 Parker MJ, Dynan Y: Is Pauwels classification still valid? *Injury* **29**: 521–3, 1998.

141 Rajan DT, Parker MJ: Does the level of an intracapsular femoral fracture influence fracture healing after internal fixation? A study of 411 patients. *Injury* **32**: 53–6, 2001.

142 Parker MJ, Pryor GA: Treatment of undisplaced subcapital fractures. *Journal of the Royal College of Surgeons of Edinburgh* **37**: 263–4, 1992.

143 Chiu FY, Lo WH: Undisplaced femoral neck fractures in the elderly. *Archives of Orthopaedic and Trauma Surgery* **115**: 90–3, 1996.

144 Raaymakers EL, Marti RK: Non-operative treatment of impacted femoral neck fractures. *Journal of Bone and Joint Surgery* [Br] **73**: 950–4, 1991.

145 Parker MJ, Handoll HH, Bhargara A: Conservative versus operative treatment for hip fractures. *Cochrane Database of Systematic Reviews* CD000337, 2000.

146 Cuckler JM, Tamarapalli JR: An algorithm for the management of femoral neck fractures. *Orthopedics* **17**: 789–92, 1994.

147 Parker MJ: Parallel Garden screws for intracapsular femoral fractures. *Injury* **25**: 383–5, 1994.

148 Levi N: Dynamic hip screw versus 3 parallel screws in the treatment of Garden 1 + 2 and Garden 3 + 4 cervical hip fractures. *Panminerva Medica* **41**: 233–7, 1999.

149 Swiontkowski MF: Intracapsular fractures of the hip. *Journal of Bone and Joint Surgery* [Am] **76**: 129–38, 1994.

150 Manninger J, Kazar G, Fekete G *et al.*: Significance of urgent (within 6 h) internal fixation in the management of fractures of the neck of the femur. *Injury* **20**: 101–5, 1989.

151 Jakob M, Rosso R, Weller K, Babst R, Regazzoni P: Avascular necrosis of the femoral head after open reduction and internal fixation of femoral neck fractures: an inevitable complication? *Swiss Surgery* **5**: 257–64, 1999.

152 Holmberg S, Dalen N: Intracapsular pressure and caput circulation in nondisplaced femoral neck fractures. *Clinical Orthopaedics and Related Research* **219**: 124–6, 1987.

153 Parker MJ: Internal fixation or arthroplasty for displaced subcapital fractures in the elderly? *Injury* **23**: 521–4, 1992.

154 Sernbo I, Fredin H: Changing methods of hip fracture osteosynthesis in Sweden. An epidemiological enquiry covering 46 900 cases. *Acta Orthopaedica Scandinavica* **64**: 173–4, 1993.

155 Schmidt AH: *Femoral neck fractures (CME)*. Medscape, 2000.

156 Clark DI, Crofts CE, Saleh M: Femoral neck fracture fixation: comparison of a sliding screw with lag screws. *Journal of Bone and Joint Surgery* [Br]: **72**: 797–800, 1990.

157 Van Audekercke R, Martens M, Mulier JC, Stuyck J: Experimental study on internal fixation of femoral neck fractures.*Clinical Orthopaedics and Related Research* **141**: 203–12, 1979.

158 Baumgaertner MR, Curtin SL, Lindskog DM, Keggi JM: The value of the tip–apex distance in predicting failure of fixation of peritrochanteric fractures of the hip. *Journal of Bone and Joint Surgery* [Am] **77**: 1058–64, 1995.

159 Madsen F, Linde F, Andersen E, Birke H, Hvass I, Poulsen TD: Fixation of displaced femoral neck fractures. A comparison between sliding screw plate and four cancellous bone screws. *Acta Orthopaedica Scandinavica* **58**: 212–16, 1987.

160 Baitner AC, Maurer SG, Hickey DG *et al.*: Vertical shear fractures of the femoral neck. A biomechanical study. *Clinical Orthopaedics and Related Research* **367**: 300–5, 1999.

161 Bray TJ: Femoral neck fracture fixation. Clinical decision making. *Clinical Orthopaedics and Related Research* **339**: 20–31, 1997.

162 Parker MJ, Pryor GA: Internal fixation or arthroplasty for displaced cervical hip fractures in the elderly: a randomised controlled trial of 208 patients. *Acta Orthopaedica Scandinavica* **71**: 440–6, 2000.

163 Chua D, Jaglal SB, Schatzker J: An orthopaedic surgeon survey on the treatment of displaced femoral neck fracture:opposing views. *Canadian Journal of Surgery* **40**: 271–7, 1997.

164 Hudson JI, Kenzora JE, Hebel JR *et al.*: Eight-year outcome associated with clinical options in the management of femoral neck fractures. *Clinical Orthopaedics and Related Research* **348**: 59–66, 1998.

165 Bray TJ, Smith-Hoefer E, Hooper A, Timmerman L: The displaced femoral neck fracture. Internal fixation versus bipolar endoprosthesis. Results of a prospective, randomized comparison. *Clinical Orthopaedics and Related Research* **230**: 127–40, 1988.

166 Jadhav AP, Kulkarni SS, Vaidya SV, Divekar MM, Suralkar SP: Results of Austin Moore replacement. *Journal of Postgraduate Medicine* **42**: 33–8, 1996.

167 Ravikumar KJ, Marsh G: Internal fixation versus hemiarthroplasty versus total hip arthroplasty for displaced subcapital fractures of femur—13 year results of a prospective randomised study. *Injury* **31**: 793–7, 2000.

168 Squires B, Bannister G: Displaced intracapsular neck of femur fractures in mobile independent patients: total hip replacement or hemiarthroplasty. *Injury* **30**: 345–8, 1999.

169 Johansson T, Jacobsson SA, Ivarsson I, Knutsson A, Wahlstrom O: Internal fixation versus total hip arthroplasty in the treatment of displaced femoral neck fractures: a prospective randomized study of 100 hips. *Acta Orthopaedica Scandinavica* **71**: 597–602, 2000.

170 Lavernia CJ: Hemiarthroplasty in hip fracture care: effects of surgical volume on short-term outcome. *Journal of Arthroplasty* **13**: 774–8, 1998.

171 Skeide BI, Lie SA, Havelin LI, Engesaeter LB: Total hip arthroplasty after femoral neck fractures. Results from the national registry on joint prostheses. *Tidsskrift for den Norske Laegeforening* **116**: 1449–51, 1996 (in Norwegian).

172 Burns RB, Moskowitz MA, Ash A, Kane RL, Finch M, McCarthy EP: Do hip replacements improve outcomes for hip fracture patients? *Medical Care* **37**: 285–94, 1999.

173 Broos PL: Prosthetic replacement in the management of unstable femoral neck fractures in the elderly. Analysis of the mechanical complications noted in 778 fractures. *Acta Chirurgica Belgica* **99**: 190–4, 1999.

174 Kyle RF: Classification and treatment of intertrochanteric fractures. *Program and Abstracts of the 14th Annual Vail Orthopaedic Symposium: Trauma Update, Vail, CO, 20–23 January 2000.*

175 Mahomed N, Harrington I, Kellam J, Maistrell, G, Hearn T, Vroemen J: Biomechanical analysis of the Gamma nail and sliding hip screw. *Clinical Orthopaedics and Related Research* **304**: 280–8, 1994.

176 Parker MJ, Handoll HH: Gamma and other cephalocondylic intramedullary nails versus extramedullary implants for extracapsular hip fractures. *Cochrane Database of Systematic Reviews* CD000093, 2000.

177 Parker MJ, Handoll HH, Chinoy MA: Extramedullary fixation implants for extracapsular hip fractures. *Cochrane Database of Systematic Reviews* CD000339, 2000.

178 Parker MJ: Failure of femoral head fixation: a cadaveric analysis of lag screw cut-out with the Gamma locking nail and the AO dynamic hip screw. *Injury* **29**: 569, 1998.

179 Parker MJ: Valgus reduction of trochanteric fractures. *Injury* **24**: 313–16, 1993.

180 Chang WS, Zuckerman JD, Kummer FJ, Frankel VH: Biomechanical evaluation of anatomic reduction versus medial displacement osteotomy in unstable intertrochanteric fractures. *Clinical Orthopaedics and Related Research* **225**: 141–6, 1987.

181 Parker MJ: Trochanteric hip fractures. Fixation failure commoner with femoral medialization: a comparison of 101 cases. *Acta Orthopaedica Scandinavica* **67**: 329–32, 1996.
182 Steinberg GG, Desai SS, Kornwitz NA, Sullivan TJ: The intertrochanteric hip fracture. A retrospective analysis. *Orthopedics* **11**: 265–73, 1988.
183 Parker MJ, Tripuraneni G, McGreggor-Riley J: Osteotomy, compression and reaming techniques for internal fixation of extracapsular hip fractures. *Cochrane Database of Systematic Reviews* CD000522, 2000.
184 Boriani S, De Iure F, Bettelli G *et al.*: The results of a multicenter Italian study on the use of the Gamma nail for the treatment of pertrochanteric and subtrochanteric fractures: a review of 1181 cases. *Chirugia degli Organi di Movimento* **79**: 193–203, 1994.
185 Hoffman CW, Lynskey TG: Intertrochanteric fractures of the femur: a randomized prospective comparison of the Gamma nail and the Ambi hip screw. *Australia and New Zealand Journal of Surgery* **66**: 151–5, 1996.
186 Bess RJ, Jolly SA: Comparison of compression hip screw and Gamma nail for treatment of peritrochanteric fractures. *Journal of the Southern Orthopaedic Association* **6**: 173–9, 1997.
187 Boriani S, De Iure F, Campanacci L *et al.*: A technical report reviewing the use of the 11-mm Gamma nail: interoperative femur fracture incidence. *Orthopedics* **19**: 597–600, 1996.
188 Lyddon DW Jr: The prevention of complications with the Gamma locking nail. *American Journal of Orthopaedics* **25**: 357–63, 1996.
189 O'Brien PJ, Meek RN, Blachut PA, Broekhuyse HM, Sabharwal S: Fixation of intertrochanteric hip fractures: Gamma nail versus dynamic hip screw. A randomized, prospective study. *Canadian Journal of Surgery* **38**: 516–20, 1995.
190 Adams CI, Robinson CM, Court-Brown CM, McQueen MM: Prospective randomized controlled trial of an intramedullary nail versus dynamic screw and plate for intertrochanteric fractures of the femur. *Journal of Orthopaedic Trauma* **15**: 394–400, 2001.
191 Osnes EK, Lofthus CM, Falch JA: More postoperative femoral fractures with the Gamma nail than the sliding screw plate in the treatment of trochanteric fractures. *Acta Orthopaedica Scandinavica* **72**: 252–6, 2001.
192 Parker MJ, Pryor GA: Gamma versus DHS nailing for extracapsular femoral fractures. Meta-analysis of ten randomised trials. *International Orthopaedics* **20**: 163–8, 1996.
193 Bellabarba C, Herscovici D Jr, Ricci WM: Percutaneous treatment of peritrochanteric fractures using the Gamma nail. *Clinical Orthopaedics and Related Research* **375**: 30–42, 2000.
194 Park SR, Kang JS, Kim HS, Lee WH, Kim YH: Treatment of intertrochanteric fracture with the Gamma AP locking nail or by a compression hip screw—a randomised prospective trial. *International Orthopaedics* **22**: 157–60, 1998.
195 Pelet S, Arlettaz Y, Chevalley F: Osteosynthesis of per- and subtrochanteric fractures by blade plate versus Gamma nail. A randomized prospective study. *Swiss Surgery* **7**: 126–33, 2001 (in French).
196 Buhl K, du Bois YD, Lamade W, Meeder PJ: The long Gamma nail—indications, technique and results. *Chirurg* **71**: 1107–14, 2000 (in German).
197 Kukla C, Heinz T, Gaebler C, Heinze G, Vecsei V: The standard Gamma nail: a critical analysis of 1000 cases. *Journal of Trauma* **51**: 77–83, 2001.

198 Sailer R, Ulmer H, Hrubesch R, Fink C, Hoser C, Rangger C: Surgical stabilization of per- and subtrochanteric femoral fractures with the Gamma nail. *Chirurg* **71**: 1380–4, 2000 (in German).

199 Valverde JA, Alonso MG, Porro JG, Rueda D, Larrauri PM, Soler JJ: Use of the Gamma nail in the treatment of fractures of the proximal femur. *Clinical Orthopaedics and Related Research* **350**: 56–61, 1998.

200 Rantanen J, Aro HT: Mechanical failure of the intramedullary hip screw in a subtrochanteric femoral fracture. *Journal of Orthopaedic Trauma* **10**: 348–50, 1996.

201 Rantanen J, Aro HT: Intramedullary fixation of high subtrochanteric femoral fractures: a study comparing two implant designs, the Gamma nail and the intramedullary hip screw. *Journal of Orthopaedic Trauma* **12**: 249–52, 1998.

202 Baixauli F, Vicent V, Baixauli E *et al.*: A reinforced rigid fixation device for unstable intertrochanteric fractures. *Clinical Orthopaedics and Related Research* **361**: 205–15, 1999.

203 Fritz T, Hiersemann K, Krieglstein C, Friedl W: Prospective randomized comparison of gliding nail and Gamma nail in the therapy of trochanteric fractures. *Archives of Orthopaedic and Trauma Surgery* **119**: 1–6, 1999.

204 Haidukewych GJ, Israel TA, Berry DJ: Reverse obliquity fractures of the intertrochanteric region of the femur. *Journal of Bone and Joint Surgery* [Am] **83**: 643–50, 2001.

205 Chinoy MA, Parker MJ: Fixed nail plates versus sliding hip systems for the treatment of trochanteric femoral fractures: a meta analysis of 14 studies. *Injury* **30**: 157–63, 1999.

206 Barquet A, Francescoli L, Rienzi D, Lopez L: Intertrochanteric-subtrochanteric fractures: treatment with the long Gamma nail. *Journal of Orthopaedic Trauma* **14**: 324–8, 2000.

207 Edwards SA, Pandit HG, Clarke HJ: The long Gamma nail: a DGH experience. *Injury* **31**: 701–9, 2000.

208 Edwards SA, Pandit HG, Clarke HJ: The treatment of impending and existing pathological femoral fractures using the long Gamma nail. *Injury* **32**: 299–306, 2001.

209 Lahoud JC, Asselineau A, Salengro S, Molina V, Bombart M: Subtrochanteric fractures. A comparative study between Gamma nail and angular osteosynthesis with lateral cortical support. *Revue de Chirurgie Orthopédique et Reparatrice de l'Appareil Moteur* **83**: 335–42, 1997 (in French).

210 Curtis MJ, Jinnah RH, Wilson V, Cunningham BW: Proximal femoral fractures: a biomechanical study to compare intramedullary and extramedullary fixation. *Injury* **25**: 99–104, 1994.

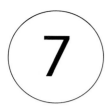

7

Criteria for primary implant selection in total hip arthroplasty: a North American perspective

Robert B. Bourne

Introduction

Total hip arthroplasty (THA) has been one of the most significant medical breakthroughs of the twentieth century, revolutionizing the care of patients with end-stage arthritic conditions of their hip joints.[1-13] Comparative clinical research has revealed that THAs, both cemented and cementless, are among the most cost-effective medical or surgical interventions utilized, are cost saving, and are durable for up to 20 or more years following implantation (Fig. 7.1).[10] Data from the Swedish Hip Registry suggest that cementless femoral components are associated with lower revision rates in patients aged less than 60 years.[14] Despite the overwhelming success of THA, variations have been noted in outcomes such as revision rates, thigh pain, and osteolysis.[15-24] This has led to considerable controversy among surgeons with regard to many significant features such as surgical technique, mode of fixation, surface finish, bearing surfaces, and implant preferences. The purpose of this chapter is to provide, as much as is possible, a North American perspective on primary THA implant selection criteria. As patient, surgical, and implant factors all play a role in prosthesis selection in North America, these aspects will be highlighted.

Patient factors

Many North American surgeons use the concept of 'demand matching' of patient factors for implant selection. Here, patient age, bone stock, activity level, type of arthritis, and cost are considered. Different patients are offered different prostheses based on these criteria. Elderly patients are more likely to receive lower-cost cemented implants based on the good clinical outcomes in published data and the belief that these devices will serve them well for their anticipated life expectancies. On the other hand, more active younger patients with a life expectancy of 20 or more years will be offered

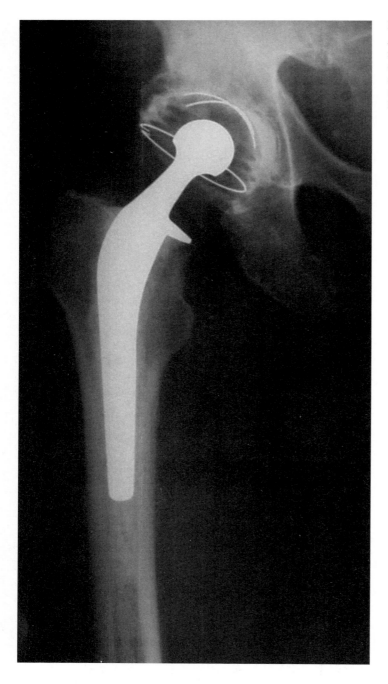

Fig. 7.1
An 18-year follow-up radiograph of a successful cemented total hip arthroplasty.
(HD-2, Howmedica, East Rutherford, NJ)

higher-demand prostheses, which are often more expensive, in the hope that these implants might offer greater durability. These high-demand implants will usually be inserted cementless and may feature ceramic femoral heads. Newer alternative bearing surfaces (i.e. metal-on-metal, ceramic-on-ceramic, or metal-on-crosslinked polyethylene) might also be considered in this patient group.

Bone stock is also considered important in guiding implant selection in North America. Dorr and coworkers have classified proximal femoral medullary shapes into types A (champagne flute shaped), B (funnel shaped), or C (cylindrical) (Fig. 7.2).[25,26] Funnel-shaped proximal femoral canals (Dorr types A and B) are more often found in younger patients and in at least 80 per cent of patients in general. The funnel-shaped femoral canal is considered ideal for cementless fixation (Fig. 7.3). Cylindrical femoral canal shapes are more often found in elderly osteoporotic patients or those with inflammatory types of arthritis (Fig. 7.4). They seem to be best suited to cemented femoral stem fixation. There is controversy regarding active patients over 70 years of age who have funnel-shaped medullary canals. Some North American surgeons prefer to use

Fig. 7.2

Radiographic examples of Dorr type A, B, and C proximal femoral morphologues.

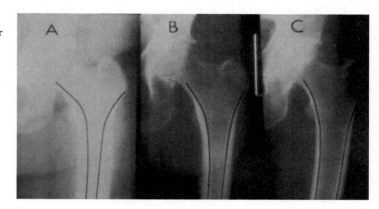

Fig. 7.3

An example of a successful cementless tapered total hip arthroplasty in a Dorr type B femur. (Synergy, Smith & Nephew, Memphis, TN)

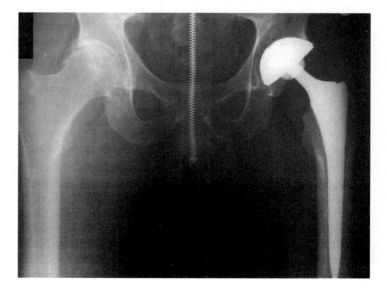

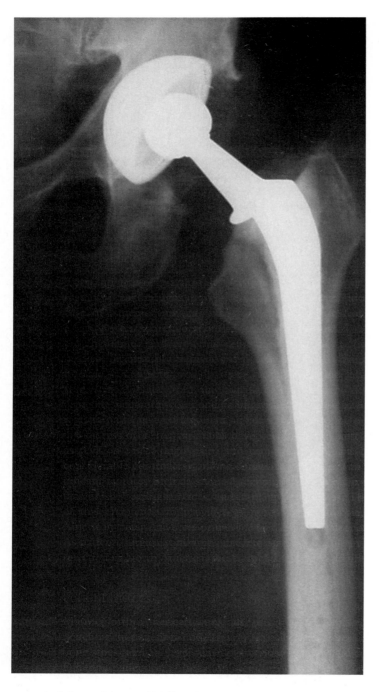

Fig. 7.4
An example of a successful cemented total hip arthroplasty in a Dorr type C femur. (Spectron/Reflection, Smith & Nephew, Memphis, TN)

cemented femoral stems in all patients aged over 70 years. They argue that the bone in elderly patients is weaker and more prone to fracture when cementless femoral stems are inserted. Others disagree with this stance and advocate the use of cementless femoral

166

stems in all funnel-shaped proximal femoral canals, regardless of whether the patients are less or more than 70 years of age.[19]

Traditionally, patients were believed to walk a million steps per year and most wear studies have been based on this premise. Recent investigations[27-29] have challenged this concept as an oversimplification. Podometry studies have revealed that, in general, patients aged less than 60 years and males have increased activity levels. However, some patients walk more than 3.5 million steps per year and age is a poor indicator of activity level in these very active individuals. These investigators have encouraged the incorporation of activity scales in prospective follow-up studies of THA outcomes, particularly wear analyses. These studies have also challenged the selection of prosthetic type only on the basis of age. As a result, many North American surgeons use cementless higher-demand implants even in very active patients aged more than 70 years.

With the ageing of the 'baby boomers' in North America and the anticipated increased demand for total hip arthroplasty, cost control will become a major issue. Total hip replacement is a high-volume high-cost procedure that has drawn much attention from the providers of health care.[5] Much as low cost hemi-arthroplasties have been used to treat low-demand elderly femoral neck fracture patients, some have suggested that this strategy be expanded to the field of THA. Less expensive low-demand hip arthroplasties have been suggested for elderly low-demand patients, reserving more expensive devices for younger more active patients. The issues of ethics and patient choice remain and, as yet, are unresolved.

Surgical factors

Surgical factors also influence total hip replacement selection. The surgeon has several choices in terms of mode of fixation, implant selection, and soft-tissue balancing of the hip. In elderly patients with poor balance, comorbid conditions, and other joint problems, the surgeon may prefer to use cement fixation, which permits immediate full weight-bearing.[1,30] The actual selection of one prosthetic type over another is influenced by many factors, including surgeon training, published results, peer pressure, ease of insertion, and cost. In cemented THA, these factors might also influence the selection of a polished versus a satin-finished versus a matt-finished stem. Considerable debate exists as to which femoral stems provide the optimal cement mantles (Fig. 7.5), but stems with rounded rectangular cross-sections both proximally and distally seem to have performed best (Fig. 7.6).[2,8,31]

In cementless THA, many stems provide durable fixation.[19,23,32-40] Training, published results, and cost are important factors which may influence the selection of an anatomic, tapered, or cylindrical femoral stem that relies on either proximal or distal

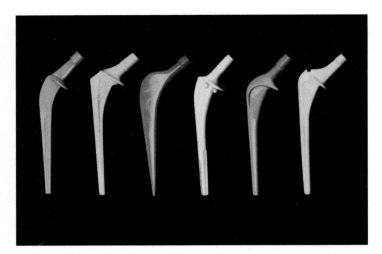

Fig. 7.5

Examples of contemporary cemented stems.

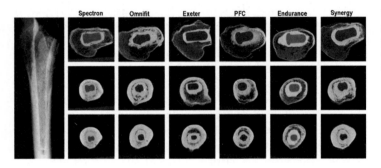

Fig. 7.6

Examples of cement mantles provided by the contemporary cemented stems highlighted in Fig. 7.5.

fixation. These stems are differentiated by the issues of stress shielding, thigh pain, and range of motion allowed.

Soft-tissue balancing of the hip during THA is another surgeon-controlled variable that may influence implant selection.[32,41,42] Restoration of femoral neck offset has been shown to affect polyethylene wear, abductor strength, limp, the need for walking aids, and the risk of postoperative dislocation.[42] The surgeon may choose a femoral component with a lower neck–shaft angle (i.e. 131° versus 135°) and more than one offset choice (i.e. standard and high offset options). The surgeon may also wish to use an acetabular socket which can be employed in a standard mode or with a lateralized option (i.e. the ability to use a socket with an extra 4 mm of thickness). This extra versatility also minimizes the surgeon's need to use skirted femoral heads when attempting to recreate the patient's leg lengths and femoral neck offset, thereby avoiding impingement and lessening the risk of postoperative dislocation (Fig. 7.7). Soft-tissue balancing of the hip is best achieved by careful preoperative planning and the use of intra-operative measurements during the performance of a total hip replacement operation.

Fig. 7.7

Intra-operative measurement of leg length and offset during a total hip replacement. (Smith & Nephew, Memphis, TN)

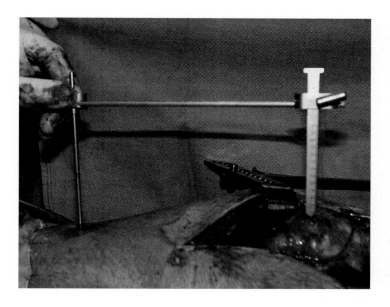

Implant factors

Acetabular components

In North America, cemented acetabular sockets are infrequently used because of the perception, right or wrong, that cementless sockets provide better outcomes, are easier to implant, add greater versatility (i.e. ability to reorient the component, to use lipped liners for enhanced stability, and to use lateralized liners to avoid the use of skirted femoral heads), and allow polyethylene exchange in the case of wear.[16,43] In fact, the use of cemented acetabular sockets is so uncommon in many parts of North America that many orthopaedic residents lack proper training in how to cement an all-polyethylene acetabular component. Therefore, they will avoid the use of cemented sockets in their own future surgical practices.

Laboratory and clinical investigations have defined the prerequisites of an acceptable cementless acetabular component. Ingrowth metal shells have been found to be superior to screw ring or hydroxyapatite-coated devices. Hemispherical polyethylene, which conforms closely to the metal shell and is securely locked to it, has been found to be very important. In addition, a polyethylene thickness of at least 6–8 mm has been found to be critical, leading to the use of thinner metal shells and smaller femoral head sizes (i.e. 22, 26, or 28 mm versus 32 mm) to achieve this. The association of osteolysis with screw holes has led many surgeons to use 'no-hole' acetabular cups, whenever possible, and even the use of 'manhole covers' to cover the central hole used by introduction tools. There also seems to be a movement towards polishing the inner surfaces of the acetabular metal shells in an effort to minimize 'backside' polyethylene debris generation. Debate still exists as to the superiority of screws, fins, spikes, dual geometry, or under-reaming in achieving optimal cementless cup fixation.

Considerable attention has been directed to improving the ultrahigh molecular weight polyethylene (UHMWPE) used in acetabular components. Quality control has led to the use of higher molecular weight (3–6 million daltons) medical-grade polyethylene. Sterilization in air with gamma irradiation is no longer used to prevent carbon-chain scission, oxidation, and increased wear. Ethylene oxide, plasma gas, or irradiation in an oxygen-free environment are now the preferred methods of UHMWPE sterilization. More recently, there has been considerable interest in and assessment of alternative acetabular bearing surfaces (i.e. cross-linked polyethylene, alumina, ceramic-on-ceramic, and metal-on-metal) (Fig. 7.8).

Femoral heads

In North America, most orthopaedic surgeons prefer to use modular rather than monoblock femoral components.[19,32,34] Surgeons seem willing to accept concerns about fretting and galvanic corrosion in exchange for the versatility provided in adjusting leg lengths, offset, and femoral head size. Morse taper sizing has also been an issue. Larger machined tapers have performed better than smaller smooth tapers. An industry-wide move to 12/14 European tapers has resulted in this becoming the industry standard. In addition, the importances of Morse taper tolerances and surface finish

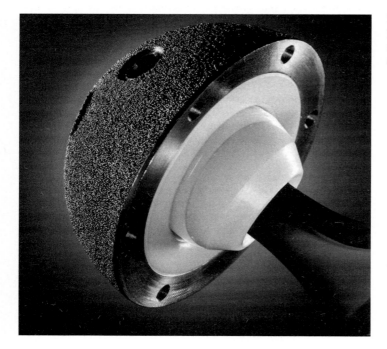

Fig. 7.8
Examples of a ceramic-on-ceramic total hip replacement.

have been recognized, particularly when utilizing ceramic femoral heads, leading to much improved quality assurance in this important area.

Controversy also surrounds the choice of material for the modular femoral head. Titanium heads have been shown to be inferior to cobalt-chrome with regard to wear characteristics.[17,32,44] Therefore cobalt-chrome has become the industry standard. Early alumina ceramic femoral heads have had an unacceptable catastrophic failure rate. Today, higher-quality alumina and zirconia femoral heads with smaller grain sizes and more rigorous factory testing have been developed with reported fracture rates of between 1 in 10 000 and 1 in 25 000. These heads have a higher polished surface and better wettability characteristics than cobalt-chrome and are being used with greater frequency in younger patients.[45]

Femoral components

Considerable improvements have been made in both cemented and cementless femoral components in terms of neck design, minimization of the need for skirted femoral heads, and the ability to 'soft-tissue balance the hip' by restoring neck–shaft offset and the centre of rotation of the femoral head.[32,42] Morse tapers have been better designed and excess taper length removed in an attempt to minimize acetabular socket–femoral component neck impingement (Fig. 7.9). To maximize THA range of motion, many manufacturers have moved from round femoral neck cross-sections to rounded-trapezoid neck designs (Fig. 7.10). These improvements have been instrumental in reducing the risk of dislocation and the production of polyethylene debris related to this impingement.

Surgeons have also been given the option to restore femoral neck–shaft offset by means of variable offset femoral stems.[32,41,42] Different manufacturers solve the offset problem in different ways. Some encourage the surgeon to restore offset by using modular femoral heads with longer neck lengths. This approach is less

Fig. 7.9

Examples of different femoral neck and Morse taper designs. Shortening the Morse taper and using a rounded rectangular neck design increase range of motion.

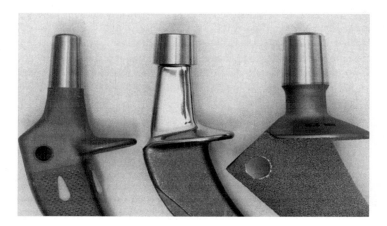

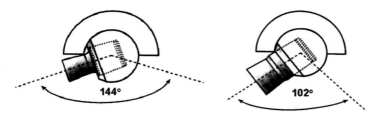

Fig. 7.10
Effect of neck design on THA range of motion.

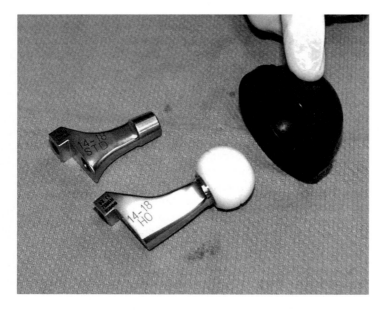

Fig. 7.11
Options available to the surgeon not only to equalize leg lengths, but also to restore offset (dual-offset femoral neck options and lateralized actabular polyethylene insert). (Synergy, Smith & Nephew, Memphis, TN)

popular, as not only offset but also leg length is increased. Other manufacturers offer the same femoral stems with one or more neck–shaft angles (i.e. 130° and 135°). This option also has the disadvantage of affecting both offset and leg length. The approach which is gaining the greatest popularity is that of lowering the femoral component neck–shaft angle on all components (i.e. 130° or 131°) and offering two or more offset stems which maintain the same neck–shaft angle, but proportionally medialize the femoral neck according to stem size in the 'high-offset' options (Fig. 7.11). The ability to 'soft-tissue balance the hip' allows the surgeon not only to equalize leg lengths, restore offset, and minimize postoperative dislocation, but also to re-establish the resting length of the abductor muscles.[42] Abductor strength is increased, which minimizes limp and the need for walking aids. It has also been demonstrated that proper restoration of offset is important in reducing the resultant force across the hip joint which affects polyethylene wear.[32] When this is combined with the use of 'lateralized acetabular polyethylene liners', the surgeon has the additional advantages of being able to restore not only offset, but also the centre of rotation of the hip joint in relation to the acetabular tear drop. All these innovations play an important role in allowing the surgeon to avoid the use of skirted femoral heads which are known to increase acetabular socket impingement, hip dislocation, and polyethylene debris formation.

Cemented

Cemented femoral components are commonly used in North America, particularly in combination with cementless acetabular implants. This combination has been called the 'hybrid THA'. There is relative consensus that cemented femoral components should be fabricated from cobalt-chrome alloy for reasons related to their biocompatibility, stiffness, and abrasion resistance.[2,30,31] Most cemented cobalt-chrome femoral stems are also forged rather than cast because of the increased fatigue strength. As cost becomes more of an issue, some 'low-demand' stems are being offered in cast cobalt-chrome alloy. In order to minimize the risk of stem fracture, these cast stems must have a minimum thickness and hence are often bulkier than stronger forged femoral implants.

In terms of cemented femoral component shape, most North American surgeons prefer a 'rounded-rectangular' cross-section along the entire length of the femoral component and the avoidance of sharp corners which might act as stress risers on the cement. North American surgeons also like cemented femoral stems with a number of size options. Less expensive 'low-demand' cemented femoral stems typically have three femoral stem sizes, whereas the more commonly used cemented implants have five or more size options[2,31] Most cemented femoral stems are also proportional in length, such that the smaller sizes are in the range of 11–12 cm long and the larger sizes are 14–15 cm long.

The surface finish of the cemented femoral stem remains a very controversial area in North America. Polished, satin, matt, rough, and pre-coat options are available. Some recent reports have implicated some precoat cemented femoral stems in premature failure.[46] The selection of a polished, satin, matt, or rough surface finish remains less clear. On the one hand, if the surgeon believes that subsidence is inevitable and that cement will be abraded by this subsidence, creating cement debris and increased third-body wear, a polished tapered cemented stem is often selected. If a polished cemented femoral stem is selected, it is usually tapered and free from grooves or ridges to allow stem subsidence without fracture of the cement mantle. On the other hand, many surgeons point to the excellent results over 10 years or more with satin, matt, and proximally roughened cemented stems, the apparent lack of subsidence, and low wear rates to justify their preference for this option.[2,30,31] It is becoming increasingly apparent that cemented femoral stems of varying surface finish can achieve excellent durable clinical results.

Cementless

Cementless femoral components are favoured in younger more active patients. These cementless stems may be tapered, anatomic, or cylindrical. Typically, tapered and anatomic cementless stems are proximally coated with a porous ingrowth surface (i.e. sintered beads or crimped wire). Hydroxyapatite fixation is available, but is not as commonly used in North America. Grit-blasted surfaces are not popular owing to the perception that a proximal ingrowth/ongrowth surface prevents the development of distal femoral osteolysis. Cylindrical cementless femoral stems are typically extensively coated with an ingrowth surface and depend on 'fit and fill', both proximally and distally, for fixation.

The various cementless femoral stem designs (i.e. tapered, anatomic, and cylindrical) have all been associated with durable fixation. Differentiating features include stress shielding and thigh pain.

All total hip replacements cause some stress shielding. However, stress shielding can be minimized by avoiding large cementless femoral components, particularly in osteoporotic femurs, using metals with a lower modulus of elasticity (i.e. titanium alloys) or using less bulky tapered cementless stems [47,48] Table 7.1 demonstrates stress shielding with the use of tapered, anatomic, and cylindrical cementless femoral components.

Pain in the thigh following total hip replacement occurs with both cemented and cementless implants, but to varying degrees. Thigh pain may be caused by poor femoral component fixation, modular mismatch, and/or endosteal irritation. In a randomized clinical trial comparing cemented with cementless tapered total hip replacements, mild thigh pain was noted in 3 per cent of patients with both cemented and cementless tapered femoral components.[10] Conversely, thigh pain has been noted to be much more frequent with anatomic cementless femoral implants, often exceeding a prevalence of 20 per cent![34,40] Similarly, disabling thigh pain has been associated with 8–15 per cent of cylindrical distal fixation femoral stems.[19]

Algorithm for femoral component selection

As a consequence of these various observations and perceptions, a 'typical' algorithm for femoral component selection in North America can be developed. Based on patient age, the shape of the proximal

Table 7.1 Algorithm for femoral component selection

	Cementless	Cemented
Age (years)	<75	>75
Metaphyseal shape	Funnel	Cylindrical
Type of arthritis	Osteoarthritis/ avascular necrosis	Inflammatory
Demand	High	Low

Table 7.2 Algorithm for acetabular component selection

	Cementless	Cemented
Age (years)	<75	>75
Host support (%)	>50	<50
Bone disease	Osteoarthritis/ avascular necrosis	Irradiated/ Paget's disease
Demand	High	Low

femoral medullary canal, the type of arthritis and patient demand, such an algorithm has proved useful in guiding femoral component selection (Table 7.1). In our centre, the use of such an algorithm has led to the use of cementless tapered devices in 75 per cent of patients.

Algorithm for acetabular component selection

Although cementless acetabular components are widely used in North America, cemented acetabular sockets may be considered in elderly patients or in association with extensive bone-grafting procedures (i.e. protrusio acetabular conditions), certain bone diseases (i.e. Paget's disease), or previously irradiated bone where bone ingrowth potential is poor or unknown.[16] Cemented acetabular components are usually applied to a clean dry acetabulum in which many cement seating holes have been prepared.[2] Cementless acetabular sockets can be fixed by screw fixation press-fitting into an under-reamed socket or with a variety of supplemental fixation devices (i.e. fins, dual geometry, or spikes).[17,19,22,23,32,34] Similar to the femoral component selection algorithm, an acetabular component selection algorithm can be developed based on patient age, host support, bone disease (i.e. prior irradiation or Paget's disease), and patient demand (Table 7.2).

Future directions supported by evidence-based practice

It is widely recognized that evidence-based decision-making criteria are often absent when selecting a primary total hip replacement. National joint replacement registries, such as Sweden, have worked effectively to reduce the number of revision arthroplasties.[8,14,21] Unfortunately, most (96 per cent) primary total hip replacements in Sweden are inserted with cement fixation. In North America, most primary acetabular and, to a lesser extent, femoral components are inserted cementless. Many of the popular cemented THRs used in Scandinavia are not used in North America. As a result, considerable efforts are under way to establish large North American joint-replacement registries. In Canada, the Canadian Joint Replacement Registry was launched in June 2000, and more extensive provincial registries, such as the Ontario Joint Replacement Registry, are starting to help monitor not only implant, surgeon, and hospital performance, but also waiting times, patient satisfaction, and annual outcomes. Such information will be welcome to patients, surgeons, hospitals, and health care providers in providing the best evidence-based total hip replacement surgery.

Conclusions

Primary total hip replacement is now growing at 8 per cent per year. As the postwar 'baby boomers' age in North America, the peak population of this age group will reach the age of 60 years in 2018 and the number of primary total hip replacements will at least double. This factor, plus the fact that patients are living longer more active lives, has stimulated considerable activity in improving the results of primary total hip replacement, especially in the areas of fixation bearing surfaces and soft-tissue balancing. Monitoring of clinical performance and evidence-based decision-making will become increasingly important in improving primary total hip arthroplasty in North America and beyond.

References

1 Bourne RB, Rorabeck CH, Laupacis A, Tugwell P, Wong C, Bullas R: Total hip replacement. The case for non-cemented femoral fixation because of age. *Canadian Journal of Surgery* **38**: 567, 1995.

2 Bourne RB, Rorabeck CH, Skutek M *et al.*: The Harris design total hip replacement fixed with so-called second generation cementing techniques. A ten to fifteen year follow-up. *Journal of Bone and Joint Surgery* [Am] **80**: 1775–80, 1998.

3 Charnley J: *Low friction arthroplasty of the hip.* Springer-Verlag, Berlin, 1979.

4 Klapach AS, Callaghan JJ, Goetz DD, Olejiniczak BA, Johnston RC: Charnley total hip arthroplasty with use of improved cementing techniques. A minimum twenty-year follow-up study. *Journal of Bone and Joint Surgery* [Am] **83**: 1840, 2001.

5 Laupacis A, Bourne RB, Rorabeck C *et al.*: The effect of elective total hip replacement on health related quality of life. *Journal of Bone and Joint Surgery* [Am] **75**: 1619, 1993.

6 Laupacis A, Bourne RB, Rorabeck C, Feeny D, Tugwell P, Sim DA: Randomized trials in orthopaedics; why, how and when? *Journal of Bone and Joint Surgery* [Am] **71**: 535, 1989.

7 Lombardi AV Jr, Mallory TH, Vaughn BJ, Drouilliard P: Aseptic loosening in total hip arthroplasty secondary to osteolysis induced by wear debris from titanium-alloy modular femoral heads. *Journal of Bone and Joint Surgery* [Am] **71**: 1337–42, 1989.

8 Malchau H, Herberts P, Ahnfelt L: Prognosis of total hip replacement in Sweden. Follow-up of 92 675 operations performed 1978–1990. *Acta Orthopaedica Scandinavica* **64**: 497–506, 1993.

9 Older J: Low friction arthroplasty of the hip. *Clinical Orthopaedics and Related Research* **211**: 36–42, 1986.

10 Rorabeck CH, Bourne RB, Laupacis A *et al.*: A double blind study of 250 cases comparing cemented to cementless total hip arthroplasty. Cost effectiveness and its impact on health related quality of life. *Clinical Orthopaedics and Related Research* **298**: 156–64, 1994.

11 Stauffer RN: Ten year follow-up study of total hip replacement. *Journal of Bone and Joint Surgery* [Am] **64**: 983–90, 1982.

12 Sutherland CJ, Wilde AH, Borden LS, Marks KE: A ten year follow-up of 100 consecutive Muller curved stem total hip replacement arthroplasties. *Journal of Bone and Joint Surgery* [Am] **64**: 970–82, 1982.

13 Wrobleski BM: Fifteen–21 year results of the Charnley low-friction arthroplasty. *Clinical Orthopaedics and Related Research* **211**: 30, 1986.

14 Malchau H, Herberts P, Soderman P: Prognosis of total hip replacement in Sweden. Presented at Canadian Orthopaedic Association Meeting, 2 June 2001.

15 Clarke IC, Gruen T, Matos, Amstutz HC: Improved methods for quantitative radiographic evaluation with particular reference to total hip arthroplasty. *Clinical Orthopaedics and Related Research* **121**: 83–91, 1976.

16 Clohisy JC, Harris WA: Matched pair analysis of cemented and cementless acetabular reconstruction in primary total hip arthroplasty. *Journal of Arthroplasty* **16**: 697, 2001.

17 Dowdy PA, Rorabeck CH, Bourne RB: Uncemented total hip arthroplasty in patients 50 years of age or younger. *Journal of Arthroplasty* **12**: 853, 1997.

18 Emerson RH Jr, Sanders SB, Head WC, Higgins L: Effect of circumferential plasma-spray porous coating on the rate of femoral osteolysis after total hip arthroplasty. *Journal of Bone and Joint Surgery* [Am] **81**: 1291–8, 1999.

19 Engh CA Jr, Culpepper WJ II, Engh CA: Long term results of use of anatomic medullary locking prosthesis in total hip arthroplasty. *Journal of Bone and Joint Surgery* [Am] **79**: 177–84, 1997.

20 Gruen JA, McNeice GM, Amstutz HC: Modes of failure of cemented stem-type femoral components. A radiographic analysis of loosening. *Clinical Orthopaedics and Related Research* **141**: 17–27, 1979.

21 Havelin LI, Espehaug B, Vollset SE, Engesaeter LB: Early aseptic loosening of uncemented femoral components in primary total hip replacement. A review based on the Norwegian Arthroplasty Register. *Journal of Bone and Joint Surgery* [Br] **77**: 11–17, 1995.

22 Hellman EJ, Capello NN, Feinberg JR: Omnifit cementless total hip arthroplasty. A 10-year average follow-up. *Clinical Orthopaedics and Related Research* **364**: 164–74, 1999.

23 Mallory TH, Lombardi AV, Leith JR *et al.*: Minimal 50-year results of a tapered cementless femoral component in total hip arthroplasty. *Journal of Arthroplasty* **16**: 49, 2001.

24 Wykman A, Lundberg A: Subsidence of porous coated noncemented femoral components in total hip arthroplasty. A roentgen stereo photogrammatic analysis. *Journal of Arthroplasty* **7**: 197–200, 1992.

25 Bourne RB, Rorabeck CH: A critical look at cementless stems. Taper designs and when to use alternatives. *Clinical Orthopaedics and Related Research* **355**: 212–23, 1998.

26 Dorr L, Faugere M, Mackel A: Structural and cellular assessment of bone quality. *Bone* **14**: 231–42, 1993.

27 Goldsmith AAJ, Dowson D, Wrobleski BM *et al.*: Comparative study of the activity of total hip arthroplasty: patients and normal subjects. *Journal of Arthroplasty* **16**: 613, 2001.

28 Schmalzried TP, Jasty M, Harris WH: Periprosthetic bone loss in total hip arthroplasty. Polyethylene wear debris and the concept of the effective joint space. *Journal of Bone and Joint Surgery* [Am] **74**: 849–63, 1992.

29 Schmalzried TP, Szuozcjewicz ES, Northfield MR *et al.*: Quantitative assessment of walking activity after total hip or knee replacement. *Journal of Bone and Joint Surgery* [Am] **80**: 54, 1998.

30 Mulroy RD, Harris WH: The effect of improved cementing techniques on component loosening in total hip replacement: an 11-year radiographic review. *Journal of Bone and Joint Surgery* [Br] **72**: 757, 1990.

31 Barrack RL, Mulroy RD, Harris WH: Improved cementing techniques and femoral component loosening in young patients with hip arthroplasty. *Journal of Bone and Joint Surgery* [Br] **74**: 385, 1992.

32 Bourne RB, Rorabeck CH, Patterson J, Guerin J: Tapered titanium cementless total hip replacements: a 10–13 year follow-up study. *Clinical Orthopaedics and Related Research* **393**: 112–20, 2001.

33 Delauncy C, Kapandji AI: Ten-year survival of Zweymuller total prostheses in primary uncemented arthroplasty of the hip. *Revue de Chirurgie Orthopédique et Reparatrice de l'Appareil Moteur* **84**: 759–61, 1998.

34 Kawamura H, Dunbar M, Murray P, Bourne R, Rorabeck C: The porous coated anatomic total hip replacement: a ten to fourteen year follow-up of a cementless total hip arthroplasty. *Journal of Bone and Joint Surgery* [Am] **83**: 1333, 2001.

35 McLaughlin JR, Lee KR: Total hip arthroplasty with an uncemented femoral component. Excellent results at ten-year follow-up. *Journal of Bone and Joint Surgery* [Br] **79**: 900–7, 1997.

36 McLaughlin JR, Lee KR: Total hip arthroplasty in young patients: 8 to 13 year results using an uncemented stem. *Clinical Orthopaedics and Related Research* **373**: 153–63, 2000.

37 Rothman RH, Cohn JC: Cemented versus cementless total hip arthroplasty: a critical review. *Clinical Orthopaedics and Related Research* **254**: 153, 1990.

38 Sakalkale DP, Engh K, Hozack WJ, Rothman RH: Minimum 10 year results of a tapered cementless hip replacement. *Clinical Orthopaedics and Related Research* **362**: 138–44, 1999.

39 Schram M, Keck F, Hohmann D, Pitto RP: Total hip arthroplasty using a cemented femoral component with taper design. Outcome at 10-year follow-up. *Archives of Orthopaedic and Traumatic Surgery* **120**: 7–8, 2000.

40 Xenos JS, Callaghan JJ, Heeken RD *et al.*: The porous coated anatomic total hip prosthesis, inserted without cement. A prospective study with a minimum of ten years of follow-up. *Journal of Bone and Joint Surgery* [Am] **81**: 74–82, 1999.

41 Davey JR, O'Connor DO, Burke DW, Harris WH: Femoral component offset. Its effect on strain in bone cement. *Journal of Arthroplasty* **8**: 23–6, 1993.

42 McGrory BJ, Morrey BF, Cahalan, LD, An KN, Cabanela ME: Effect of femoral offset on range of motion and abductor muscle strength after total hip arthroplasty. *Journal of Bone and Joint Surgery* [Br] **77**: 865–9.

43 Willert HG, Bertram H, Buchhorn GH: Osteolysis in allo arthroplasty of the hip. The role of ultra-high molecular weight polyethylene wear particles. *Clinical Orthopaedics and Related Research* **258**: 95–107, 1990.

44 Puolakka TJ, Pajamaki KJ, Pulkkinen PO, Nevalainen JK: Poor survival of cementless Biomet total hip: a report on 1047 hips from the Finnish Arthroplasty Register. *Acta Orthopaedica Scandinavica* **70**: 425–9, 1999.

45 Urban JA, Garvin KL, Boese CK *et al.*: Ceramic-on-polyethylene bearing surfaces in total hip arthroplasty. Seventeen to twenty-one year results. *Journal of Bone and Joint Surgery* [Am] **83**: 1688, 2001.

46 Sylvain GM, Kassab S, Coutts R, Santore R: Early failure of a roughened surface, precoated femoral component in total hip arthroplasty. *Journal of Arthroplasty* **15**: 141, 2001.

47 Mulliken BD, Bourne RB, Rorabeck CH, Nayak NN: A tapered titanium femoral stem inserted without cement in a total hip arthroplasty. Radiographic evaluation and stability. *Journal of Bone and Joint Surgery* [Am] **78**: 1214–25, 1996.

48 Mulliken BD, Bourne RB, Rorabeck CH, Nayak NN: Results of the cementless Mallory head primary total hip arthroplasty: a 5 to 7 year review. *Iowa Orthopaedic Journal* **16**: 20–34, 1996.

8

Criteria for implant selection in revision total hip arthroplasty: a North American perspective

David A. Parker and Cecil H. Rorabeck

Introduction

Total hip arthroplasty (THA) has become one of the most successful and cost-effective orthopaedic interventions.[1] However, despite improved long-term results, the large number of arthroplasties performed has predictably led to an increased number of revision procedures which make up a significant proportion of all THA surgery (60).[2] Therefore the arthroplasty surgeon is obliged to be familiar with the appropriate techniques to optimize the success of revision surgery as this will inevitably become an increasingly significant part of any arthroplasty practice.

The main goal of revision surgery, as in primary surgery, is to achieve a stable prosthesis with good pain relief, function, and longevity. Goals more specific for revision surgery include wide exposure, atraumatic removal of the original prostheses, restoration of bone stock, and minimizing operative complications, which are more prevalent than in primary surgery. Difficulties encountered more often in revision include bone and soft-tissue defects, trochanteric non-union, periprosthetic fractures, and infection. Any one of these complications can significantly decrease the chance of achieving a successful implant.

Optimizing chances of success requires a clear understanding of the reasons for the original failure and an appreciation of which particular technique is most likely to succeed in each particular situation. Careful preoperative planning should identify reasons for the failure of the primary implant, exclude infection, identify the previous surgical approach, plan for prosthetic removal, and determine the degree of bone-stock loss. Bone defects can be classified using a number of systems,[3-9] and it is important that the surgeon choose a system which can clearly guide subsequent management.

There are a multitude of prosthetic designs available for use in revision surgery and implant choice is integral to the success of the procedure. Choosing the most appropriate design for a particular revision requires careful preoperative planning coupled with a knowledge of the likelihood of success of each design in any particular revision procedure. As the number of revision procedures increases, so does the available literature on the success of the various designs in each specific indication for revision surgery.

The earliest reported series of revision total hip arthroplasties from North America appeared in the literature over 20 years ago.[10,11] In more recent times, as revision hip procedures have become more common, the literature devoted to reporting the results of revision THA have increased exponentially. In earlier reports, the operative techniques and implants used were significantly less variable than the vast spectrum of procedures and implants used today. The earlier reports also tended to have less favourable results than those published today. Certainly, an additional 20 years of experience has led to a greater understanding of the appropriate methods for achieving successful results, and has seen certain trends evolve for implant and procedure selection for different scenarios.

In this chapter we consider the various implants and techniques that are available, and review the North American literature to analyse the reported results. Analysing results across the available literature poses the ongoing problem of different classification systems for preoperative assessment of bony defects and different outcome measures. However, re-revision rate and radiographic loosening are measures used consistently across the studies, the combination of which gives an overall mechanical failure rate. This universally reported outcome measure allows comparisons between different centres and techniques, and the literature review will be followed by an amalgamation of these findings into treatment recommendations based around a classification of bone defects encountered in revision arthroplasty.

Femoral revision

Cementless revision

Although both cemented and cementless implants have been used for revision THA by several centres across North America, contemporary surgical practice has resulted in the majority using cementless implants. High failure rates with cemented revision procedures initially led to increased use of cementless prostheses, with encouraging results.[12-14] The theoretical advantages of cementless prostheses include long-term stability via biological fixation, reconstitution of bone stock, and avoidance of the suboptimal fixation obtained using cement in a sclerotic or damaged cortical tube. The types of cementless stem used tend to fall into two main categories, depending on whether they rely on proximal or distal fit for stability. Specialized modular systems also exist, providing the surgeon with increased flexibility which may prove useful when performing cementless hip revision in certain scenarios, as discussed below.

Extensively porous-coated implants

Extensively porous-coated implants (Table 8.1) generally consist of a long cobalt-chrome stem which has a porous coating along its entire length. The most widely reported results are those of the Anatomic Medullary Locking (AML) stem[12-18] with a smaller subgroup reporting on results of the Solution stem.[16] Several designs are currently available (Fig. 8.1), with the philosophy essentially the same for all. That is, bony deficiencies present in the revision femur usually preclude good proximal fill, thus making a revision implant reliant on distal stability. These implants aim to bypass proximal bony deficiencies by obtaining an isthmic fit distal to the defects, utilizing a porous coating which allows for long-term biological fixation and stability (Fig. 8.2). Excellent long-term results of the AML stem are available in the primary arthroplasty,[19,20] and the same principles have been applied to the revision scenario.

The longest reported follow-up to date is that of Paprosky et al.[16] who reported on 170 patients at an average of 13.2 years postoperatively. The overall mechanical failure rate was 4.1 per cent, and failure was correlated to both canal fill and bony defects. Stable stems had a 92 per cent canal fill, and failure of fixation occurred more commonly with more severe defects, particularly those with less than 4 cm of diaphyseal isthmus. Paprosky and coworkers concluded that a minimum 4 cm of tight distal fit was required. Thigh pain, a frequently quoted concern in this type of prosthesis, was said to be significant in 9 per cent of patients. Stress shielding, another concern, was reported in association with these cases but was not considered to be a cause of subsequent problems. Glassman and Engh[15] reviewed 154 cases at an average of 9.2 years, 75 per cent of whom had significant metaphyseal bone loss, with a mechanical failure rate of 6.6 per cent. Other authors

Fig. 8.1

Extensively porous-coated stems. These straight stems have porous coating along their length, with a polished bullet-shaped tip. A range of stem lengths, diameters, and calcar-replacing options are available.

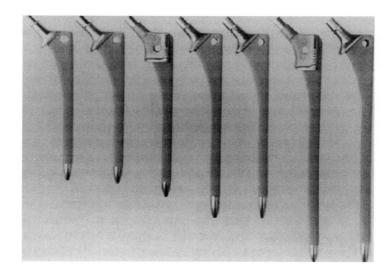

Table 8.1 Results of femoral revision with extensively porous-coated implants

	Stem type	No. of cases	Mean follow-up (years)	% revised (loosening)	Additional radiological loosening (%)	Defects and comments
Krishnamurthy et al.[12]	AML	297	8.3	1.6	0.7	Loosening correlated with < 75% canal fill and worst segmental defects
Lawrence et al.[13]	AML	160	7.4	3.5	3.4	Mild, 25% Moderate, 53% Severe, 22% Loosening correlated with defects
Glassman and Engh[15]	AML	154	9.2	3.3	3.3	Mild, 25% Moderate, 46% Severe, 29% Loosening correlated with defects
Paprosky et al.[16]	AML or Solution	170	13.2	3.5	0.6	Type I, 11% Type II, 30% Type III, 59% Stability correlated with canal fill and defects
Moreland and Bernstein[14]	AML	175	5	2.3	0.6	Stability correlated with canal fill and defects
Engh et al.[17]	AML	22	6.3	0	0	All cavitary defects
Lawrence et al.[18]	Mostly AML	83	9	8.4	1.2	No comment

Fig. 8.2

Femoral revision using an extensively
porous-coated stem. (a) Preoperative
radiograph shows a loose cemented stem
with significant bony deficiencies proximally.
(b) Revision using a long extensively
porous-coated stem to bypass the proximal
defects. This has been reinforced laterally
with a cortical strut allograft which was
incorporated after follow-up for 1 year.

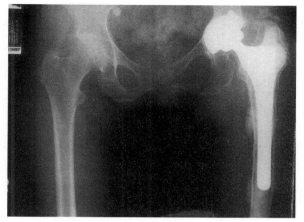

a

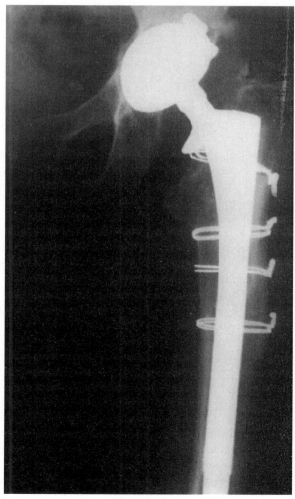

b

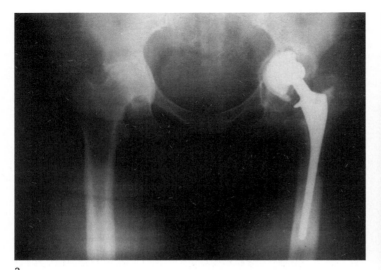

a

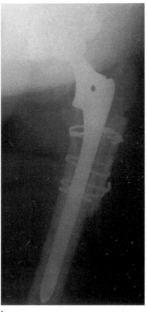

b

have reported similarly excellent results with average follow-up ranging from 5 to 8.3 years and overall mechanical failure ranging from zero to 5.7 per cent.[12,13,17,18,21]

The results of these stems have been excellent at long-term follow-up, but their insertion is not always uncomplicated. A significant incidence of fracture has been reported by several authors.[16,17,22] Egan and Di Cesare[22] reported specifically on complications associated with these stems, finding a combined incidence of complications of 44 per cent, with the likelihood correlated with stem length and diameter as well as with worsening bone quality. In their series of 135 cases, they reported eccentric reaming in 27 per cent, femoral perforation in 17 per cent, and femoral fracture in 20 per cent, all of which can signficantly add to the morbidity of the procedure. However, the incidence of complications decreased throughout the period of the study. This finding, coupled with the lower complication rate reported by other authors with extensive experience, suggests that these complications can certainly be kept to an acceptably low level.

More recent developments in surgical approach and prosthetic design are also likely to improve the outcome of this approach. Use of an extended trochanteric osteotomy can facilitate the removal of well-fixed prostheses and/or cement plugs whilst, with appropriate planning, still allowing for good distal fixation.[23] Newer design features such as distal slots, fluting, and bullet-shaped ends may allow a reduction in intra-operative complications such as fracture and perforation, and may also decrease the incidence of thigh pain in the long term (Fig. 8.3).

Therefore extensively porous-coated implants do seem to provide a revision option with the capacity to deal with most scenarios and

Fig. 8.3

Revision of both components. (a) Preoperative radiograph shows loose cemented components with migration of the acetabular component and a large segmental femoral defect laterally. (b) Revision using cementless acetabular component and extensively porous-coated femoral calcar-replacing femoral component with a lateral cortical strut allograft.

unequalled long-term results. It must be kept in mind, however, that the majority of the results cited above have come from two main specialist arthroplasty units, reflecting that these results are probably optimized in this setting and not necessarily transferable to the general orthopaedic community.

Proximally porous-coated implants

The use of proximally porous-coated implants in primary THA has been associated with good short- to intermediate-term results,[24] providing support for their ongoing use in this scenario. However, application of these stems to revision arthroplasty has not met with the same success. There is a large volume of literature reporting results with these prostheses (Table 8.2), but the follow-up at this stage remains intermediate term at best, with most reports covering 5 years or less. In one of the larger studies, Berry et al.[32] reported the Mayo Clinic experience with several designs at an average follow-up of 4.7 years, but with some of up to 9 years. For those patients with 8 year follow-up the survivorship free of revision for aseptic femoral failure was only 58 per cent, and surviving prostheses showed a radiological loosening of 41 per cent and subsidence greater than 5 mm in 42 per cent. Bone loss correlated with the likelihood of prosthetic loosening and subsidence, and they concluded that this prosthetic design should not be recommended in revision surgery.

Other authors have reported similarly disappointing results (Table 8.2). Peters et al.[28] reported results for the BIAS stem at an average follow-up of 5.5 years, with 4 per cent re-revision for loosening and 45 per cent incidence of progressive subsidence or definite loosening. They also found a correlation between proximal bone loss and subsidence, and concluded that this design was not appropriate for revision with moderate to severe bone loss. Mulliken et al.[29] reported results for the Mallory–Head stem at an average of 4.6 years, with 10 per cent re-revision and a further 14 per cent loose, again finding worse results with more extensive bone loss, particularly if the cavitary defects extended beyond the porous coat. Certainly it appears that prostheses designed to achieve proximal stability can be significantly compromised in this capacity in the presence of proximal bone defects, which are common in revision surgery. The proximal–distal mismatch commonly found in revision arthroplasty may be beyond the capacity of most proximally coated implants, which are more suited to the primary arthroplasty. A high incidence of intra-operative fracture (up to 45 per cent) has also been reported by several authors,[21,29,30,40] and higher subsequent failure rates have been reported for these cases in some series.[21]

However, there have been some reports of more favourable results with this type of prosthesis, albeit with quite short-term

Table 8.2 *Results of femoral revision with proximally porous-coated stems*

	Stem type	No. of cases	Mean follow-up (years)	% revised (loosening)	Additional radiological loosening (%)	Defects and comments
Head et al.[25]		174	3	3	0	Calcar replacement stem with strut allografts
Gustilo and Pasternak[26]	BIAS	57	2.8	7	1.8	All loose stems undersized
Buoncristiani et al.[27]	APR	66	4.7	4.5	0	Results not related to defects; better results with HA
Peters et al.[28]	BIAS	49	5.5	4	45	Subsidence correlated with bone defects
Mulliken et al.[29]	Mallory–Head	52	4.6	10	14	Type I, 29% Type II, 42% Type III, 25% Type IV, 4% Worst results in types III and IV and when cavitary defect beyond coating
Woolson and Delaney[30]	HG	25	5.5	16	45	Type I, 68% Type II, 28% Type III, 4% No bulk allografts No relation to failure
Bargar et al.[31]	Custom made	45	2.5	2.2	4.4	Cavitary, 30% Combined, 70%
Berry et al.[32]	Multiple stems	375	4.7	15.7	41	Mild, 16% Moderate, 58% Severe, 10% Correlated with loosening Significant failures with each stem

Malkani et al.[21]	Osteonics	69	3	7.5	20	Type I, 31% / Type II, 19% / Type III, 50% / Increased failure with intra-operative fractures
Hozack et al.[33]	Bi-metric Mallory–Head	59	2.6	0	0	Select group with focal osteolytic defects: 18% stabilize; 42% regress; 40% healed
Hussamy and Lachiewicz[34]	BIAS	41	5	0	4.9	Mild, 12% / Moderate, 19.5% / Severe, 68.5%
Meding et al.[35]	PCA Bi-metric	32	3.6	0	0	Pedestal in 53% (considered stable)
Hedley et al.[36]	PCA	42	1.7	2.4	7	No segmental allografts
Chandler et al.[37]	S-ROM*	52	3	3.8	5.8	44% required allografts 27% required PFA
Smith et al.[38]	S-ROM*	66	3.5	0	10	Type I, 7.5% / Type II, 24% / Type III, 67% / Type IV, 3% / Type V, 1.5% / Type VI, 1.5%
Cameron[39]	S-ROM*	91	3.8	0	2.6	29 primary and 62 revision (longer and curved) stems

*Stems with a proximal coat but relying on distal rather than proximal stability.

results. Head et al.[25] reported a re-revision rate of only 3 per cent at 3 years in 174 patients. A proximally coated titanium stem with strut allografts was used in this study, and the authors stressed the importance of the calcar replacement proximal load-bearing design to avoid proximal bone resorption. Buoncristiani et al.[27] reported 66 cases at an average of 4.7 years with a 3 per cent re-revision rate for stem loosening and no additional cases of radiographic loosening. Interestingly, they found no relation to bone defects and had improved results in prostheses with HA coating. Meding et al.[35] had no cases of loosening at 3.6 years using PCA and Bi-Metric stems. Bargar et al.[31] used a custom-made implant reported only 2 per cent re-revision at 2.5 years, but with significant subsidence (>3 mm) in 15 per cent. Hozack et al.[33] looked specifically at osteolytic defects after revision with Bi-metric or Mallory–Head stems and, finding no progression of defects and no re-revision, concluded that this technique was good for restoring bone stock. However, these results are very short term and thus cannot currently be used as the basis for recommending these implants for revision surgery.

Use of a modular prosthesis attempts to overcome the mismatch between metaphyseal defects and better preserved diaphysis distally. The most reported example of this is the S-ROM prosthesis,[37–39] with a wide range of proximal components allowing proximal fill in combination with distal fixation from a modular stem. Cameron[39] reported on 91 revision arthroplasties with 62 using revision S-ROM stems and 29 using primary stems at an average follow-up of 4 years and 3.5 years respectively. There was a 3.8 per cent incidence of radiographic loosening in the revision stems but none required re-revision, and no cases of loosening occurred with the primary stem. Thigh pain was only present in one patient, which is another potential advantage of a titanium stem compared with the stiffer extensively coated chrome-cobalt stems in which the incidence of significant thigh pain is reported to be 8–9 per cent.[14,16] Chandler et al.[37] found a 4 per cent incidence of thigh pain with the S-ROM, with stems greater than 17 mm having a positive correlation with thigh pain. Less favourable reports of S-ROM stems include a 12.4 per cent. mechanical failure at 5 years[38] and a 10 per cent loosening rate at 3 years.[37] However, these reports included a high percentage of patients with major bony defects.

The results reported with proximally coated stems cover a wide spectrum of outcomes from high to relatively low failure rates. This probably reflects, at least in part, the severity of bony defects in each series, as well as definitions of failure and the invariably short-term follow-up. Stems which were originally intended for primary arthroplasty seem to have a high risk of failure as they are designed to obtain proximal fit for stability, which is often not possible in the presence of significant defects (Fig. 8.2). Therefore obtaining distal stability is essential and is often beyond the standard proximally coated stems. Modular systems which allow independent matching of metaphysis and diaphysis can certainly overcome this problem and have had good early results. These stems have the theoretical advantages over extensively coated stems of decreased thigh pain and easier re-revision should this be necessary. Longer-term follow-up is essential before these stems can be recommended over the extensively porous-coated stems which have now been followed up for over 10 years.

Cemented revision

Cemented revision components (Table 8.3) have the theoretical advantages of immediate stability and the ability to deal with wide variations in femoral anatomy and defects. Long-stem femoral components have been developed specifically for cemented revision (Fig. 8.4). Mann *et al.*[61] tested cemented stems of different lengths *in vitro*, finding that a stem extending two femoral diameters beyond the area of a cancellous defect was most effective in minimizing stresses and motion that may be associated with subsequent loosening. However, in the revision scenario the endosteal surface is frequently smooth and sclerotic which greatly compromises the potential for cement interdigitation. Dohmae *et al.*[62] reported reduction of shear strength in revision to 20.6 per cent of a primary replacement and to 6.8 per cent after the second revision. Other potential problems include difficulties with cement pressurization in long-stem components and additional bone loss if such an implant loosens and requires re-revision.

The earlier studies of cemented femoral revision yielded generally disappointing results. Callaghan *et al.*[56] reported re-revision of 4.4 per cent and progressive radiolucencies in a further 25 per cent at only 3.6 years follow-up. Kavanagh *et al.*[54] had similarly disappointing results, with 4 per cent re-revision and 44 per cent of femurs probably loose at 4.5 years. Other early series had similar failure rates.[41,42,52,53] With time, cementing techniques became more refined, including the introduction of systematic canal preparation and cement pressurization. This led to an improvement in results but failure rates still remained relatively high, particularly as the follow-up became longer. Mulroy and Harris[46] reported on 35 hips using second-generation cementing techniques at an average of 15 years; overall loosening was 26 per cent. They also found a significantly higher failure rate in patients having their second or third revisions. Katz *et al.*[48] followed 42 hips with minimum 10 year follow-up, with 26 per cent loosening. Iorio *et al.*[63] found 99 per cent survivorship at 5 years but this dropped markedly to 77 per cent at 10 years, suggesting that short-term results may not be a reliable indicator of long-term prognosis. The best results of cemented femoral revision are those of Ash *et al.*[64] in revisions of cup arthroplasties, with overall loosening of 2 per cent

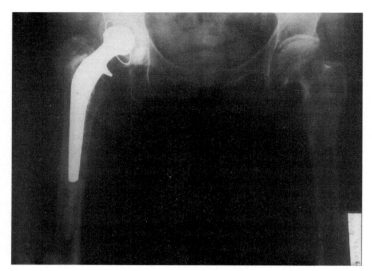

a

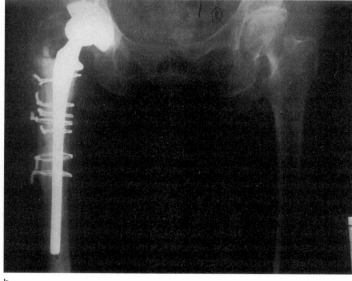

b

Fig. 8.4
Revision of both components.
(a) Preoperative radiograph
shows loose cemented femoral
and acetabular components.
(b) Revision using cementless
acetabular component and
cemented femoral component.
The femoral side has been
reinforced with cortical strut
allograft which is well
incorporated.

at minimum 10-year follow-up. In this scenario bone stock is effectively equivalent to a primary arthroplasty, and the improved results over other revision studies illustrate the importance of relatively good bone stock for the success of cemented stems.

Two separate studies[65,66] looked at the results of cement-within-cement revision, i.e. the femoral stems are recemented into intact cement mantles. The advantages of this technique include avoiding the need for cement removal with its associated morbidity and the preservation of a good-quality cement mantle which would be difficult to reproduce after removal of the original mantle and the

Table 8.3 Results of femoral revision with cemented implants

	Stem type	No. of cases	Mean follow-up (years)	% revised (loosening)	Additional radiological loosening (%)	Defects and comments
Rubash and Harris[41]	HD2 CR	43	6	2	9	Medial calcar defect, 39% Good bone stock, 61%
Turner et al.[42]		110	6.7	3	7	Long-stem component
Pierson and Harris[43]	Several long stems	29	8.5	6.9	3.4	Osteolysis: focal, 10%; multifocal, 41%; diffuse and focal, 45%; ectasia, 3%
Estok and Harris[44]	HD2 CR	38	11.7	10.5	10.5	Type I, 34% Type II, 47% Type III, 19% No correlation with result
Pierson and Harris[45]	Several stems	46	8.8	7	6	Type I, 35% Type II, 30% Type III, 35% Results related to mantle quality but not defects
Mulroy and Harris[46]	Several stems	35	15.1	16	10	Results not related to defects or mantle quality Poorer results in multiple revisions
McLaughlin and Harris[47]	CR stems	38	10.8	21	11	Type I, 58% Type II, 32% Type III, 8% Type IV, 2% Defects not related to result

193

Table 8.3 (Continued)

	Stem type	No. of cases	Mean follow-up (years)	% revised (loosening)	Additional radiological loosening (%)	Defects and comments
Katz et al.[48]	Mostly Iowa and Charnley stems	42	11.9	9.5	16.6	Results related to mantle quality but not defects
Ballard et al.[49]	Iowa stem	25	5	0	0	All patients were over 80 years old
Weber et al.[50]	Iowa stem	48	6.2	3	5	Type I, 15% Type II, 25% Results not related to defects or mantle quality 8-year survival, 81%
Iorio et al.[51]	Charnley	107	7.7	7.6	12	Type I, 1% Type II, 7% Type III, 1% Results not related to grafting 5-year survival, 99%; 10-year survival, 77%
Pellicci et al.[52]		99	8.1	18	6	Progressive lucency in further 12%; related to poor prognosis
Hoogland et al.[53]		32	3.2	8.3	4.2	
Kavanagh et al.[54]	Mostly Charnley	135	4.5	3.7	40.6	Loosening most likely in revisions for loosening

Kavanagh and Fitzgerald[55]	Mostly Charnley	45	3	6.7	18	All patients with multiple revisions; subgroup of series above
Callaghan et al.[56]		136	3.6	4.4	13	Further 26% with progressive lucencies / Related to defects and poor bone quality
Meding et al.[57]	CPT stem*	34	2.5	6		Allograft incorporated in 94% / 38% subsidence (average 10 mm) / Subsided stems stabilized / Only recommended if cementless stem not possible
Leopold et al.[58]	Harris CDH precoat*	25	5.2	4	4	Type I, 7% / Type II, 62% / Type III, 28% / Type IV, 3% / Only recommended if cementless stem not possible
Capello[59]	CR stem*	172 (minimum)		0	0	
Elting et al.[60]	CPT stem*	56	2.6	0	2	Type I, 13% / Type II, 43% / Type III, 31% / 48% subsidence (average 2.8 mm)

*Impaction grafting.

adjacent cancellous bone. Both studies had a follow-up of 5 years with no re-revisions for loosening and radiographic loosening of zero and 5 per cent. This technique requires an intact mantle with no cracks beyond the proximal 2 cm and should be used with smooth stems. Greenwald et al.[67] demonstrated that it was important for the cement to be dry and rasped, and that this technique involved only a 6 per cent reduction in shear strength. Although this may seem an attractive alternative to more conventional techniques, longer-term clinical follow-up is necessary before this can be generally recommended.

A technique that has gained more popularity in the United Kingdom than in North America is the use of impaction allografting with cemented stems (Fig. 8.5). This technique has been popularized by Gie et al.[68] for cavitary defects and good results have been reported. The theoretical basis for the technique is very attractive, in that the sclerotic interface is replaced by a cancellous one that is more amenable to cement fixation and restoration in bone stock is possible, which is particularly useful in younger patients. Malkani et al.[69] performed an in vitro study using cadaver femora, comparing impaction grafting with the primary cementing technique, and found mean subsidences of less than 1 mm in both groups and no difference in the mean torque to failure. In another in vitro study,[70] it was found that using an extended osteotomy did not adversely affect the initial mechanical stability of the implant. Other studies[71,72] have demonstrated stable initial fixation and subsequent good graft incorporation histologically.

Clinical studies have all been relatively short term with follow-up ranging from 2 to 5 years and with variable results. Meding et al.[57] found 38 per cent subsidence averaging 10 mm but only 6 per cent re-revision at 2.5 years. Leopold et al.[58] found 92 per cent survival at 6 years. Both of these groups recommended this technique only for extensive bone loss which would preclude a long-stem cementless component. Eldridge et al.[73] also reported 11 per cent massive early subsidence, with a further 11 per cent of patients having lesser degrees of subsidence. However, Elting et al.[60] reported no re-revisions for loosening at 31 months and found that subsidence was not associated with poor results. There is a significant incidence of fracture with this technique[57,58] which can be associated with subsequent failure. Impaction grafting may prove to be a very useful technique for specific scenarios, but at this stage longer follow-up is necessary before it can be recommended over other techniques such as cementless stems.

Revision for periprosthetic fracture

There have been few studies looking specifically at the results of revision for periprosthetic fracture, although the presentation of a

Fig. 8.5

Femoral impaction allografting. (a) Preoperative radiograph showing a loose cemented bipolar prosthesis secondary to infection. (b) First-stage revision using an antibiotic-impregnated cement spacer; note the capacious femoral canal with no residual isthmus available, making cementless distal fixation impossible.

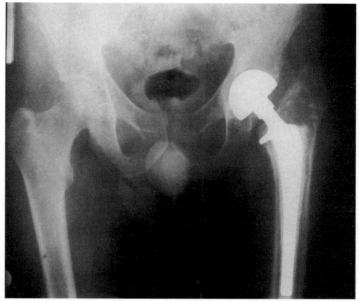

a

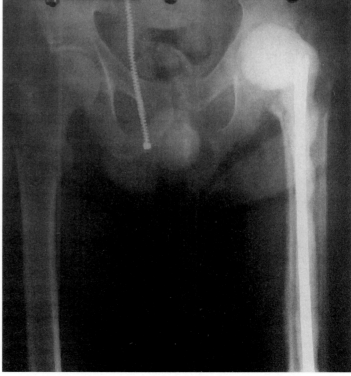

b

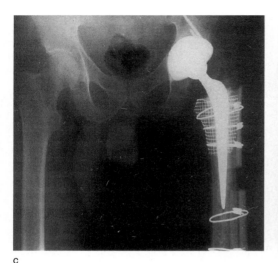
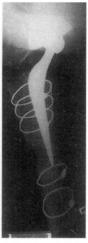

c

Fig. 8.5
(c) Second-stage revision using femoral impaction allografting reinforced with cortical strut allografts.

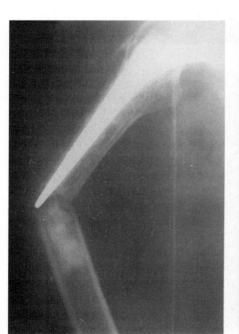
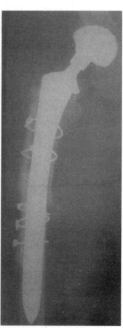

Fig. 8.6
Revision for periprosthetic fracture. Fracture has occurred around the tip of a cemented stem and has been revised with a large extensively porous-coated stem reinforced with cortical strut allograft.

patient with a fracture through an osteolytic defect is not uncommon (Fig. 8.6). The topic of this chapter limits this discussion to those fractures which necessitate revision, notably those which are associated with an unstable implant with or without significant bone defects. Incavo *et al.*[74] reported on 14 cases of fracture through osteolytic defects, 12 of which were managed with various types of long-stem cementless prostheses; the other two were managed with proximal femoral allografts (PFAs). Strut allografts were used in 50 per cent of the prostheses. Ninety-two per cent of fractures healed and although there was an overall failure rate of 36 per cent, no loosening occurred in stems with distal porous coating. The resultant preferred option was for distal fixation, usually with an extensively porous-coated stem, in combination with wires and possibly strut allografts. If distal fixation was compromised then a PFA was recommended.

In a smaller study, Moran[75] used extensively porous-coated stems to manage fractures through osteolytic defects in four patients. All fractures healed and all stems were stable at 2.7 years, lending support to the above recommendations. Although there is minimal literature specifically on this topic, it is reasonable to extrapolate the findings of the previous discussions on the various options for femoral revision to this scenario, coupled with appropriate stabilization of the fracture and allograft supplementation of bone defects if necessary.

Revision in significant bone-stock loss

The availability of allograft material has enhanced the orthopaedic surgeon's capacity to deal with the bone defects encountered in revision hip arthroplasty, The allografts can generally be divided into morsellized bone, which is generally used to fill cavitary defects, and structural graft, which is used either to support or to replace completely areas of segmental or combined defects. Structural allografts for the femur include cortical struts, which are usually used to add strength to segmental or large cavitary or combined defects, and PFAs, which are used to replace the proximal femur when the defects are so severe as to preclude the residual femur supporting any type of implant.

Strut allografts

Cortical strut allografts are now widely employed to supplement the structurally deficient femur in revision surgery (Figs 8.2, 8.3, 8.5, and 8.7). This can add to the strength of the initial construct as well as counteracting the proximal stress shielding that can occur when implants relying on distal fixation are used. The results of these allografts, in terms of union and incorporation (Fig. 8.2), are nearly universally favourable across the literature.[76-78] Head and Malinin[77] reported on the use of freeze-dried strut allografts in 251 revision cases associated with cavitary and segmental defects. They used these struts in combination with cementless proximal-load-bearing implants, and achieved a union rate of 100 per cent and subsequent complete incorporation. They suggested that freeze-drying was the appropriate treatment for these grafts as it allowed preservation of bone morphogenic protein.

Pak et al.[78] used cortical struts in 95 cases of revision with an extensively porous-coated stem and obtained a union rate of 93 per cent. The 7 per cent of grafts that did not unite and resorbed were

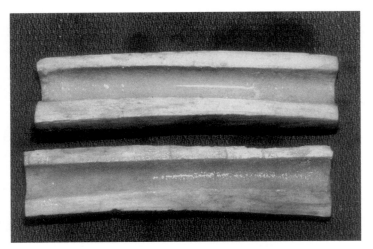

a

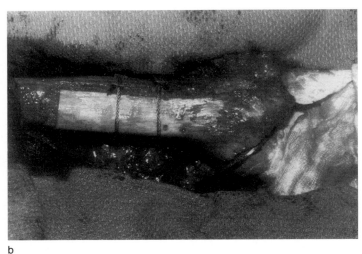

b

Fig. 8.7
Cortical strut allografts.
(a) Segments of frozen strut allografts ready for use.
(b) Implanted strut secured with cables.

all associated with undersized stems, leading to the conclusion that femoral implant stability is important for graft incorporation. Therefore Pak *et al.* recommended the use of an extensively porous-coated stem for this purpose. In the same study they looked at the results of 18 calcar grafts, which were less successful, with 61 per cent resorption thought to be associated with inhibition of proper loading of the graft by distal fixation. Allan *et al.*[79] also had poor results with short-segment calcar grafts, leading them to abandon their use, whilst their results with struts were excellent with 100 per cent union and no structural failures. The use of cortical strut allografts certainly appears to be a reliably good form of structural supplementation for the markedly deficient proximal femur, providing long-term restoration of proximal bone stock and possibly making up for the stress shielding often seen with implants relying on distal stability.

Proximal femoral allografts

Circumferential defects of the proximal femur can be a technically difficult problem to manage with standard revision prostheses. Defects of up to 3 cm can usually be dealt with using calcar replacement prostheses, but defects larger than this require custom implants such as tumour prostheses or the use of PFAs. Potential advantages of this technique include restoration of bone stock with a normal gradation of forces from implant to bone, early weight-bearing, a good interface for cementing, and the possibility of further revisions if necessary.[7,80] Potential disadvantages are inherent in the use of allograft bone. The risk of disease transmission is present, but this is minimized if American Association of Tissue Banks guidelines are followed, reducing risk of HIV to less than one in a million.[81] Allograft bone is also not as biologically active as autograft, with increased risk of non-union, but this can be decreased by using autograft at host–allograft junctions and achieving rigid fixation. Resorption of allografts can also occur and can lead to implant failure.[7]

Reports of PFA use have come mainly from specialist centres which perform this technique more frequently, suggesting that it is probably best reserved for these centres if results are to be optimized. Gross et al.[82] reported on 168 cases at 5-year follow-up, all of which had circumferential bone loss in excess of 3 cm. Purpose-designed long-stem femoral components were used. These implants were cemented into the allograft bone and then press-fitted distally into host bone. There was a 10 per cent re-revision rate, and only 4 per cent non-union and 4 per cent graft resorption. Overall success in 130 grafts with minimum 2-year follow-up was 85 per cent. In another large series, Head et al.[83] reported on 164 cases, also with an 85 per cent success rate. Haddad et al.[84] reported on 55 cases, with a longer follow-up of 9 years; the overall re-revision rate was 11 per cent, for infection, allograft fracture, or non-union. They found a high incidence of trochanteric non-union which was related to subsequent instability. Significant resorption occurred in 20 per cent of cases, all of which used cement into the host bone and discarded the residual proximal femur, but this did not lead to structural failure in any case. The subsequent recommendations were to avoid cement distally, to preserve any residual proximal femur, and to use extended rather than conventional trochanteric osteotomy. Barrack et al.[85] have described the use of a distal femoral allograft in cases where the diameter of the distal canal exceeds that of any available PFA (Fig. 8.8). The size of the distal femoral allograft is chosen to allow for an adequate cement mantle, and again the preference is to press-fit the stem distally, with cementing reserved for elderly patients with limited longevity

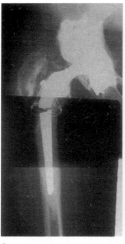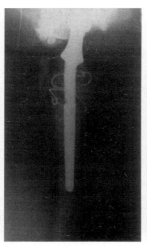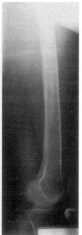

a

Fig. 8.8
Revision using distal femoral
allograft. (a) Preoperative
radiograph shows a fracture
cemented stem, trochanteric
non-union, and a large
combined proximal bony
femoral defect. (b) The frozen
distal femoral segment prior to
preparation.

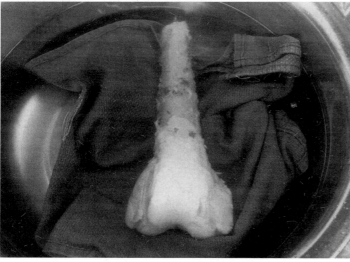

b

only. Although only a relatively short-term follow-up of 4 years is
reported for only nine patients, the results thus far have been pleas-
ing, with all graft–host junctions uniting and no components
revised.

Use of a proximal or distal femoral allograft to reconstruct the
severely deficient proximal femur certainly has a number of theoretical advantages as listed above. The results from major centres performing this procedure lend strong support to this technique, which
when performed by experienced surgeons for appropriate indications can provide a predictably good result for a difficult problem
with the added advantage of long-term restoration of bone stock.

Fig. 8.8

(c) A proximal 5-cm segment has been fashioned and the prosthesis cemented within this; note the 7–8 cm of porous coating distally to achieve fixation distal to the allograft. (d) Postoperative radiograph with trochanter rewired.

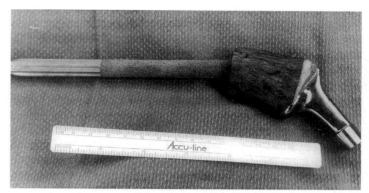

c

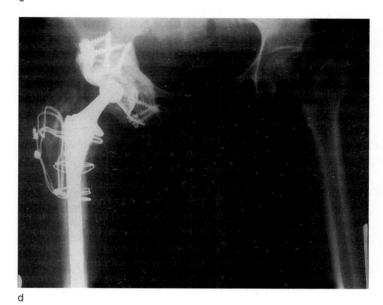

d

Acetabular revision

Follow-up studies on acetabular components in primary THA are now sufficiently long term to demonstrate an improved survival rate of cementless implants over their cemented counterparts. Hence these are the implants currently favoured by most surgeons in North America for primary arthroplasty. Likewise, in revision surgery cemented implants have had largely poor results (Table 8.4) and cementless implants are generally favoured as long as sufficient acetabular bone is present to support the implant in a similar manner to primary arthroplasty. Wide variations in acetabular defects dictate a need for a correspondingly wide variety of surgical techniques and implants, as the following review of the literature will demonstrate.

Cementless revision

POROUS-COATED CUPS

The most widely reported revision acetabular component in the literature is the Harris–Galante (HG) cup, which is used in combination with screw fixation. This is a porous-coated multi-hole cup, the original version of which has been superseded by a new implant with a larger screw diameter and more screw holes, as well as a thicker shell and more tines for liner fixation (27).[86] Other reported cups are similar hemispheric porous-coated designs with multiple screw holes. All are available in larger diameters, the so called 'jumbo cups', to obtain a satisfactory rim fit in the relatively larger cavities remaining after removal of primary components. In a study of 109 cases at an average follow-up of 10.5 years, Leopold et al.[87] reported no cases of re-revision for loosening and only 2 per cent were loose radiographically. They found a partial non-progressive radiolucency in 52 per cent of cups and questioned the prognostic significance of this finding. However, they did find a 10 per cent incidence of osteolysis greater than 2 cm and a 3 per cent incidence of screw osteolysis. Dorr and Wan[88] reported on 139 cases at an average of 4.3 years, with only 14 per cent re-revision for loosening and a 20 per cent incidence of radiolucent lines in components judged to be stable.

Other authors have had similarly good results (Table 8.5), with several reporting no re-revisions at follow-up of 4 to 10.5 years and others all reporting rates of less than 10 per cent for follow-up of up to 10 years (Fig. 8.9). Additional patients with radiographic loosening are generally no more than a further 3 per cent. Worse results do tend to occur in those patients with more severe defects, as shown by Woolson and Adamson[91] who reported a re-revision rate of 9.4 per cent at 6 years in patients with type III or type IV defects. Most authors stress the need for a good rim fit, morsellized allograft to fill cavitary defects, and screws to supplement initial fixation. It is hoped that more modern implants, with features such as improved locking mechanisms and increased polyethylene thickness, will result in further improvements in the results obtained for cementless cups in revision THA.

Threaded cups

Little literature is available on the use of threaded cups in revision THA in North America. More et al.[99] reported a re-revision rate of 44 per cent for loosening in 29 hips at 2.5 years, with a further 24 per cent loose on radiographs. Approximately half of these patients were said to have severe bone-stock deficiency. Engh et al.[95] also had a high failure rate using threaded cups, with an overall mechanical failure rate of 41 per cent at 4.4 years. Other authors have had similarly disappointing results.[100] Whilst there is not a large volume of literature on this type of cup, the results are

Table 8.4 Results of acetabular revision with cemented implants

	No. of cases	Mean follow-up (years)	% revised (loosening)	Additional radiological loosening (%)	Defects and comments
Weber et al.[50]	56	6.5	9	21	Type I, 27% Type II, 15% Type III, 4% 8-year survival, 36%
Callaghan et al.[56]	76	3.6	0	9	Additional 35% with progressive lucencies Related to bone quality
Katz et al.[48]	40	11.9	27.5	37.5	Not recommended No relation to defects
Kavanagh et al.[54]	81	4.5	3.7	20.1	Worst results in revisions for cup loosening
Iorio et al.[63]	85	7.7	3.8	13	Type I, 3% Type II, 20% Type III, 6% 5-year survival, 95%; 10-year survival, 74% Not related to bone grafting
Kavanagh and Fitzgerald[55]	45	3	6.7	18	Patients with multiple revisions
Pellicci et al.[52]	99	8.1	7	8	Progressive lucencies related to poor prognosis

Table 8.5 Results of acetabular revision with cementless implants

	Cup type	No. of cases	Mean follow-up (years)	% revised (loosening)	Additional radiological loosening (%)	Defects and comments
Lawrence et al.[18]	Depuy porous	43	9	4.6	4.6	9% bulk allograft; 35% screws Bulk allograft use not related to failure
Chareancholvanich et al.[89]	HG	40	8	5	0	Type I, 15% Type II, 75% Type III, 7.5%
Dorr and Wan[88]	APR	139	4.3	1.4	0	Type I, 9% Type II, 67% Type III, 23% Type IV, 1% 20% radiolucent lines but judged stable
Silverton et al.[90]	HG	115	8.2	0	2	Type I, 9% Type II, 73% Type III, 8% Type IV, 2%
Leopold et al.[87]	HG	109	10.5	0	1.8	Screw osteolysis, 3% Thin radiolucent lines not significant
Woolson and Adamson[91]	HG	32	5.8	9.4	3	Type III, 97% Type IV, 3%
Lachiewicz and Poon[92]	HG	57	7	0	0	Type I, 12% Type II, 40% Type III, 37% 19% bulk allograft—all healed
Dearborn and Harris[86]	HG	46	10.4	2.2	3.8	High hip centre used in all with no problem

the high hip centre contributed to these poor results, it appears that most surgeons prefer a more anatomical reconstruction of the hip centre if possible.

Bilobed/eccentric cups

The use of eccentric cups is another technique for managing large superior segmental defects. The superior half of an oblong cup rather than structural allograft is used to fill the defect. There have been relatively few reports of the use of this design in revision arthroplasty.[96,97,103] The indications have generally been large superior segmental defects, with the cited advantage being restoration of the hip centre without the need for structural grafts. However, the corollary to this is that bone stock is not restored, which may prove significant if further surgery becomes necessary.

Chen et al.[96] reported 37 cases using a bilobed component in cases in which a standard hemispherical component would have contacted less than 50 per cent of the host bone. At an average of 3.4 years there was a 60 per cent re-revision rate and another 18 per cent were unstable, with all loosening in defects with superior migration of more than 2 cm. Chen et al. concluded that this cup is contraindicated in superior migration of greater than 2 cm in combination with a medial wall defect, but could be recommended for mild to moderate superior bone loss, or for severe superior loss in combination with an intact medial wall. Berry et al.[97] reported 38 cases, also with a bilobed component used for mostly large superior lateral segmental defects. At 3 years one patient whose cup was supported by more than 50 per cent allograft required re-revision but all other cups were reported stable, giving an overall success rate of 97 per cent. They concluded that a bilobed cup was appropriate for large superolateral segmental deficiencies but cautioned that the procedure was technically difficult. Bilobed cups offer an alternative option for cases with superolateral defects, but the literature currently available is only short term and comes from a small number of large specialist centres. Therefore at present it is difficult to endorse their widespread use outside these specialist centres.

Allograft reconstruction

As with PFAs, a large proportion of this work has been performed in a small number of specialist centres. Although early results for structural allografts revealed high failure rates,[104-106] later reports have shown improved outcomes as indications for different techniques become clearer (Fig. 8.11). Gross and coworkers have reported extensively on the use of allograft in acetabular revision.[107-110] In their study,[110] the type of reconstruction used was dictated by whether defects were contained or uncontained, and whether more or less than 50 per cent of the acetabulum was involved. Morsellized graft was used for contained defects, in combination with a cementless cup if more than 50 per cent host

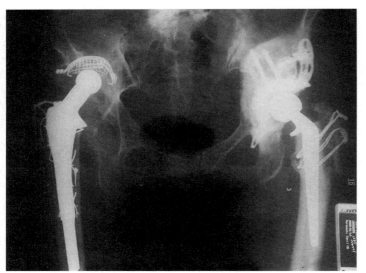

a

Fig. 8.11
Acetabular revision using structural allograft.
(a) Preoperative radiograph shows loose components with a large proximal acetabular defect, but intact posterior column. (b) Postoperative radiograph shows revision of both components. The acetabulum has been revised using a structural allograft fashioned from a femoral head and secured with screws to fill the proximal defect in combination with a reinforcement ring with cemented acetabular component.

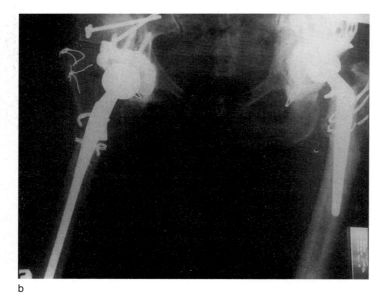

b

support was present or with a reinforcement ring and cemented cup if less support was present. If all quadrants were involved, a reconstruction ring was used.

The success rates at 6.8 years were 92 per cent for cementless cups and 100 per cent for reinforcement rings. Shelf allograft with either cementless or cemented cups was used in uncontained defects with more than 50 per cent host support, whereas those with less than 50 per cent support were managed with acetabular allografts, reconstruction rings, and cemented cups. At 7.1 years the shelf allografts had a success rate of 86 per cent, but the major allografts were less successful at 55 per cent. Failure of these major allografts only occurred when the cup was inserted directly into the allograft, supporting the use of a reconstruction ring in these cases. Even in the cases of graft union but cup failure there has been a successful restoration of bone stock, making further revisions potentially less demanding.

Paprosky and Magnus[111] looked at the results of revision in defects with more than 2 cm superior migration. Those in which Kohler's line was intact were managed with either femoral heads or distal femur allograft in combination with an cementless cup, with only 7 per cent failure at 5 years, all of which had used femoral heads rather than distal femur to fill the segmental defect. Those in which Kohler's line was not intact were managed with proximal femur or whole acetabular allograft, in combination with cementless cups or cemented cups respectively. These had a higher failure rate of 29 per cent, all in patients with more than 60 per cent contact of porous cups with allograft. Several studies have supported the finding of an increased failure rate when cementless cups are supported by less than 50 per cent of host bone,[105,112,113] and this has become a frequently quoted limit for the use of cementless cups. Chandler[112] stressed that structural grafts should be of good quality, fit the defects accurately, and have trabeculae and fixation oriented in line with weight-bearing forces. Heekin et al.[114] in a retrieval analysis on morsellized allograft from three patients, showed that graft incorporation took several years and was not accurately predicted by radiographs. Structural grafts have rates of union varying from 94–97 per cent[6,115] for minor allografts to 75 per cent for massive allografts.[6,116]

The use of rings and cages has generally met with favourable results.[110,117] Metal rings are fixed to the pelvis, usually over bone graft, with multiple screws and provide a stable interface into which a cup can be cemented. Reinforcement rings (Fig. 8.11) can be used for cavitary defects and less severe segmental defects in which proximal screw fixation of the ring provides a stable construct. Reconstruction rings (Fig. 8.12) allow for both proximal fixation in the ilium and distal fixation at the level of the ischium, which are necessary when there are extensive unstable deficiencies such as a pelvic discontinuity. Schatzker and Wong[117] reported on 95 revisions with these devices in association with bone grafting, with 12.5 per cent failure of reinforcement rings at 8.3 years and 54 per cent failure of reconstruction rings at 6.6 years. There was consistent graft incorporation and the failures of reinforcement rings were thought to be related to their use in patients with medial deficiencies in whom reconstruction rings would have been preferable. They listed the advantages of this technique as restoration of hip centre and bone stock, a large contact area between the implant and host bone, and protection of graft during incorporation. Certainly,

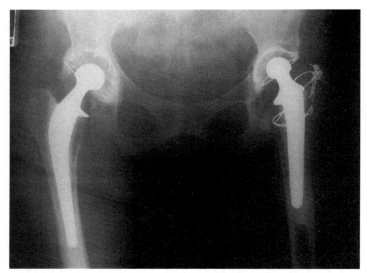

a

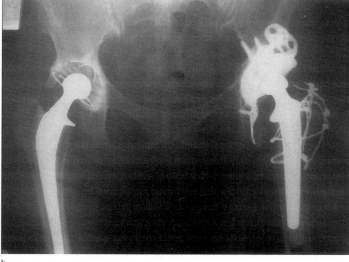

b

Fig. 8.12
Acetabular revision using
a reconstruction ring.
(a) Preoperative radiograph
shows a loose cemented
component with possible
pelvic discontinuity.
(b) Postoperative radiograph
shows revision using a
reconstruction ring. Multiple
screws are used superiorly and
the inferior flange is secured
into the ischium.

rings provide a method for achieving a stable implant in the face of severe bone loss, with generally good results.

Berry *et al.*[118] reported on the Mayo Clinic experience in the management of pelvic discontinuity in 31 hips at an average of 3 years. Best results were achieved in patients without severe segmental bone loss, and the worst results occurred if severe segmental or combined loss was present or in patients with previous irradiation. Reconstruction rings achieved 85 per cent success, whereas cups placed against structural graft failed. Berry *et al.* recommended a systematic approach involving stabilization and bone

Fig. 8.12

(c) Intra-operative picture shows placement of the ring with screws through the superior flange into the ilium and cemented component *in situ*.

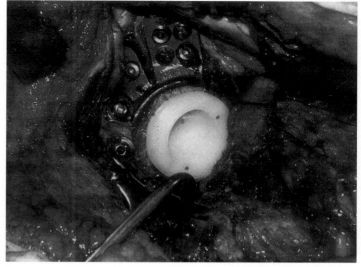

c

grafting of the discontinuity, treatment of bony defects, and placement of a stable cup. Plate stabilization and cementless implants are advised in patients with good bone stock, whereas the preferred option in patients with less than 50 per cent host bone support or previous irradiation is a reconstruction ring with a cemented cup.

Bipolar prostheses

Bipolar prostheses provide an alternative to acetabular reconstruction, but they have not achieved consistently good results and are rarely used today. In a study of 101 hips, Murray[119] used bipolar prostheses for acetabular salvage in association with allograft. At a mean follow-up of 3 years there was a 12 per cent incidence of re-revision for migration, subluxation, or dislocation of the bipolar implant, and the average superior migration was 2.4 mm. Murray concluded that this remained a viable option in selected cases, but warned of limited function and the need for permanent external support. Roberson and Cohen[120] used bipolar implants in 27 patients either for recurrent dislocation or when stable cementless fixation was not possible. At 2–6 years there was only one re-revision, for dislocation, but 26 per cent of patients had moderate or severe pain.

Cameron and Jung[121] compared the use of bipolar implants in cavitary and segmental defects, finding worse results with segmental defects but claiming excellent results with cavitary defects. However, follow-up was short term and the number of cases was quite small. In the study by Garbuz *et al.*[116] of massive column allografts supporting more than 50 per cent of the cup, results with bipolar prostheses were worse than those with reinforcement rings and with cementless cups. Bipolar implants certainly seem to have

215

a limited role in revision surgery today, especially when options with more stable and durable constructs are available to deal with all types of acetabular defects.

Isolated femoral or acetabular revision

It is not uncommon to encounter cases in which one component is clearly unstable and requires revision, whereas the other appears radiologically stable (Figs 8.2, 8.9, and 8.12). There is certainly a greatly reduced morbidity when revising one component than when revising both, but does this compromise the long-term outcome of the procedure? More commonly, acetabular components have loosened in the presence of stable femoral components, and a number of studies[93,94,122] have reported the results of isolated acetabular revision in this circumstance. Peters et al.[122] looked at 37 hips at an average of 5.5 years with an overall failure of 22 per cent. There was no difference in the time from the primary surgery in loose stems compared with stable stems, but stems that failed had a greater tendency towards varus alignment. Peters et al. recommended leaving well-fixed stems in situ, as did authors of two similar but separate studies[93,94] with stem loosening of 3 per cent and 5 per cent at 5 years and 4 years respectively.

In a study of 26 patients with isolated femoral revision in the presence of stable cemented acetabular components, Berger et al.[123] found only 77 per cent cup revision at an average of 8.4 years, with an additional 7.7 per cent loose radiographically. No cup with an acceptable cement mantle loosened, and loose cups tended to have been implanted for a shorter period of time than those which remained stable. They recommended retention of stable cemented cups as long as the position, orientation, cement mantle, and wear were acceptable.

Cost analysis

Cost analysis is not a commonly cited criterion when choosing implants for surgery, but it is currently a very topical issue that can have a significant influence on these decisions. Several studies have looked at this issue, comparing primary with revision surgery[51,124,125] and examining changes in the costs of revision surgery over the last decade.[126] Iorio et al.[51] found that, whilst primary THA made a net profit for the hospital, revision surgery resulted in a net loss and they concluded that, despite cost-containment measures, revision THA was not a profitable procedure.

Lavernia et al.[125] compared costs of primary and revision hip and knee arthroplasty, and found that revision THA had the highest costs, not comparable to the other procedures. They concluded that revision THA could be a financial liability to the hospital and thus open to limitation by administrators. They also found that prosthetic costs made up 45 per cent of the total billed costs, indicating that this may need consideration when choosing implants. Barrack and coworkers[126,127] also analysed costs of primary and revision surgery, finding that the reimbursement schedule offered a disincentive to both surgeon and hospital to support revision surgery. Although not the main focus of this chapter, these findings need to be considered when making decisions such as implant choice if revision THA is to be a viable procedure for hospitals and surgeons to undertake in the future.

Recommendations for implant selection

The above literature review gives an overall impression of the North American experience with the use of the many available surgical techniques and implants available for revision THA, and of the success of each in the various scenarios encountered. Therefore it can be used as a guide to the formulation of an algorithm to provide recommendations for implant selection for each scenario. As the bone defects present in each case tend to be the main determinant of which implant and which technique are the most appropriate, a classification system of these defects can be used as the basis for this algorithm. Many classification systems have been described, but perhaps the most widely used one currently in North America is that of the AAOS.

The AAOS classification system for acetabular defects was described by D'Antonio et al.[4] in 1989 and was an attempt to provide a standard nomenclature which could be used as a guide to management. They described radiographic determination of bone defects, but advised that ultimate determination occurred intraoperatively. The two main categories are segmental (type I) and cavitary (type II), with the former being any complete loss of bone in the supporting hemisphere including the medial wall, and the latter being contained volumetric bone loss with an intact rim. Both are also divided into peripheral and central subgroups. Further categories are combined cavitary and segmental (type III), discontinuity (type IV), and arthrodesis (type V), with the last category not being a true defect but more representational of a significant degree of technical difficulty.

The femoral classification system[5] was described in 1993 and is based on similar categories. Segmental defects (type I) refer to cortical loss and are divided into partial, intercalary, and proximal (greater trochanter). Cavitary defects (type II) represent a contained excavated lesion with an intact outer cortical shell, and are divided into cancellous, cortical, and ectasia. Combined defects (type III) are a combination of types I and II, and a further three categories exist for malalignment (type IV), stenosis (type V), and discontinuity (type VI), which refers to a fracture with or without an implant present. All categories are further subdivided by level and location. The many possible permutations are beyond the scope of this chapter, but the main categories allow construction of a framework for management.

Femoral implant selection

The literature review above demonstrated clearly superior long-term survival for extensively porous-coated implants over all other options for most revision scenarios, making this often the implant of choice. Bony deficiencies and other factors such as patient age and functional demand play a major role in implant choice. Defects are largely proximal, necessitating distal fixation. This is well illustrated by the poor results obtained with implants relying on proximal fit for stability, making it difficult to recommend these implants for any revision scenario with bone-stock loss. Cementless implants relying on distal stability are usually preferable in younger patients with good bone stock, whereas elderly patients often have grossly ectatic femora, making distal cementless fixation impossible and cemented fixation preferable. Use of a cementless implant requires a minimum of 4–6 cm of endosteal contact distal to bony defects to achieve stability, and the ability to attain this determines whether or not this type of implant can be used.

Type I (segmental) defects encompass a wide range of patterns of bone-stock loss. If good cortical contact can be achieved distal to bony defects, an extensively coated stem should be used together with strut allografting proximally. Calcar replacement prostheses may be required if the segmental loss results in significant shortening, and this should be predicted with preoperative templating. If there is extensive segmental loss beyond the capacity for replacement with a calcar replacement component (>3 cm), use of a PFA may need to be considered. This seems to have best results when purpose-designed long-stem components are cemented to the allograft but not to the host femur. Other desirable technical points include preservation of residual proximal femur, use of an extended trochanteric osteotomy with secure fixation, and strut allografting of the host allograft junction. This should be reserved for specialist centres who are most familiar with the technique. Use of long-stem cemented stems together with strut allograft reinforcement of the proximal femur should be considered if poor distal bone quality precludes good distal fixation, or if a PFA is not technically possible at the treating centre.

Type II defects can be managed using the same principles. If good fixation is possible distal to the cavitary defect, an extensively coated stem is recommended. If the cavitary defects are corticocancellous or involve a degree of femoral ectasia, the best recommendation is probably impaction grafting. This is recommended with some reservation, however, as the results are rather short term and would not be preferred over the extensively coated stem if this latter option was possible. The other option that can be considered is a modular stem which has proximal coating but allows for distal stability, such as the S-ROM component. This has the theoretical advantages over extensively coated stems of lower incidence of stress shielding and thigh pain, but long-term follow-up is required before this can be strongly recommended. Use of all options should be combined with strut grafting if there is a thin cortical tube with compromise of structural integrity.

Type III defects are again managed similarly, and if good distal fit is possible, an extensively coated stem is preferred. Strut allografting of proximal defects should be included, and large segmental loss may require the use of a PFA. Type IV and V defects largely relate to technical aspects of the revision surgery rather than implant selection specifically. The type VI defect essentially refers to a periprosthetic fracture. This is best managed with an extensively coated stem achieving fixation distal to the fracture, which should be reinforced with strut allografts and cerclage wires. Again, if the femoral anatomy precludes distal fixation, the cortical tube should be reconstituted, with the help of strut allograft if necessary, and a long-stem femoral component should then be cemented into the tube.

Acetabular implant selection

From the above literature review it is clear that cementless porous-coated hemispherical cups with supplementary screw fixation have achieved the best long-term results given the appropriate setting. The requirements for good results with this implant have been satisfactory rim contact and greater than 50 per cent of the support for the cup coming from host bone. If these criteria are not met, a different construct is necessary to improve the stability. Reinforcement rings with cemented cups have produced good results when dealing with defects too extensive to support a cementless implant, and reconstruction rings are necessary if a discontinuity is present in association with significant defects. Threaded components certainly have no role, and there is no clear indication of where bipolar implants would be the best option.

Management of type I (segmental) defects depends largely on their size and location. Most of the reports of successful cementless implants include a significant number of type I defects. Requirements for these implants include a satisfactory rim fit and greater than 50 per cent host contact. If greater than 50 per cent host support is present, the defect can be filled with a structural allograft, allowing use of a cementless implant with screws. Defects involving more than 50 per cent of the acetabulum should be grafted, taking care to achieve the appropriate biomechanical alignment of the graft and fixation. A reinforcement ring can then be secured to host bone and allograft and a cup cemented into the ring. Major segmental defects involving all quadrants require the use of large structural allografts such as whole acetabulae or distal femora, together with a reconstruction ring and cemented cup. Large medial segmental defects should also be managed with a reconstruction ring. This technique obviously requires expertise and is probably best done at specialist centres to optimize chances of success.

Type II (cavitary) defects can generally be filled with morsellized graft, after which a cementless cup can be implanted as there is usually good stability from an intact rim. This contained defect is the most common defect reported in series of successful cementless cups, suggesting that it can usually be managed with this technique. If the defects are so extensive that allograft bone is supporting more than 50 per cent of the cup, then, although good stability is achieved from the rim, the potential for good ingrowth from a mostly avascular surface is minimal and possibly compromises long-term stability. In this scenario it may be preferable to graft the defects and then use a reinforcement ring with a cemented cup.

Type III defects combine cavitary and segmental deficiencies and essentially follow the same general guidelines as outlined above for the separate defects. Type IV defects also follow the same principles but require stabilization of the discontinuity as a primary concern. If there is no major bone defect, the discontinuity can be plated and grafted and a cementless cup implanted, but if there is significant bone-stock loss, reducing host support to less than 50 per cent, a reconstruction ring and cemented cup should be used after grafting. Most of the large series of cementless cups have only small numbers of type IV defects; thus if there is any doubt in the surgeon's mind the preference is to err on the side of the reconstruction ring. This provides a very stable construct which has had the most reliable results in this setting.

In revision surgery for both isolated acetabular or femoral loosening there is good evidence that well-fixed components in good alignment and with minimal wear should be left *in situ* as long as they do not compromise the revision of the loose component. This greatly reduces the morbidity of the revision procedure and does not seem to compromise the eventual outcome.

Conclusion

A number of techniques for revision THA have been reported in North America in over 20 years of extensive literature, and over this time period the results appear to have significantly improved. This is due partly to greater technical expertise on the part of the surgeons, but also to the development of new implants and more importantly to the recognition of which implants and surgical techniques are most likely to succeed in each revision scenario. In this chapter we have aimed to provide a comprehensive review of the results for each implant and associated techniques, and ultimately use this to formulate an evidence-based algorithm for the appropriate selection of implants for the many scenarios encountered in revision THA.

References

1 Rorabeck CH, Bourne RB, Laupacis A *et al*: A: double-blind study of 250 cases comparing cemented with cementless total hip arthroplasty. Cost-effectiveness and its impact on health-related quality of life. *Clinical Orthopaedics and Related Research* **298**: 156–64, 1994.

2 Herberts P, Malchau H: Long-term registration has improved the quality of hip replacement: a review of the Swedish THR Register comparing 160 000 cases. *Acta Orthopaedica Scandinavica* **71**, 111–21, 2000.

3 Aribindi R, Barba M, Solomon M, Arp P, Paprosky W: Bypass fixation. *Orthopedic Clinics of North America* **29**: 319–29, 1998.

4 D'Antonio J, Capello W, Borden L *et al*.: Classification and management of acetabular abnormalities in total hip arthroplasty. *Clinical Orthopaedics and Related Research* **243**: 126–37, 1989.

5 D'Antonio J, McCarthy J, Bargar W *et al*.: Classification of femoral abnormalities in total hip arthroplasty. *Clinical Orthopaedics and Related Research* **296**: 133–9, 1993.

6 Garbuz D, Morsi E, Mohamed N, Gross AE: Classification and reconstruction in revision acetabular arthroplasty with bone stock deficiency. *Clinical Orthopaedics and Related Research* **324**: 98–107, 1996.

7 Gross AE, Allan DG, Leitch KK, Hutchison CR: Proximal femoral allografts for reconstruction of bone stock in revision arthroplasty of the hip. *Instructional Course Lectures* **45**: 143–7, 1996.

8 Mallory T: Preparation of the proximal femur in cementless total hip revision. *Clinical Orthopaedics and Related Research* **235**: 47–60, 1988.

9 Paprosky W, Lawrence J, Cameron H: Classification and treatment of the failed acetabulum: a systematic approach. *Contemporary Orthopaedics* **22**: 121, 1991.

10 Goetz DD, Capello WN, Callaghan JJ, Brown TD, Johnston RC: Salvage of a recurrently dislocating total hip prosthesis with use of a constrained acetabular component. A retrospective analysis of fifty-six cases. *Journal of Bone and Joint Surgery* [Am] **80**: 502–9, 1998.

11 Hunter GA, Welsh RP, Cameron HU, Bailey WH: The results of revision of total hip arthroplasty. *Journal of Bone and Joint Surgery* [Br] **61**: 419–21, 1979.

12 Krishnamurthy AB, MacDonald SJ, Paprosky WG: 5 to 13 year follow-up study on cementless femoral components in revision surgery. *Journal of Arthroplasty* **12**: 839–47, 1997.

13 Lawrence JM, Engh CA, Macalino GE: Revision total hip arthroplasty. Long-term results without cement. *Orthopedic Clinics of North America* **24**: 635–44, 1993.

14 Moreland JR, Bernstein ML: Femoral revision hip arthroplasty with uncemented, porous-coated stems. *Clinical Orthopaedics and Related Research* **319**: 141–50, 1995.

15 Glassman AH, Engh CA: Cementless revision for femoral failure. *Orthopedics* **18**: 851–3, 1995.

16 Paprosky WG, Greidanus NV, Antoniou J: Minimum 10-year-results of extensively porous-coated stems in revision hip arthroplasty. *Clinical Orthopaedics and Related Research* **369**: 230–42, 1999.

17 Engh CA, Culpepper WJ II, Kassapidis E: Revision of loose cementless femoral components to larger porous coated components. *Clinical Orthopaedics and Related Research* **347**: 168–78, 1998.

18 Lawrence JM, Engh CA, Macalino GE, Lauro GR: Outcome of revision hip arthroplasty done without cement. *Journal of Bone and Joint Surgery* [Am] **76**: 965–73.

19 Engh CA Jr, Culpepper WJ II, Engh CA: Long-term results of use of the anatomic medullary locking prosthesis in total hip arthroplasty. *Journal of Bone and Joint Surgery* [Am] **79**: 177–84, 1997.

20 Engh CA Sr, Culpepper WJ, II: Femoral fixation in primary total hip arthroplasty. *Orthopedics* **20**: 771–3, 1997.

21 Malkani AL, Lewallen DG, Cabanela ME, Wallrichs SL: Femoral component revision using an uncemented, proximally coated, long stem prosthesis. *Journal of Arthroplasty* **11**: 411–18, 1996.

22 Egan KJ, Di Cesare PE: Intraoperative complications of revision hip arthroplasty using a fully porous-coated straight cobalt-chrome femoral stem. *Journal of Arthroplasty* **10** (Supplement): 545–51, 1995.

23 Taylor JW, Rorabeck CH: Hip revision arthroplasty. Approach to the femoral side. *Clinical Orthopaedics and Related Research* **369**: 208–22, 1999.

24 Mallory TH, Head WC, Lombardi AV Jr, Emerson RH Jr, Eberle RW, Mitchell MB: Clinical and radiographic outcome of a cementless, titanium, plasma spray-coated total hip arthroplasty femoral component. Justification for continuance of use. *Journal of Arthroplasty* **11**: 653–60, 1996.

25 Head WC, Wagner RA, Emerson RH Jr, Malinin TI: Revision total hip arthroplasty in the deficient femur with a proximal load-bearing prosthesis. *Clinical Orthopaedics and Related Research* **298**: 119–26, 1994.

26 Gustilo RB, Pasternak HS: Revision total hip arthroplasty with titanium ingrowth prosthesis and bone grafting for failed cemented femoral component loosening. *Clinical Orthopaedics and Related Research* **235**: 111–19, 1988.

27 Buoncristiani AM, Dorr LD, Johnson C, Wan Z: Cementless revision of total hip arthroplasty using the anatomic porous replacement revision prosthesis. *Journal of Arthroplasty* **12**: 403–15, 1997.

28 Peters CL, Rivero DP, Kull LR, Jacobs JJ, Rosenberg AG, Galante JO: Revision total hip arthroplasty without cement: subsidence of proximally porous-coated femoral components. *Journal of Bone and Joint Surgery* [Am] **77**: 1217–26, 1995.

29 Mulliken BD, Rorabeck CH, Bourne RB: Uncemented revision total hip arthroplasty: a 4- to 6-year review. *Clinical Orthopaedics and Related Research* **325**: 156–62, 1996.

30 Woolson ST, Delaney TJ: Failure of a proximally porous-coated femoral prosthesis in revision total hip arthroplasty. *Journal of Arthroplasty* **10** (Supplement): 522–8, 1995.

31 Bargar WL, Murzic WJ, Taylor JK, Newman MA, Paul HA: Management of bone loss in revision total hip arthroplasty using custom cementless femoral components. *Journal of Arthroplasty* **8**: 245–52, 1993.

32 Berry DJ, Harmsen WS, Ilstrup D, Lewallen DG, Cabanela ME: Survivorship of uncemented proximally porous-coated femoral components. *Clinical Orthopaedics and Related Research* **319**: 168–77, 1995.

33 Hozack WJ, Bicalho PS, Eng K: Treatment of femoral osteolysis with cementless total hip revision. *Journal of Arthroplasty* **11**: 668–72, 1996.

34 Hussamy O, Lachiewicz PF: Revision total hip arthroplasty with the BIAS (Biologic Ingrowth Anatomic System) femoral component. Three to six-year results. *Journal of Bone and Joint Surgery* [Am] **76**: 1137–48, 1994.

35 Meding JB, Ritter MA, Keating EM, Faris PM: Clinical and radiographic evaluation of long-stem femoral components following revision total hip arthroplasty. *Journal of Arthroplasty* **9**: 399–408, 1994.

36 Hedley AK, Gruen TA, Ruoff DP: Revision of failed total hip arthro-
    plasties with uncemented porous-coated anatomic components.
    Clinical Orthopaedics and Related Research **235**: 75–90, 1988.
37 Chandler HP, Ayres DK, Tan RC, Anderson LC, Varma AK: Revision
    total hip replacement using the S-ROM femoral component.
    Clinical Orthopaedics and Related Research **319**: 130–40, 1995.
38 Smith JA, Dunn HK, Manaster BJ: Cementless femoral revision arthro-
    plasty. 2 to 5 year results with a modular titanium alloy stem.
    Journal of Arthroplasty **12**: 194–201, 1997.
39 Cameron HU: The two to six year results with a proximally modular
    noncemented total hip replacement used in hip revisions. *Clinical
    Orthopaedics and Related Research* **298**: 47–53, 1994.
40 Morrey BF, Kavanagh BF: Complications with revision of the femoral
    component of total hip arthroplasty. Comparison between cemented
    and uncemented techniques. *Journal of Arthroplasty* **7**: 71–9, 1992.
41 Rubash HE, Harris WH: Revision of non-septic, loose, cemented
    femoral components using modern cementing techniques. *Journal of
    Arthroplasty* **3**: 241–8, 1988.
42 Turner RH, Mattingly DA, Scheller A: Femoral revision total hip
    arthroplasty using a long-stem femoral component. Clinical and
    radiographic analysis. *Journal of Arthroplasty* **2**: 247–58, 1987.
43 Pierson JI, Harris WH: Cemented revision for femoral osteolysis in
    cemented arthroplasties: results in 29 hips after a mean 8.5 year
    follow-up. *Journal of Bone and Joint Surgery* [Br] **76**: 40–4, 1994.
44 Estok DM, II, Harris WH: Long term results of cemented femoral
    revision surgery using second-generation techniques: an average
    11.7 year follow-up evaluation. *Clinical Orthopaedics and Related
    Research* **299**: 190–202, 1994.
45 Pierson JL, Harris WH: Effect of improved cementing techniques on the
    longevity of fixation in revision cemented femoral arthroplasties.
    Average 8.8 year follow-up period. *Journal of Arthroplasty* **10**:
    581–91, 1995.
46 Mulroy WF, Harris WH: Revision total hip arthroplasty with use of
    so-called second-generation cementing techniques for aseptic
    loosening of the femoral component. A fifteen-year-average follow-up
    study. *Journal of Bone and Joint Surgery* [Am] **78**: 325–30, 1996.
47 McLaughlin JR, Harris WH: Revision of the femoral component of a
    total hip arthroplasty with the calcar-replacement femoral compon-
    ent. Results after a mean of 10.8 years postoperatively. *Journal of
    Bone and Joint Surgery* [Am] **78**: 331–9, 1996.
48 Katz RP, Callaghan JJ, Sullivan PM, Johnston RC: Long-term results
    of revision total hip arthroplasty with improved cementing tech-
    nique. *Journal of Bone and Joint Surgery* [Br] **79**: 322–6, 1997.
49 Ballard WT, Callaghan JJ, Johnston RC: Revision of total hip arthro-
    plasty in octogenarians. *Journal of Bone and Joint Surgery* [Am] **77**:
    585–9, 1995.
50 Weber KL, Callaghan JJ, Goetz DD, Johnston RC: Revision of a failed
    cemented total hip prosthesis with insertion of an acetabular com-
    ponent without cement and a femoral component with cement. A
    five to eight year follow-up study. *Journal of Bone and Joint Surgery*
    [Am] **78**: 982–94, 1996.
51 Iorio R, Healy WL, Richards JA: Comparison of the hospital cost of
    primary and revision total hip arthroplasty after cost containment.
    Orthopedics **22**: 185–9, 1999.
52 Pellicci PM, Wilson PD Jr, Sledge CB *et al.*: Long-term results of revi-
    sion total hip replacement. A follow-up report. *Journal of Bone and
    Joint Surgery* [Am] **67**: 513–16, 1985.

53 Hoogland T, Razzano CD, Marks KE, Wilde AH: Revision of Mueller total hip arthroplasties. *Clinical Orthopaedics and Related Research* **161**: 180–5, 1981.

54 Kavanagh BE, Ilstrup DM, Fitzgerald RH Jr: Revision total hip arthroplasty. *Journal of Bone and Joint Surgery* [Am] **67**: 517–26, 1985.

55 Kavanagh BE, Fitzgerald RH Jr: Multiple revisions for failed total hip arthroplasty not associated with infection. *Journal of Bone and Joint Surgery* [Am] **69**: 1144–9, 1987.

56 Callaghan JJ, Salvati EA, Pellicci PM, Wilson PD Jr, Ranawat CS: Results of revision for mechanical failure after cemented total hip replacement, 1979 to 1982. A two to five-year follow-up. *Journal of Bone and Joint Surgery* [Am] **67**: 1074–85, 1985.

57 Meding JB, Ritter MA, Keating EM, Faris PM: Impaction bone-grafting before insertion of a femoral stem with cement in revision total hip arthroplasty. A minimum two-year follow-up study. *Journal of Bone and Joint Surgery* [Am] **79**: 1834–41, 1997.

58 Leopold SS, Berger RA, Rosenberg AG, Jacobs JJ, Quigley LR, Galante JO: Impaction allografting with cement for revision of the femoral component. A minimum four-year follow-up study with use of a precoated femoral stem. *Journal of Bone and Joint Surgery* [Am] **81**: 1080–92, 1999.

59 Capello WN: Impaction grafting plus cement for femoral component fixation in revision hip arthroplasty. *Orthopedics* **17**: 878–9, 1994.

60 Elting JJ, Mikhail WEM, Zicat BA, Hubbell JC, Lane LE, House B: Preliminary report of impaction grafting for exchange femoral arthroplasty. *Clinical Orthopaedics and Related Research* **319**: 159–67.

61 Mann KA, Ayers DC, Damron TA: Effects of stem length on mechanics of the femoral hip component after cemented revision. *Journal of Orthopaedic Research* **15**: 62–68, 1997.

62 Dohmae Y, Bechtold J, Sherman R: Reduction of cement–bone interface shear strength between primary and revision arthroplasty. *Clinical Orthopaedics and Related Research* **236**: 214–20, 1988.

63 Iorio R, Eftekhar NS, Kobayashi S, Grelsamer RP: Cemented revision of failed total hip arthroplasty. Survivorship analysis. *Clinical Orthopaedics and Related Research* **316**: 121–30, 1995.

64 Ash SA, Callaghan JJ, Johnston RC: Revision total hip arthroplasty with cement after cup arthroplasty. Long-term follow-up. *Journal of Bone and Joint Surgery* [Am] **78**: 87–93, 1996.

65 Lieberman JR, Moeckel BH, Evans BG, Salvati EA, Ranawat CS: Cement-within-cement revision hip arthroplasty. *Journal of Bone and Joint Surgery* [Br] **75**: 869–71, 1993.

66 Nabors ED, Liebelt R, Mattingly DA, Bierbaum BE: Removal and reinsertion of cemented femoral components during acetabular revision. *Journal of Arthroplasty* **11**: 146–52, 1996.

67 Greenwald A, Narten N, Wilde A: Points in the technique of recementing in the revision of an implant arthroplasty. *Journal of Bone and Joint Surgery* [Br] **60**: 107–10, 1978.

68 Gie G, Linder L, Ling R, Simon J, Slooff T, Timperley A: Impacted cancellous allografts and cement for revision total hip arthroplasty. *Journal of Bone and Joint Surgery* [Br] **1**: 14–21, 1993.

69 Malkani AL, Voor MJ, Fee KA, Bates CS: Femoral component revision using impacted morsellised cancellous graft. A biomechanical study of implant stability. *Journal of Bone and Joint Surgery* [Br] **78**: 973–8, 1997.

70 Chassin EP, Silverton CD, Berzins A, Rosenberg AG: Implant stability in revision total hip arthroplasty: allograft bone packing following

extended proximal femoral osteotomy. *Journal of Arthroplasty* **12**: 863–8, 1997.

71 Berzins A, Sumner DR, Wasielewski RC, Galante JO: Impacted particulate allograft for femoral revision total hip arthroplasty. *In vitro* mechanical stability and effects of cement pressurization. *Journal of Arthroplasty* **11**: 500–6, 1996.

72 Nelissen RG, Bauer TW, Weidenhielm LR, LeGolvan DP, Mikhail WE: Revision hip arthroplasty with the use of cement and impaction grafting. Histological analysis of four cases. *Journal of Bone and Joint Surgery* [Am] **77**: 412–22, 1995.

73 Eldridge JD, Smith EJ, Hubble MJ, Whitehouse SL, Learmonth ID: Massive early subsidence following femoral impaction grafting. *Journal of Arthroplasty* **12**: 535–40, 1997.

74 Incavo SJ, Beard DM, Pupparo F, Ries M, Wiedel J: One-stage revision of periprosthetic fractures around loose cemented total hip arthroplasty. *American Journal of Orthopedics* **27**: 35–41, 1998.

75 Moran MC: Treatment of periprosthetic fractures around total hip arthroplasty with an extensively coated femoral component. *Journal of Arthroplasty* **11**: 981–8, 1996.

76 Emerson RH Jr, Malinin TI, Cuellar AD, Head WC, Peters PC: Cortical strut allografts in the reconstruction of the femur in revision total hip arthroplasty. A basic science and clinical study. *Clinical Orthopaedics and Related Research* **285**: 35–44, 1992.

77 Head WC, Malinin TI: Results of onlay allografts. *Clinical Orthopaedics and Related Research* **371**: 108–12, 2000.

78 Pak JH, Paprosky WG, Jablonsky WS, Lawrence JM: Femoral strut allografts in cementless revision total hip arthroplasty. *Clinical Orthopaedics and Related Research* **295**:172–8, 1993.

79 Allan DG, Lavoie GJ, McDonald S, Oakeshott R, Gross AE: Proximal femoral allografts in revision hip arthroplasty. *Journal of Bone and Joint Surgery* [Br] **73**: 235–40, 1991.

80 Gross AE, Hutchison CR: Proximal femoral allografts for reconstruction of bone stock in revision hip arthroplasty. *Orthopedics* **21**: 999–1001, 1998.

81 Gross AE, Hutchison CR: Proximal femoral allografts for reconstruction of bone stock in revision arthroplasty of the hip. *Orthopedic Clinics of North America* **29**: 313–17, 1998.

82 Gross AE, Hutchison CR, Alexeeff M, Mahomed N, Leitch K, Morsi E: Proximal femoral allografts for reconstruction of bone stock in revision arthroplasty of the hip. *Clinical Orthopaedics and Related Research* **319**: 151–8, 1995.

83 Head WC, Emerson RH, Malinin TI: Structural bone grafting for eemoral reconstruction. *Clinical Orthopaedics and Related Research* **369**: 223–29, 1999.

84 Haddad ES, Spangehl MJ, Masri BA, Garbuz DS, Duncan CP: Circumferential allograft replacement of the proximal femur. *Clinical Orthopaedics and Related Research* **371**: 98–107, 2000.

85 Barrack RL, Wolfe MW, Michas P, Frentz B: Distal femoral allograft for massive proximal femoral deficiency. *Acta Orthopaedica Scandinavica* **71**: 90–4, 2000.

86 Dearborn JT, Harris WH: High placement of an acetabular component inserted without cement in a revision total hip arthroplasty. Results after a mean of ten years. *Journal of Bone and Joint Surgery* [Am] **81**: 469–80, 1999.

87 Leopold SS, Rosenberg AG, Bhatt RD, Sheinkop MB, Quigley LR, Galante JO: Cementless acetabular revision. *Clinical Orthopaedics and Related Research* **369**: 179–86, 1999.

88 Dorr LD, Wan Z: Ten years of experience with porous acetabular components for revision surgery. *Clinical Orthopaedics and Related Research* **319**: 191–200, 1995.

89 Chareancholvanich K, Tanchuling A, Seki T, Gustilo RB: Cementless acetabular revision for aseptic failure of cemented hip arthroplasty. *Clinical Orthopaedics and Related Research* **361**: 140–9, 1999.

90 Silverton CD, Rosenberg AG, Sheinkop MB, Kull LR, Galante JO: Revision total hip arthroplasty using a cementless acetabular component. Technique and results. *Clinical Orthopaedics and Related Research* **319**: 201–8, 1995.

91 Woolson ST, Adamson GJ: Acetabular revision using a bone-ingrowth total hip component in patients who have acetabular bone stock deficiency. *Journal of Arthroplasty* **11**: 661–7, 1996.

92 Lachiewicz PF, Poon ED: Revision of a total hip arthroplasty with a Harris–Galante porous- coated acetabular component inserted without cement. A follow-up note on the results at five to twelve years. *Journal of Bone and Joint Surgery* [Am] **80**: 980–4, 1998.

93 Poon ED, Lachiewicz PF: Results of isolated acetabular revisions: the fate of the unrevised femoral component. *Journal of Arthroplasty* **13**: 42–9, 1998.

94 Moskal JT, Danisa OA, Shaffrey CI: Isolated revision acetabuloplasty using a porous-coated cementless acetabular component without removal of a well-fixed femoral component. A 3 to 9 year follow-up study. *Journal of Arthroplasty* **12**: 719–27, 1997.

95 Engh CA, Glassman AH, Griffin WL, Mayer JG: Results of cementless revision for failed cemented total hip arthroplasty. *Clinical Orthopaedics and Related Research* **235**: 91–110, 1988.

96 Chen W, Engh CA, Hopper RH, MeAuley JP, Engh CA: Acetabular revision with use of a bibobed component inserted without cement in patients who have acetabular bone-stock deficiency. *Journal of Bone and Joint Surgery* **82**: 197–206, 2000.

97 Berry DJ, Sutherland CJ, Trousdale RT et al.: Bilobed oblong porous coated acetabular components in revision total hip arthroplasty. *Clinical Orthopaedics and Related Research* **371**: 154–60, 2000.

98 Padgett DE, Kull L, Rosenberg A, Sumner DR, Galante JO: Revision of the acetabular component without cement after total hip arthroplasty. Three to six-year follow-up. *Journal of Bone and Joint Surgery* [Am] **75**: 663–73, 1993.

99 More RC, Amstutz HC, Kabo JM, Dorey FJ, Moreland JR: Acetabular reconstruction with a threaded prosthesis for failed total hip arthroplasty. *Clinical Orthopaedics and Related Research* **282**: 114–22, 1992.

100 Shaw JA, Bailey JH, Bruno A, Greer RBD: Threaded acetabular components for primary and revision total hip arthroplasty. *Journal of Arthroplasty* **5**: 201–15, 1990.

101 Lombardi AV Jr, Mallory TH, Kraus TJ, Vaughn BK: Preliminary report on the S-ROM constraining acetabular insert: a retrospective clinical experience. *Orthopedics* **14**: 297–303, 1991.

102 Kelley SS: High hip center in revision arthroplasty. *Journal of Arthroplasty* **9**: 503–10, 1994.

103 Sutherland CJ: Treatment of type III acetabular deficiencies in revision total hip arthroplasty without structural bone-graft. *Journal of Arthroplasty* **11**: 91–8, 1996.

104 Jasty M, Harris WH: Salvage total hip reconstruction in patients with major acetabular bone deficiency using structural femoral head allografts. *Journal of Bone and Joint Surgery* [Br] **72**: 63–67, 1990.

105 Kwong LM, Jasty M, Harris WH: High failure rate of bulk femoral head allografts in total hip acetabular reconstruction at 10 years. *Journal of Arthroplasty* **8**: 341–6, 1993.

106 Wilson MG, Nikpoor N, Aliabadi P, Poss R, Weissman BN: The fate of acetabular allografts after bipolar revision arthroplasty of the hip. A radiographic review. *Journal of Bone and Joint Surgery* [Am] **71**: 1469–79, 1989.

107 Gross AE, Lavoie MV, McDermott P, Marks P: The use of allograft bone in revision of total hip arthroplasty. *Clinical Orthopaedics and Related Research* **197**: 115–22, 1985.

108 Gross AE, Allan DG, Catre M *et al.*: Bone grafts in hip replacement surgery: the pelvic side. *Orthopedic Clinics of North America* **24**: 679–95, 1993.

109 Gross AE, Garbuz D, Morsi ES: Acetabular allografts for restoration of bone stock in revision arthroplasty of the hip. *Instructional Course Lectures* **45**: 135–42, 1996.

110 Gross AE: Revision arthroplasty of the acetabulum with restoration of bone stock. *Clinical Orthopaedics and Related Research* **369**: 198–207, 1999.

111 Paprosky WG, Magnus RE: Principles of bone grafting in revision total hip arthroplasty. Acetabular technique. *Clinical Orthopaedics and Related Research* **298**: 147–55, 1994.

112 Chandler HP: Structural grafting of the acetabulum. *Orthopedics* **18**: 863–4.

113 Hooten JP Jr, Engh CA, Jr, Engh CA Eailure of structural acetabular allografts in cementless revision hip arthroplasty. *Journal of Bone and Joint Surgery* [Br] **76**: 419–22, 1994.

114 Heekin RD, Engh CA, Vinh T: Morselized allograft in acetabular reconstruction. *Clinical Orthopaedics and Related Research* **319**: 184–90, 1995.

115 Woodgate IG, Saleh KJ, Jaroszynski G, Agnidis Z, Woodgate MM, Gross AE: Minor column structural acetabular allografts in revision hip arthroplasty. *Clinical Orthopaedics and Related Research* **371**: 75–85, 2000.

116 Garbuz D, Morsi E, Gross AE: Revision of the acetabular component of a total hip arthroplasty with a massive structural allograft. Study with a minimum five-year follow-up. *Journal of Bone and Joint Surgery* [Am] **78**: 693–7, 1996.

117 Schatzker J, Wong M: Acetabular revision. The role of rings and cages. *Clinical Orthopaedics and Related Research* **369**: 187–97, 1999.

118 Berry DJ, Lewallen DG, Hanssen AD, Cabanela ME: Pelvic discontinuity in revision total hip arthroplasty. *Journal of Bone and Joint Surgery* [Am] **81**: 1692–1702, 1999.

119 Murray WR: Acetabular salvage in revision total hip arthroplasty using the bipolar prosthesis. *Clinical Orthopaedics and Related Research* **251**: 92–9, 1990.

120 Roberson JR, Cohen D: Bipolar components for severe periacetabular bone loss around the failed total hip arthroplasty. *Clinical Orthopaedics and Related Research* **251**: 113–18, 1990.

121 Cameron HU, Jung YB: Acetabular revision with a bipolar prosthesis. *Clinical Orthopaedics and Related Research* **251**: 100–3, 1990.

122 Peters CL, Kull L, Jacobs JJ, Rosenberg AG, Galante JO: The fate of well-fixed cemented femoral components left in place at the time of revision of the acetabular component. *Journal of Bone and Joint Surgery* **79**: 701–6, 1997.

123 Berger RA, Quigley LR, Jacobs JJ, Sheinkop MB, Rosenberg AG, Galante JO: The fate of stable cemented acetabular components

retained during revision of a femoral component of a total hip arthroplasty. *Journal of Bone and Joint Surgery* [Am] **81**: 1682–91, 1999.

124 Barrack RL: Economics of revision total hip arthroplasty. *Clinical Orthopaedics and Related Research* **319**: 209–14, 1995.

125 Lavernia CJ, Drakeford MK, Tsao AK, Gittelsohn A, Krackow KA, Hungerford DS: Revision and primary hip and knee arthroplasty. A cost analysis. *Clinical Orthopaedics and Related Research* **311**: 136–41, 1995.

126 Barrack RL, Sawhney J, Hsu J, Cofield RH: Cost analysis of revision total hip arthroplasty. A 5-year followup study. *Clinical Orthopaedics and Related Research* **369**: 175–8, 1999.

127 Barrack RL: The evolving cost spectrum of revision hip arthroplasty. *Orthopedics* **22**: 865–6, 1999.

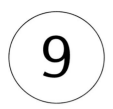

9

Criteria for implant selection in revision total hip arthroplasty: a European perspective

H. Wagner and M. Wagner

Introduction

Loosening of a hip joint prosthesis involves bone loss as a result of bone resorption in the prosthesis bed, which can make the fixation of a new prosthesis at the old site difficult or impossible. When prostheses are changed, the new prosthesis must be stably anchored, which means that the choice of implant and operation technique must be adapted to the state of the bone.

If the bone in the old prosthesis bed is still in relatively good condition and the patient is elderly, a new prosthesis can be fixed at the old site with bone cement. This is a simple operative technique, although cement fixation of a replacement prosthesis is less stable than in primary implantation because of the smooth inner surface of the medullary cavity, so that a shorter lifespan may be expected. The medullary cavity at the old prosthesis site becomes wider as a result of the loosening and bone resorption and must be filled with a larger quantity of cement. On further loosening, the bone defect will be even greater.

With a replacement prosthesis involving a titanium implant without bone cement, part of the bone defect is filled with new vital bone substance by osseo-integration.

If the bone damage in the old prosthesis bed is so severe that the bone can no longer support a load, femoral prostheses with a long stem should be used to bridge the old prosthesis bed and be fixed distally in the intact medullary cavity. The SL femur revision prosthesis has been used for the past 14 years for this purpose and for stabilizing difficult complex post-traumatic conditions.[1-8] This prosthesis, which is made from titanium–aluminium–niobium alloy and has a conical stem lined with sharp longitudinal ribs, is inserted into the conically reamed medullary cavity. The sharp longitudinal ribs cut into the bone, thus providing a high degree of rotational stability. Therefore thigh pain is extremely rare. Very effective osseo-integration is obtained from the coarse-blasted titanium surface.

Statement of the problem

In aseptic loosening of a total hip prosthesis, there is almost always some bone loss due to bone resorption, foreign body granulomas, and movement relative to the bone site, which results in weakening of the femur in the area of the prosthesis bed. This is the main problem in the case of a replacement prosthesis because stable fixation of a new prosthesis at the old site can be difficult or even impossible as a result of the loss of bone substance. Where septic prosthesis loosening is involved, there is also the problem of bacterial infection in the old prosthesis bed. Very careful debridement and effective local antisepsis combined with systemic antibiotic treatment is required before a new prosthesis can be implanted.

The most important condition to be met in the case of a replacement prosthesis is the fixation of a new prosthesis which must be sufficiently stable for the patient to be able to walk again immediately. In addition, an optimal solution must be found to ensure the longest possible lifespan for the new prosthesis. A suitable new implant and an appropriate operating technique are the most important preconditions.

Replacement prosthesis with cement

Many surgeons still opt for a replacement prosthesis with bone cement. When only minor bone loss has occurred on loosening of the prosthesis and the proximal end of the femur still exhibits good bone quality, this method may be considered, particularly for elderly patients. A replacement prosthesis with cement, like all other techniques, has advantages and disadvantages. The indisputable advantage of the revision prosthesis with cement is that it is a technically simple procedure with which all hip surgeons are familiar and in which the early results at least are almost always very good. The decision is more difficult if the patient still has a long life expectancy. The disadvantages of the procedure then come into play.

Loosening of the prosthesis enlarges the bone cavity as a result of bone resorption and relative movement, and the larger cavity must be filled with methacrylate cement. The foreign body that is implanted is necessarily be larger than the primary implant and the larger bone cavity in the old prosthesis bed cannot become smaller again—'the defect remains a defect'.

The high stability of primary implantations with bone cement is due in large part to the fact that the bone cement penetrates the small indentations in the bone in the plastic phase in the coarse inner surface of the medullary cavity and creates a fixed coral-shaped interdigitation. This is not possible in revision prostheses with cement because the inner surface of the medullary cavity is smooth due to bone resorption and relative movement between the loosened prosthesis and the bone which prevents interdigitation of the cement with the bone (Fig. 9.1). Fixation is based simply on the complete filling of the bone cavity with the cement (fit and fill). Therefore this fixation is less stable than in the primary implantation so that a shorter lifespan must be expected.[9,10,11,12]

Therefore, although a replacement prosthesis with cement is a simpler surgical intervention, a larger foreign body mass with poorer stability and a shorter lifespan is used in a larger bone defect. On subsequent loosening the bone defect will become even larger and the surgical problem more difficult. Whether this is of major clinical significance depends on the patient's life expectancy.

Surgeons should be aware of these problems and weigh them up against other possibilities when choosing the procedure for a revision prosthesis. If the bone defect is so substantial that the proximal femur segment can no longer load-bear, the proximal end of the femur should not be stabilized with large metal assemblies on the surface of the bone in order to allow a replacement prosthesis with cement. This procedure requires excessive surgical intervention with a dubious result. In such difficult cases, including elderly patients, it is better and safer to use longer prostheses to bridge the defect with a stable fixation distal to the old prosthesis bed in the healthy medullary cavity. Experience has shown that spontaneous bone formation also occurs in the proximal femoral segment following distal fixation and this fills the defect with vital bone substance.

Cementless replacement prosthesis

Since it was discovered that osseo-integration takes place on the coarse-blasted surfaces of titanium alloy implants, i.e. new bone tissue is deposited directly on the metal without an intervening layer

Fig. 9.1

(a) The cement mantle after primary implantation shows a coral-shaped interdigitation. (b) The cement mantle after cemented revision shows a relatively smooth surface. Anchorage of the prosthesis is achieved by 'fit and fill' only.

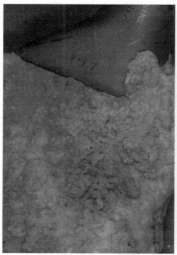
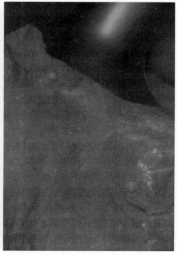

a

b

of connective tissue, new prospects for endoprosthetics have opened up (Fig. 9.2). The unavoidable precondition for this formation of new bone is the high primary stability of the prosthesis fixation, where rotational stability is of particular importance.[13]

Replacement prosthesis with short femoral stem

In cementless replacement prostheses, preference should be given to titanium implants to promote osseo-integration. There is no osseo-integration in implants made from other metal alloys, even with a coarse or granulated surface. At best, there is an ingrowth of bone tissue into the structured surface, which also results in a firm fixation. However, in this case the metal surface is lined with connective tissue. This can result in relatively small movements which cause the typical thigh pain of these prostheses without any negative findings being detectable on radiography. A further advantage of the titanium alloy is that the prosthesis stems are rather more elastic than those made from chromium–cobalt alloys, which is beneficial for the physiology of the bone.

When preparing for a cementless revision prosthesis, an implant should be chosen which can fit into the bone defect with the minimum of bone resection. Prosthesis stems with a conical configuration have the advantage that they can attach firmly to bone with only slight impaction. It is easy to select a suitable prosthesis model using the available planning templates.

The site for the new prosthesis in the bone is prepared by reaming and rasping. This must allow firm fixation for the new prosthesis because the load on the prosthesis must be transferred to vital bone in the femur and not to non-vital bone shavings. The essential precondition for a successful revision is stable fixation of the new implant. In the case of titanium prostheses, spontaneous bone

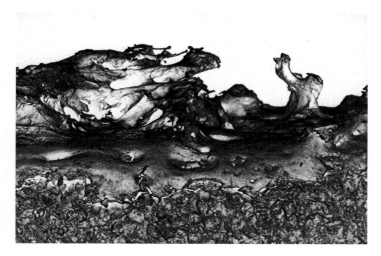

Fig. 9.2

Osseo-integration on titanium alloy. New bone tissue is deposited directly on the coarse-blasted surface of the titanium alloy (below) without an intervening fibrous tissue (scanning electron microscope).

formation from the neighbouring tissue is so active that painstaking filling of all small bone fissures with bone shavings is unnecessary. The insertion of bone shavings may be useful when there are large gaps (>10 mm), but experience has shown that this is not absolutely neccessary in the case of stable fixation because of the good spontaneous bone formation (Fig. 9.3).

An important condition for a change of prosthesis is high rotational stability. A new prosthesis of normal length is only inserted when the bone quality of the proximal femoral segment is still relatively good. In this case, good rotational stability can be achieved for the new prosthesis in the configuration of the trochanter and the calcar femorale.

Femur revision prosthesis with long stem

As the proximal end of the femur becomes further weakened and no longer possesses appreciable load-bearing capacity, the damaged proximal femoral segment with the old prosthesis bed must be bridged and a new prosthesis with a long stem fixed distally to the old bed in the intact medullary cavity. In this situation there is no longer the option of ensuring rotational stability in the area of the trochanter. This must also be done in the distal medullary cavity.

PRINCIPLE

To achieve this we have developed a femoral prosthesis with a long stem which satisfies both conditions: high stability with a vertical

Fig. 9.3
Revision of a loosened femoral prosthesis through the closed medullary cavity using a short uncemented conical prosthesis. (a) Left hip of a man age 61. Prosthesis loosening, subsidence and pain 1 year after cemented revision. (b) Six years after second revision with a short uncemented femoral prosthesis without removing the cement-tap. The radiograph shows continuous osseo-integration of the prosthetic shaft.

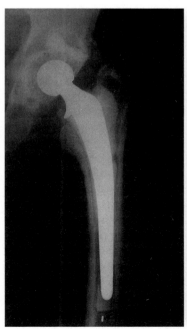
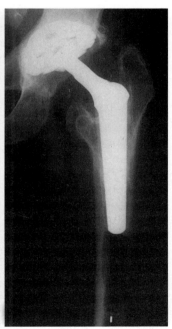

a   b

load and high rotational stability.[7] The SL femur revision prosthesis is made from a titanium–aluminium–niobium alloy and has
a coarse-blasted surface to promote osseo-integration. The stem is
conical, with a cone angle of $2°$, and is lined with eight relatively
sharp longitudinal ribs distributed evenly over the whole circumference of the stem (Fig. 9.4).

The prosthesis is available in six different lengths in 40-mm
sections (Fig. 9.5) so that it can be adapted to the extent of the bone
defect. In the standard variant the neck of the prosthesis has a CCD
angle of $145°$ with an offset of 36 mm, and in the lateralization variant
it has a CCD angle of $135°$ and an offset that increases gradually up
to 46 mm with increasing stem diameter (Fig. 9.6).

For the implantation of the conical stem, the cylindrical
medullary cavity must be enlarged with a conical reamer. With a
cone angle of $2°$ only very little bone substance need be removed;
a layer of only about 2 mm of bone at the opening of the medullary
cavity distal to the old prosthesis bed is sufficient (Fig. 9.7). When
the prosthesis is impacted into the medullary cavity, the sharp longitudinal ribs bite about 0.5 mm deep into the bone and as a result
give the implant a very high degree of rotational stability. This
explains why almost no thigh pain is observed with this fixation
principle.

Using this conical stem fixation, a conical implant is positioned
in the conically reamed medullary cavity with continuous contact
along the whole length of the conical connection and this accord-
ingly results in continuous load transfer. Under these conditions,
the size of the mechanical load transferred depends on the size of
the contact area. Since the size of the surface area per unit of
length increases with the diameter in the case of a conical stem, a
greater load is transmitted in the proximal part of the stem where
the diameter is larger than distally where it is smaller.[14] Thus, for

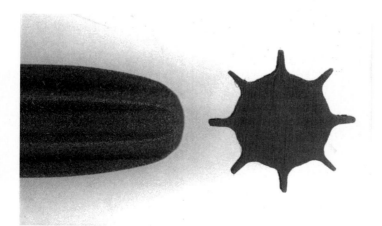

Fig. 9.4
Revision femoral prosthesis.
Left: the tip of the shaft shows
the conical shape and the
rough blasted metal surface.
Right: the cross-section shows
the eight relatively sharp
longitudinal ribs arranged
evenly over the whole
circumference.

Fig. 9.10

Planning template for the
revsion femoral prosthesis
standardized to an
enlargement factor of 1:15:1.

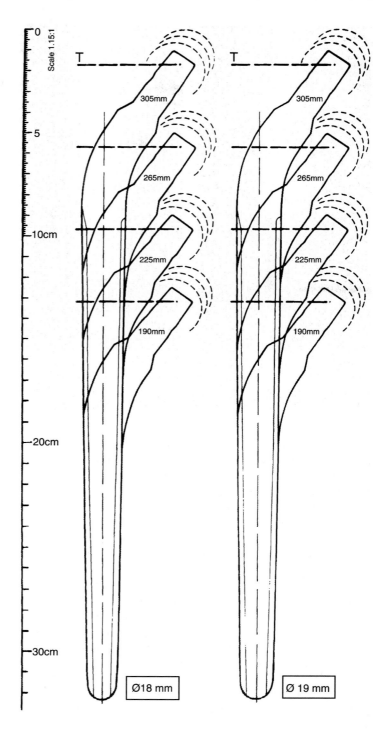

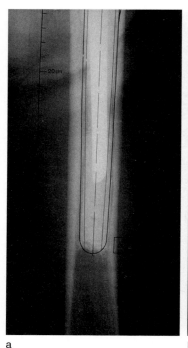 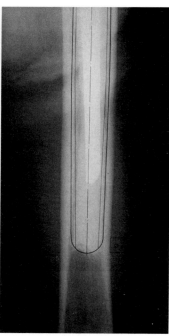

a   b

Fig. 9.11
Selection of the correct stem diameter. (a) If the planning template is laid on the original radiograph and the outline of the template fits exactly over the outline of the cortical bone, the diameter of the stem is too thin and the prosthesis will subside. (b) In order to determine the correct stem diameter the outlines of the template must overlap the outlines of the cortical bone by 1 mm on both sides.

medullary cavity with the conical reamers, a sufficiently long conical bed should be created, ideally 10 cm and a minimum of 7 cm. Reaming is continued using increasing diameters until strong frictional resisance is felt and the graduation on the reamer for the selected prosthesis length is on a level with the tip of the greater trochanter. When the last two reamers are carefully withdrawn from the bone, it is possible to determine from the adherent bone shavings whether the conical bed in the bone has reached the desired length of 7–10 cm. To avoid incurring unnecessary costs, the implant should not be taken from the sterile packaging until the correct diameter of the prosthesis stem has been confirmed with the reamers.

In order to check the depth of penetration of the reamer, and subsequently of the prosthesis, the tip of the greater trochanter is generally used as a reference point. However, there may also be (anatomical) situations in which it is necessary to deviate from this. Thus the check must be made from a different reference point established during preoperative planning (Fig. 9.12).

Surgical approaches

When replacing a prosthesis, as well as removing the loosened prosthesis, the bony prosthesis bed must also be carefully revised. Granulation and scar tissue, foreign body granulomas, and cement

Fig. 9.12

Preoperative plan with the outline drawing of the bone and the implant including the measurements of the essential distances. This gives a reliable orientation during surgery.

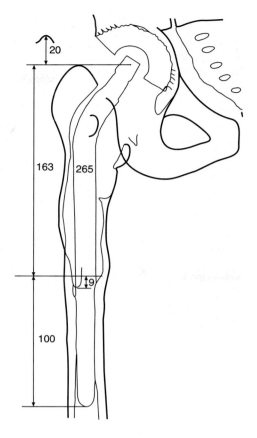

fragments must be completely removed. Thus a careful inspection of the medullary cavity is necessary. Cold light probes or arthroscopes can be useful for this purpose. In general, the operative approach used in the primary implantation should be adopted. Occasionally an exception has to made to this rule in order to obtain a good view of the medullary cavity. A temporary osteotomy of the greater trochanter should be avoided for reasons of stability.

In replacing short prostheses, the posterior approach with the patient in the lateral position is very effective because it is possible to see deep into the medullary cavity with the hip and knee joint flexed without obstruction from the surrounding soft tissues.

The transfemoral approach

Specific conditions arise when the bone in the old prosthesis bed is so severely damaged that the proximal femur segment no longer has any mechanical load-bearing capacity or when long prostheses have to be removed. In this case, it is often impossible to avoid unwanted perforation of the cortical bone or uncontrolled fractures when scraping out the medullary cavity. The same applies when long firmly seated cement plugs are encountered which cannot be removed through the closed medullary cavity. In addition, inspection of the closed medullary cavity is only possible to a limited depth, which is often not sufficient.[7,15]

When these problems are present, the transfemoral approach is indicated. With the patient in the lateral position, the femur is exposed behind the vastus lateralis muscle at the linea aspera and opened like a door, so that the loosened prosthesis with cement and granuloma tissue becomes directly accessible. Obviously, opening the femur also stimulates callus formation, so that particularly active bone formation is observed following a transfemoral approach.[7,16,17] In the lateral position, gravity causes the soft tissues and venous blood to descend, which is particularly welcome in obese patients.

Sectioning of the skin is started two fingerbreadths behind the greater trochanter and routed distally in the direction of the lateral epicondyle of the femur. The length of the skin section is determined during preoperative planning and depends essentially on the length of the loosened prosthesis.

After lengthwise sectioning of the fascia lata, the vastus lateralis muscle is dissected free from the lateral intermuscular septum and the linea aspera is exposed. With careful preparation, no muscle tissue is sacrificed. A Steinmann pin is inserted at the tip of the greater trochanter as a reference point for the subsequent measurements. The preplanned length of the transfemoral approach is measured from this point in a distal direction and marked with a fine osteotome. At the site marked, and only at that site, the muscle is released subperiosteally to a width of 2 cm around half the circumference of the femoral shaft .

At the site marked, two drill holes of diameter 3.2 mm are created to delineate the subsequent semicircular transverse osteotomy, one directly on the linea aspera and the second about 120° further ventrally. The distance between the two drill holes determines the width of the bony lid through which the medullary cavity is opened (Fig. 9.13).

A semicircular transverse osteotomy is performed between the two drill holes using fine chisels. Oscillating saws generate heat, contaminate the Haversian vascular channels, and disperse cement particles into the wound. This is avoided if chisels are used. In addition, by using a hammer and chisel, the operator obtains a better feeling for the layer thickness and strength of the bone.

Starting from the dorsal drill hole, the femoral shaft is split proximally along the linea aspera, while the overlying muscle is spared. Proximally to the tuberculum innominatum, the osteotomy is gently routed ventrally so as to preserve a strong strip of bone at the posterior edge of the greater trochanter for subsequent suturing. The osteotomy is then extended to the tip of the greater trochanter and continued a further 3 cm by scalpel in the direction

Fig. 9.13

Different steps in the transfemoral approach, which are explained in the text.

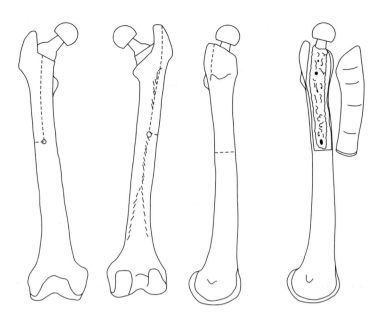

of the fibres of the tendon of the gluteus medius muscle. The superior gluteal nerve crosses about 4 cm proximally from the tip of the trochanter and must be spared.

For a straight-line limitation of the anterior border of the bony lid, several puncture osteotomies are performed in continuation of the ventral drill hole. If the longitudinal osteotomy at the linea aspera has resulted in the cortical bone being thin and flexible, the bony lid can be slightly raised and the puncture osteotomies performed through the medullary cavity.

The bony lid is loosened with flat chisels and then raised with fragment spreaders, so that the prosthesis and cement mantle are exposed over their entire length. After removal of the prosthesis, all foreign bodies, and all scar and granulation tissue, the conical site for the new prosthesis can be prepared distally to the old prosthesis bed. If as a result of the antecurvatum of the femur the medial cortical bone prevents the use of a straight reamer, the antecurvatum of the cortical bone can be reduced by osteotomy.

The transfemoral approach can also be used to replace a loosened acetabular prosthesis between the two parts of the greater trochanter. In this way the joint capsule remains intact, which contributes to the stability of the prosthetic joint.

After the cement residue from the femur has been removed, the conical site for the stem is prepared with reamers of gradually increasing diameter. The necessary depth of penetration of the reamer is assessed during preoperative planning: the conical bed in the bone should ideally be 10 cm long, and no less than 7 cm, with the necessary diameter. In most cases, the tip of the greater trochanter can no longer be used to measure the depth of penetration of the reamer once the femur has been opened. However, the distance of the transverse osteotomy of the transfemoral approach from the tip of the trochanter is known. Therefore the depth of penetration can be measured on the graduations on the reamer from the distance to the transverse osteotomy.

Reaming is continued with increasing diameters until a strong frictional resistance occurs and the graduation on the reamer has reached the required distance to the transverse osteotomy. By carefully withdrawing the last reamer, the length of the conical bone site can be determined from the attached bone shavings and extended by further drilling.

A cerclage immediately distal to the transverse osteotomy can be used to strengthen the femoral shaft and prevent the risk of a longitudinal fracture when the conical prosthesis stem is impacted. Cerclage also has an important psychological effect because it gives the operator a greater feeling of safety when forcefully impacting the prosthesis. Studies in the biomechanical laboratory have shown that a double cerclage with 1.5-mm diameter steel wire applied in two loops around the bone is particularly beneficial. The cerclage should be tautened with special tension forceps before it is twisted. Tautening at the time of twisting produces less tension and risks fracturing the wire.

After these preparations, the selected revision prosthesis is inserted into the medullary cavity. Marked resistance occurs about 3 cm before the definitive position. The angle of anteversion to the axis of the lower leg can be checked by flexion of the knee joint at right angles. The prosthesis is then hammered a further 1.5 cm approximately into the medullary cavity until the fixation can sustain a trial reduction. The final fixation depth should not be achieved immediately as it can be very tiresome to loosen the prosthesis again if the trial reduction has shown that the rotation needs to be corrected.

The trial reduction is performed with the shortest trial head because the prosthesis has not yet reached its final depth. With the hip in flexion and in internal rotation, the stability of the prosthetic joint and the tension of the soft tissues are tested and, if necessary, corrected. Following redislocation of the prosthesis, the final fixation is carried out; the prosthesis is impacted with regular taps and its progression is observed at the edge of the osteotomy. With each tap, the prosthesis is impacted a little further into the medullary cavity and the tapping is continued with equal force until the prosthesis no longer moves. The sound also changes, which is a good indication of the stability of the prosthesis fixation. A modular prosthetic head is then applied and the prosthesis is repositioned. By applying 15 kg of longitudinal traction to the extended leg, the tension of the soft tissues is tested. The prosthesis joint must not open more than 8 mm under this traction. If the joint opens further, a longer prosthetic head must be used to safeguard against dislocation.

Wound closure begins with the repositioning of the bony lid in the transfemoral approach and firm suturing of the split greater trochanter. Insertion of bone shavings is generally not necessary because vital spontaneous bone formation occurs rapidly with the transfemoral approach. Fine bone shavings should only be inserted if there are bone defects laterally on the surface of the femur or a diastasis at the transverse osteotomy, since otherwise bony consolidation may be delayed. Conversely, even relatively large bone defects on the medial surface of the femur do not require insertion of bone shavings because spontaneous ossification occurs more rapidly here than on the lateral surface.

The bony lid is generally fixed by tightening the overlying muscle on the lateral surface of the prosthesis. Occasionally, however, the bony lid has a tendency to slip onto the anterior surface of the prosthesis. This phenomenon should always be checked. If the position is unstable, the bony lid must be fixed with sutures or with a wire cerclage. After insertion of suction drains, the fascia lata is tightly closed. The leg is then placed in a foam splint. To relax the soft tissues, the leg should be placed in slight external rotation during the first 10 days and the hip flexed at no more than 60°.

Postoperative treatment is the same as after a primary implantation. From the first day the patient is seated beside the bed three times daily, from the third day walking exercises with two elbow crutches are instituted, and after 2 weeks stair-climbing is practised. Depending on the radiograph findings, load-bearing is increased after 6–8 weeks and normal load-bearing begins after 10–12 weeks (Fig. 9.14).

Results

Even with major bone defects in the femur, the rapid restoration of function and bone defect is very impressive, even in elderly

Fig. 9.14

Typical example of a femoral revision in a 59-year-old female. (a) Loosening of the femoral prosthesis 5 years after cemented revision. (b) Three weeks after second revision through the transfemoral approach using an uncemented femoral revision prosthesis. (c) Three years after the second revision. The radiographs in two planes demonstrate the amount of spontaneous bone repair.

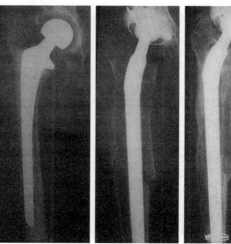
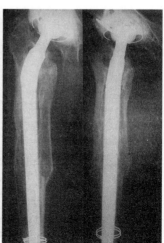

a   b   c

patients. Complications are rare. One important precondition is careful preoperative planning involving the selection of the correct prosthesis size. The determination of the correct stem diameter, in particular, is of major significance in conical fixation to prevent the prosthesis from subsiding. It should be realized that the subsidence of a conical prosthesis stem is nearly always the result of undersizing the stem diameter. If one is aware of this phenomenon, subsidence can be reliably avoided.

The findings in patients on whom we have operated show such a wide range of variation, both as far as the bone defect is concerned, which ranges from slight to excessive, and the general medical status in younger and very old subjects, that it is not possible to compare all the results with one another. Therefore, in evaluating the results, we have only included those parameters that are important for assessing a cementless replacement prosthesis (Table 9.1).

Between 1986 and 1994, we implanted 389 revision prostheses. An analysis has been carried out on our first closed series of 76 hips, operated upon between 1989 and 1992 using the same surgical technique, so as to ensure a sufficiently long postoperative observation period.

In 41 of the 76 hips, the change in prosthesis was undertaken by the transfemoral approach. Subsidence of the prosthesis was not a major problem. In 69 of the 76 hips, no subsidence was measured, four prostheses showed subsidence of less than 5 mm, and three showed subsidence of more than 5 mm. Therefore in this first series, before we had acquired any long-term experience, a total of seven prostheses were subject to subsidence. Subsequently, subsidence has been more infrequent.

Complications

The most common general surgical complication (Table 9.2) was haematoma formation (seven cases). Two patients suffered a reversible partial paralysis of the peroneal nerve. One old patient sustained a fracture of the lateral femoral condyle following a fall and required surgical treatment. In one patient, despite heparin prophylaxis and early mobilization, a pulmonary embolism occurred without sequelae. All operations were carried out in a sterile cabin under vertical airflow and no wound infections occurred. There were no fatal complications.

Table 9.1 Hip revisions between 1989 and 1992 ($n = 76$)

Transfemoral approach	41 hips
Subsidence	
0 mm	69 hips
<5 mm	4 hips
>5 mm	3 hips

Table 9.2 Surgical complications in hip revisions between 1989 and 1992 ($n = 76$)

Haematoma aspiration	7
Peroneal nerve paralysis	2
Fall: fracture of lateral femoral condyle	1
Pulmonary embolism	1
Wound infection	0
Lethal complications	0

Table 9.3 Prosthetic complications in hip revisions between 1989 and 1992 ($n = 76$)

Subsidence	7
Delayed consolidation with the transfemoral approach	4
Ectopic ossification	3
Dislocation	2

The most common complication related to the prosthesis (Table 9.3) was subsidence of the stem (discussed above), which occurred in seven cases. Delayed bone consolidation, which was obviously due to insufficient fixation of the bony lid, was observed in four hips with the transfemoral approach, but ultimately consolidation was obtained without any further measures being taken. Dislocation of the prosthesis occurred in two hips in the second postoperative week in two excessively active patients. This condition was corrected by a single closed repositioning in each case. Brooker class II ectopic ossification occurred in three hips in which there was no soft-tissue ossification before the revision.

References

1 Grunig R, Morscher E, Ochsner PE: Three- to 7-year results with the uncemented SL femoral revision prosthesis. *Archives of Orthopaedic and Traumatic Surgery* **116**: 187–97, 1997.
2 Hartwig CH, Böhm P, Czech U, Reize P, Küsswetter W: The Wagner revision stem in alloarthroplasty of the hip. *Archives of Orthopaedic and Traumatic Surgery* **115**: 5–9, 1996.
3 Kolstad K: Revision THR after periprosthetic femoral fractures. An analysis of 23 cases *Acta Orthopaedica Scandinavica* **65**: 505–8, 1994.
4 Michelinakis E, Papapolychronolon T, Vafiadis J: The use of a cementless femoral component for the management of bone loss in revision hip arthroplasty. *Bulletin of the Hospital for Joint Disease* **55**: 28–32, 1996.
5 Ponziani L, Rollo G, Bungaro P, Pascarella R, Zinghi GF: Revision of the femoral prosthetic component according to the Wagner technique. *Chirurgia degli Organi di Movimento* **80**: 385–9, 1995.
6 Stoffelen DV, Broos PL: The use of the Wagner revision prosthesis in complex (post) traumatic conditions of the hip. *Acta Orthopaedica Belgica* **61**: 135–9, 1995.

7 Wagner H: Revisionsprothese für das Hüftgelenk. *Orthopäde* **18**: 438–53, 1989.

8 Wehrli U: Wagner-Revisionsprothesenschaft. *Zeitschrift für Unfallchirurgie, Versicherungsmedizin und Berufskrankheiten* **84**: 216–24, 1991.

9 Engelbrecht DJ, Weber FA, Sweet MBE, Jakim I: Long term results of revision total hip arthroplasty. *Journal of Bone and Joint Surgery* [Br] **72**: 41–5, 1990.

10 Franzén H, Mjöberg B, Önnerfält R: Early loosening of femoral components after cemented revision. *Journal of Bone and Joint Surgery* [Br] **74**: 721–4, 1992.

11 Retpen JB, Varmarken J-E, Röck ND, Jensen JS: Unsatisfactory results after repeated revision of hip arthroplasty. *Acta Orthopaedica Scandinavica* **63**: 120–7, 1992.

12 Strömberg CN, Herberts P, Palmertz B: Cemented revision hip arthroplasty. *Acta Orthopaedica Scandinavica* **63**: 111–19, 1992.

13 Schenk RK, Wehrli U: Zur Reaktion des Knochens auf eine zementfreie SL-Femur-Revisionsprothese. Histologische Befunde an einem fünfeinhalb Monate postoperationem gewonnenen Autopsiepräparat. *Orthopäde* **18**: 454–62, 1989.

14 Wagner H, Wagner M: Conical stem fixation for cementless hip prostheses for primary implantation and revisions. In *Endoprosthetics* (ed. EW Morscher), pp. 258–67. Springer-Verlag, Berlin, 1995.

15 Rinaldi E, Marenghi P, Vaienti E: The Wagner prosthesis for femoral reconstruction by transfemoral approach *Chirurgia degli Organi di Movimento* **79**: 353–6, 1994.

16 Kolstad K, Adalberth G, Mallmin H, Milbrink J, Sahlstedt B: The Wagner revision stem for severe osteolysis. 31 hips followed for 1.5–5 years. *Acta Orthopaedica Scandinavica* **67**: 541–4, 1996.

17 Weill D, Scarlat M: La prothèse fémorale de révision de Wagner: à propos d'une série personnelle de 40 implantations. *Annales Orthopédiques de l'Ouest* **27**: 105–8.

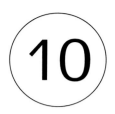

Bearing surfaces in total hip replacements: state of the art and future development

Harry A. McKellop

Mechanisms, damage, and modes of wear

To understand and compare the wear performance of bearing materials, it is convenient to define some key terms relating to the tribology of artificial joints. For joint replacements, it is most meaningful to define wear as the *removal* of material from the bearing surfaces in the form of wear particles, since the intensity of the biological reaction is a function of the rate of release of this debris. This is to distinguish wear from damage, which, in the orthopaedic literature, typically refers to visible changes in the surface of the bearings ('polishing', 'scratching', etc.)[1,2] which may or may not be accompanied by actual wear (Fig. 10.1). Wear is caused by fundamental mechanisms which include adhesion, abrasion, and fatigue.[3]

Adhesive wear occurs if the bond strength of microcontacts (e.g. between the polyethylene of the cup and the metal of the ball) exceeds the inherent strength of either material. Typically, polyethylene is pulled from the surface, forming fibrils and/or small pits. When adhesive wear occurs on a micron or submicron scale, the bearing surface still can appear highly polished to the eye.[4-7] Nevertheless, the billions of wear particles that are released into the tissues annually[6,8] are the driving force behind progressive osteolysis.[9-13]

Abrasive wear occurs when a hard projection on one surface cuts a scratch on the opposing surface during sliding. These projections can include the edge of an existing scratch, protruding carbides, embedded third-body particles, or even original contaminants that were exposed by the wear process itself. As with adhesive wear, abrasive scratching may be visible to the eye. However, if it occurs on a microscopic scale, the surfaces may appear very smooth (i.e. 'undamaged'), even though substantial wear has occurred. This is analogous to sanding a piece of wood with very fine sandpaper. The wood appears progressively smoother precisely because of the substantial amount of abrasive wear occurring.

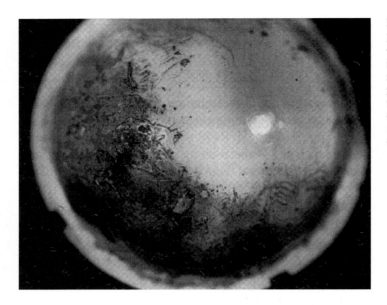

Fig. 10.1
Polyethylene acetabular cup worn *in vivo* (stained with ink to emphasize the morphology), showing highly polished area corresponding to high wear but low visible damage, and damaged area (scratches, pits, etc.) corresponding to low wear.

Fatigue wear is cracking, pitting, and/or delamination caused by cyclic stresses applied to the bearing surface. Again, this can occur on a micron scale, when it is almost invisible to the eye, or on a millimeter scale, resulting in visible damage to the implant.

Corrosion of a metal component and **oxidation** of a polyethylene component are not wear mechanisms *per se*, but they can substantially lower the wear resistance of the material.

Any number of these wear mechanisms may operate while the prosthesis is functioning in one of the following four distinct wear modes.[3,6]

- Mode 1 corresponds to articulation between two bearing surfaces only, which is necessary for the prosthesis to function.
- Mode 2 corresponds to articulation between a bearing surface and a non-bearing surface, for example, if the femoral ball penetrates the polyethylene liner (after excessive mode 1 wear) and contacts the metal backing.
- Mode 3 wear corresponds to motion between two bearing surfaces, but with third-body abrasive contaminants present.
- Mode 4 wear corresponds to motion between two non-bearing surfaces, such as 'backside' wear between the inside of a metal acetabular shell and the outside of the polyethylene liner, or fretting of the Morse taper junction between the ball and the stem.

Porous coated prostheses which tend to shed particles are particularly susceptible to mode 3 wear, and the loaded interfaces between the components of a modular prosthesis provide additional opportunities for mode 4 wear. Furthermore, the debris produced in mode

4 wear may induce local osteolysis, or it can migrate to the bearing surfaces, initiating mode 3 wear. Ideally, bearing surfaces for prosthetic joints should have high wear resistance under both ideal conditions (mode 1) and adverse conditions (modes 2, 3, and 4).

Metal–metal bearings

The first widely used total hip replacements featured cobalt–chromium alloy bearing against itself, primarily the McKee–Farrar design[14], as well as the Mueller, Ring, and other designs.[15–18] Owing to a relatively high rate of early failure, the first-generation metal–metal hips were largely supplanted by the Charnley prosthesis, which featured a stainless-steel ball and a polyethylene socket.[19] However, in hindsight, it has become apparent that a large percentage of the early failures of the McKee–Farrar hips occurred in implants from a single supplier, and involved relatively thin acetabular shells and a small ball–cup clearance, possibly leading to distortion of the cups under physiological loading, jamming, excessively high frictional torque, and rapid wear.[15,16,20–22] Disregarding the early failures, the long-term survivorship of the early metal–metal designs has been comparable to that of the metal–polyethylene Charnley prosthesis.[15,16,23,24] In particular, the steady state wear rates have been of the order of a few microns per year[17,25,26] compared with an average of $100-200$ μm of polyethylene wear per year typically reported for metal–polyethylene hips.[27–32]

In view of the growing awareness of the problem of extensive osteolysis caused by polyethylene wear debris, a number of second-generation metal–metal implants have been developed, including conventional total hips and surface replacements.[33–35] The first to be widely used clinically was the Metasul™ hip,[16,36–38] which recently received US Food and Drug Administration (FDA) approval for use in the USA. Hip simulator studies[39,40–42] and clinical retrievals[37,43,44] of modern metal–metal bearings also have typically shown steady state wear rates of the order of a few microns per million cycles (with a million cycles being the equivalent of about a year's use in a patient of average activity[45]). It is also apparent that metal–metal bearings have the ability to 'self-heal', i.e. to polish out isolated surface scratches caused by third-body particles or subluxation damage.[26,46] The overall clinical performance of second-generation metal–metal hips to date has been comparable with that of conventional metal–polyethylene hips, and somewhat better than that of first-generation metal–metal hips.[37,47]

Clinical and laboratory wear studies have indicated that metal–metal bearings often exhibit 10 to 20 times greater 'wear-in' during the initial 1–2 years of clinical use (Fig. 10.2), or one to two million cycles in a hip simulator.[37,39,40,41,43] In addition, some first- and second-generation metal–metal bearings have exhibited

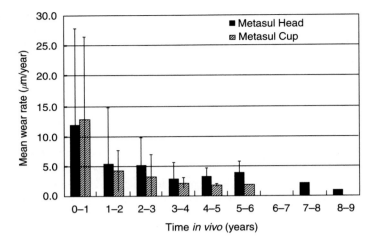

Fig.10.2

Wear rate for retrieved second-generation metal–metal hip prostheses.[43] The decrease in wear rate after the initial wear-in phase has also been observed in hip simulator studies of metal–metal bearings (see text).

extensive surface micropitting, possibly due to a fatigue-corrosion mechanism associated with the smaller carbides.[43,46,48] Although the high wear-in rate is a transitory phenomenon and the presence of the micropits does not appear to be associated with a high wear rate,[43] they represent areas for potential improvement of metal–metal implants.

Ceramic–ceramic bearings

Alumina–alumina bearings

As with metal–metal bearings, the earliest designs of alumina–alumina hip bearings often had unacceptably high wear rates.[49–55] The American experience with ceramic–ceramic bearings primarily involved the Autophor and Xenophor prostheses, which were first developed and used in Europe by Mittlemeier.[50] The clinical results with the Autophor were subject to greater problems of pain, neck–socket impingement, ceramic fracture, and component loosening than were experienced with contemporary metal–polyethylene designs, and ceramic–ceramic implants were never widely used in the USA.[52,56] The causes of high wear included poor-quality ceramic (by today's standards), edge contact of the cup on the ball due to inadequate range of motion and/or vertical cup placement, and other design shortcomings. For example, hips with a lateral opening of less than 30° or more than 55° and/or a high neck–shaft angle (i.e. more than about 140°) were at greater risk for neck–socket impingement and/or high wear as a result of increased contact stress.[57]

Fortunately, the past two decades have seen substantial improvement in prosthesis design, implantation technique, and, most importantly, the quality of the alumina.[53,57,58,59] Changes in the latter have included higher purity, finer grain structure, and improved sintering techniques. Hip simulator studies and clinical retrievals have indicated that the steady state wear rate of alumina–alumina bearings can be as low as 1–2 μm per year, i.e. even lower than for metal–metal bearings.[60–64]

However, modern alumina–alumina bearings are not immune from high wear.[65–67] For example, one study[68] recently reported severe wear and osteolysis in 22 per cent of patients after an average of only 7.7 years follow-up. While the causes of such unusually rapid wear in alumina–alumina bearings are the subject of continuing study,[57,69] these results emphasize the importance of observing proper operative technique with ceramic–ceramic bearings.[53,58] For example, edge-chipping of ceramic balls or cups during insertion can be avoided by careful alignment of the components prior to assembly.[67,70]

Gross fracture of a ceramic bearing component in the patient is a catastrophic failure, and the surgeon performing the revision procedure can be faced with a difficult decision. If a new ceramic ball is placed on a damaged Morse taper, there is a much greater chance of fracture of the new ball.[71,72] On the other hand, if a metal ball is used in the revision, fragments of ceramic that are left in the tissues may subsequently become trapped between the ball and cup and initiate extremely rapid wear of the ball and massive metallosis.[71,73,74] From the perspective of preventing wear, the safest option is to replace the femoral stem and use a new ceramic ball on a new taper; however, this can also be problematic if the stem is well fixed in the femur.

Fortunately, improvements in the quality of the alumina ceramic, particularly through hot isostatic pressing (Table 10.1), have lead to a reduction in the rate of fracture to as low as one or two in 10 000 patients,[53,75,76] a risk which must be weighed against the potential benefits of the very low wear and high biocompatability of alumina–alumina bearings.

Ceramic–ceramic bearings involving zirconia

As the outside diameter of a femoral ball is reduced (e.g. from 32 to 28 to 22 mm), it becomes progressively thinner adjacent to the Morse taper. Thus, many surgeons are reluctant to use 22-mm

Table 10.1 Physical properties of alumina and zirconia

Property	Alumina (sintered in air)	Alumina (hipped)	Zirconia (Y-TZP)
Grain size (μm)	3	1.8	<0.5
Density (g/cm³)	≥3.96	≥3.98	>6.00
Modulus (GPa)	380	380	210
Bending strength (MPa)	>500	>500	>950
Fracture toughness (MPa m$^{1/2}$)	4	4	8

Data from Früh et al.[85]

alumina balls. Owing to its finer grain structure, yttria-stabilized zirconia ceramic (Y-TZP, where TZP refers to tetragonal zirconia polycrystals) is about 73 per cent stronger than alumina (Table 10.1) and therefore provides a greater margin of safety, particularly with the smaller-diameter balls.[77-79] For example, one survey reported only two fractures of zirconia balls out of 300 000 implanted.[80] However, at high temperatures in a wet environment, Y-TZP zirconia can undergo a phase transformation that substantially weakens the material and roughens the surface, degrading its wear properties.[81-83] Thus, although zirconia is highly stable at physiological temperatures,[80,84] Y-TZP zirconia components should not be steam autoclaved.

To date, zirconia has been used primarily as a femoral ball articulating against a polyethylene acetabular cup (see below). The advisability of using Y-TZP zirconia balls against alumina or zirconia cups is a subject of controversy. Laboratory studies using a washer-on-flat test configuration have reported severe wear of zirconia–zirconia and zirconia–alumina pairs,[85,86] possibly due to a temperature-induced degradation of the zirconia. In contrast, other investigators using pin-on-disk machines and hip simulators[87,88] have observed very low wear of zirconia–alumina and zirconia–zirconia combinations. It seems likely that the differences in outcome of these studies were related to differences in the specimen configuration, the access of the lubricant to the bearing surfaces, and the type of lubricant used, resulting in substantial differences in the maximum temperatures generated. In particular, tests run in water gave severe wear of the zirconia, whereas tests run in serum did not. Thus the clinical use of Y-TZP zirconia bearing against alumina or itself remains controversial, as do the optimal conditions for laboratory wear testing of ceramic–ceramic bearings.

Most recently, ceramics have been fabricated using a mixture of zirconia and alumina in various ratios. The resultant mixed-oxide materials appear to combine the high strength of zirconia with the thermal stability of alumina, and preliminary wear tests on a pin-on-disk machine and a hip joint simulator have indicated excellent wear resistance.[89-91] Although clinical trials of alumina–alumina bearings have been underway in the USA for several years, none of the ceramic–ceramic bearing combinations have yet received FDA approval.

Materials bearing against polyethylene

Metal–polyethylene bearings

The metals used in conjunction with polyethylene have principally included stainless steel, cobalt–chromium alloy (in the vast majority), and titanium alloy. In some cases, the metal components have been surface hardened by, for example, nitriding or ion implantation. In general, the wear rate of polyethylene against stainless steel has been comparable with that against cobalt–chrome alloy in both laboratory tests[92,93] and clinical use.[94-97] In contrast, while the wear rate of polyethylene against titanium alloy under *clean* conditions appears to be comparable with that of the other metals,[98,99] the greater vulnerability of titanium alloy to abrasion by entrapped third-body particles can cause severe runaway wear.[100-102] Hardening of the surface of the titanium alloy by techniques such as gas nitriding, solution nitriding, or ion implanting can markedly improve its resistance to abrasion by third-body particles, and good 10-year results have been reported for titanium-nitride-hardened titanium–aluminium–niobium alloy balls used with polyethylene cups.[103] Nevertheless, if a hardened surface is eventually penetrated, severe wear of the underlying alloy still can be triggered.[102,104-106] Consequently, even hardened titanium alloys have seen limited clinical use as bearing surfaces.

The vast majority of metal–polyethylene bearings used in hip prostheses have involved cobalt–chrome alloy femoral balls, including cast or forged alloys, and the wear rate of this combination now forms the clinical baseline against which potentially improved bearing combinations are evaluated. As noted above, the *average* wear rate of the polyethylene against cobalt–chrome alloy is typically reported to be in the range of 0.1–0.2 mm per year. However, it should be noted that this average includes those implants which have accelerated wear rates due to excessive third-body damage to the bearing surfaces, radiation-induced oxidative degradation of the polyethylene, or other causes.[106,107] Thus, the *inherent* wear rate of a polyethylene cup with a cobalt–chrome alloy ball under clean conditions (as are usually modelled in a hip simulator) is probably somewhat below the clinical average wear rate, possibly as low as 0.05 mm per year.

Ion implanting and other surface-hardening techniques have also been applied to cobalt–chromium alloy. Laboratory tests of hardened cobalt–chromium alloy have reported both markedly reduced wear and increased wear of the opposing polyethylene,[106] and clinical results are not yet sufficient to resolve this contradiction. While it seems likely that surface hardening of cobalt–chrome may improve its resistance to moderate amounts of third-body abrasion, the uncertainty of the advantage in general has limited its clinical application.

Ceramic–polyethylene bearings

Alumina and zirconia femoral balls have been widely used as bearing surfaces against polyethylene cups, and the majority of clinical studies have shown substantially lower polyethylene wear rates than with metal balls, with wear ratios ranging from 0.75 to as low as 0.25 with alumina balls,[53,106] and a comparable advantage reported with zirconia against polyethylene.[108] However, one recent radiographic study reported little difference in the wear of polyethylene with alumina or metal balls,[97] as did one study of four retrieved alumina implants.[109] Another study reported unacceptably high rates of polyethylene wear, lysis, and loosening with an early type of zirconia ball.[83] Similarly, while the majority of the laboratory tests have indicated lower wear of polyethylene with alumina or zirconia than with metal,[106] one hip simulator study reported slightly greater polyethylene wear with alumia balls, but less with zirconia balls.[110]

Although the reasons for this disagreement among both clinical and laboratory studies are not clear, it may be due in part to the influence of third-body particles. That is, the greater hardness of ceramic balls renders them more resistant than metal balls to scratching by entrapped abrasive contaminants which can, in turn, accelerate the wear of the opposing polyethylene cup (mode 3 wear). Therefore the differences in the relative wear rates in the various clinical studies might reflect differences in the amount of third-body contamination, with those studies having relatively little such contamination showing comparable polyethylene wear rates for ceramic or metal balls (as in the laboratory tests run under clean conditions). Nevertheless, contamination by metal particles may be detrimental even with a ceramic ball, since the particles can adhere to the surface of the ceramic, effectively roughening it and thereby increasing abrasion of the polyethylene. Metal can also be transferred to the ceramic by contact against metallic components or instruments during surgery.[61] Regardless of the bearing material used, care must be taken to minimize the formation of abrasive contaminants *in vivo*, such as avoiding those porous coatings that are prone to shed particles.

Improved polyethylenes

Historical polyethylenes and the effects of air sterilization by gamma radiation

The ultrahigh molecular weight polyethylenes (UHMWPEs) that were used for acetabular cups implanted during the past 30 years were fabricated from raw powder (or 'resin') from a variety of manufacturers. At present, there are just two suppliers (Table 10.2).[111-113] The powder is converted to solid form using one of three distinct methods. In the **extrusion** process, the polyethylene powder is driven by a ram through a heated nozzle, fusing the flakes into a continuous bar typically several inches in diameter. The components are machined from the bar stock. In **bulk compression moulding**, the powder is placed in a large mould and heated under pressure to fuse it into a block or sheet, from which the final components are machined. In **net-shape moulding**, the powder is placed in a metal mould having the desired shape of the implant and then fused under heat and pressure, so that little or no final machining is required.

Table 10.2 UHMWPE resins presently available

Type	Supplier	Average molecular weight ($\times 10^6$ g/mol)	Contains calcium stearate?
GUR 1150	Ticona*	5.5–6	Yes
GUR 1050	(Germany)	5.5–6	No
GUR 1120		3.5	Yes
GUR 1020		3.5	No
1900	Montell	4.4–4.9	No
1900H	(USA)	>4.9	No

*Ticona was formerly known as Hoechst, and the Hoechst UHMWPEs produced in the USA prior to 1998 were GUR 4150/4050/4120/4020, with properties corresponding to the first four entries in the table respectively. *Data from* Kurtz et al.[113]

Whichever fabrication process is used, the final step is sterilization. Although ethylene oxide sterilization was used initially, and gas plasma more recently,[114–116] the great majority of polyethylene components implanted during the past 25 years or more were sterilized by exposure to gamma radiation, at a dose somewhere between 2.5 and 4 Mrad, and were sealed in air during irradiation and subsequent storage. Ethylene oxide and gas plasma sterilization have relatively little effect on the physical properties of polyethylene. In contrast, an extensive amount of research, particularly during the past 5 years, has shown that both gamma sterilization in air and extended storage in air have a marked effect on the physical properties of UHMWPE components (Fig. 10.3). Near the surface of the component, free radicals generated by the radiation combine with oxygen that has diffused into the polymer during the period between fabrication and irradiation. Depending on how much oxygen is present, there may be immediate oxidative degradation and very little cross-linking of the surface layer. Beneath the level of diffused oxygen, free radicals that are generated by the radiation in the amorphous regions of the polyethylene rapidly combine to form cross-links. In contrast, free radicals generated in the crystalline regions are far less mobile but can eventually migrate to the amorphous regions and combine with any oxygen that has diffused to that depth. This oxidative degradation of the polyethylene could continue for years during shelf-storage and, to a lesser extent,[117,118] during use *in vivo*. Oxidation leads to extensive chain scission, weakening and embrittling the polyethylene and directly reduces its resistance to wear, delamination, and fracture. In addition, oxidation can indirectly reduce wear resistance by reducing the level of cross-linking.[119]

While, as discussed below, gamma-induced cross-linking can markedly improve the wear resistance of UHMWPE (Fig. 10.4), excessive cross-linking can adversely affect other physical properties

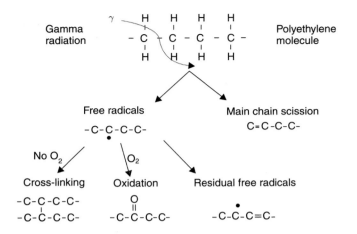

Fig. 10.3

Effect of radiation on the UHMWPE molecule. The radiation (gamma or electron-beam) causes chain scission and creates free radicals. In the absence of oxygen, the free radicals tend to form cross-links between adjacent molecules in the amorphous regions, improving wear resistance. Oxygen molecules present in the polyethylene, particularly near the surface, can combine with free radicals to cause chain scission, decreasing the strength, toughness, and wear resistance. Free radicals can remain trapped in the crystalline regions of the polyethylene for many years, eventually migrating to the amorphous regions and contributing to oxidative degradation. Free radicals can be neutralized very rapidly by heating above the 'melt' temperature (crystalline–amorphous transition), or much more slowly by annealing below the melt temperature.

such as ultimate strength, elongation, and fracture toughness.[120–123] However, studies of retrieved implants have demonstrated that weakening of the polyethylene due to immediate and long-term oxidation could be substantially greater than that due to the moderate level of cross-linking induced by the 2.5–4 Mrad of irradiation used for routine sterilization.[117,124–129] Consequently, alterations in the methods for fabricating and sterilizing UHMWPE components in the past few years have been directed at minimizing oxidative degradation while simultaneously optimizing the level of cross-linking to improve wear resistance.

Alternative sterilization techniques

In one approach to minimizing oxidative degradation, some manufacturers now sterilize the polyethylene components *without* irradiation, using either ethylene oxide or gas plasma.[113] Since these methods do not generate free radicals in the polyethylene, they completely avoid the potential for immediate and long-term oxidative degradation of the mechanical properties and wear resistance. However, since ethylene oxide or gas plasma do not induce cross-linking, they do not take advantage of its potential for improving the wear resistance of the polyethylene.

Other manufacturers continue to sterilize their implants with gamma radiation, but with the polyethylene components sealed in some type of low-oxygen atmosphere, including vacuum[130] and inert gas,[131] or with an oxygen scavenger.[132] In addition, one manufacturer anneals the polyethylene acetabular cups *after* sterilization by heating them in the nitrogen packaging at 37–50 °C (i.e. well below the melt temperature of 135 °C to avoid distorting the components) for about 6 days to reduce the level of residual free radicals induced by the gamma radiation.[133] These approaches can markedly reduce but not necessarily eliminate the oxidation that would otherwise occur during gamma sterilization and subsequent

Fig. 10.4

Reduction in wear with increased level of cross-linking. The curves for the two gamma cross-linked polyethylenes were produced on hip joint simulators in two different laboratories.[120,121] The curves for the two electron-beam cross-linked polyethylenes were produced on a bi-directional pin-on-disk machine in a third laboratory.[122,154] Since two wear machines may produce different wear magnitudes for the same material, for example due to differences in the applied load and/or the sliding distance per cycle, the original data were normalized by dividing by the wear rate for zero radiation (no cross-linking) obtained in each test.

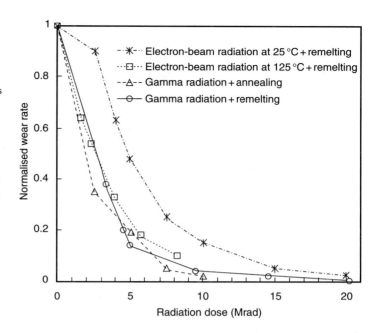

shelf-storage,[129,134] and the remaining free radicals may induce some oxidation during long-term use *in vivo*. Furthermore, since the level of cross-linking is limited to the 2.5–4 Mrad gamma dose used to sterilize the components, the improvement in wear resistance (as exhibited in laboratory wear tests) relative to non-cross-linked polyethylene ranges from about 30 to 50 per cent, compared to the reduction of 85 per cent or more achieved with elevated cross-linking doses, as described below.

In retrospective studies of shelf-stored and/or retrieved implants, some sets of components which were fabricated from block-moulded or net-shape-moulded polyethylene, gamma sterilized, and stored in air have undergone substantially lower levels of oxidation than similarly treated extruded–machined components. It has been suggested that the moulded polyethylene was more completely fused than typical extruded material, rendering it more resistant to diffusion of oxygen and therefore more resistant to immediate and long-term oxidative degradation, despite the presence of free radicals.[127,135] Consequently, several suppliers have reintroduced net-shape moulding of components. Specialized moulding techniques include hot isostatic pressing of the polyethylene powder in an argon atmosphere[136] and special moulding protocols which can provide polyethylene with a specified crystallinity and stiffness.[113,137] However, manufacturers no longer irradiate and store polyethylene in air, and so the marked differences in oxidation levels that occurred between moulded and extruded–machined components in the past may not exist under current techniques of manufacturing

259

and use. Furthermore, while moulded polyethylene may have superior resistance to oxidation, this fabrication technique alone does not address cross-linking of the polyethylene to improve its wear resistance.

Clinical studies of polyethylenes with elevated levels of cross-linking

As noted above, the moderate level of cross-linking present in the vast majority of UHMWPE components implanted over the past three decades was an *unintentional* byproduct of the 2.5–4 Mrad of gamma radiation used to sterilize the components. Nevertheless, *intentional* cross-linking has long been used to improve the wear resistance of polyethylene in industrial applications (e.g. in linings for coal chutes). In addition, polyethylene acetabular cups that had been intentionally cross-linked at levels much higher than occurs with routine sterilization have been used in three clinical studies performed over the past 25 years. Grobbelaar and colleagues[138,139] cross-linked finished polyethylene acetabular cups by exposing them to 10 Mrad of gamma radiation. By irradiating the cups while they were immersed in acetylene gas, cross-linking in the outermost 300 μm was increased substantially above what would normally occur at 10 Mrad. No post-irradiation thermal processing was done to reduce the residual free radicals. In anticipation of a lower wear rate, the cross-linked polyethylene was used with femoral balls of diameter 30 mm to reduce the incidence of dislocation which the investigators had experienced with 22-mm diameter heads. In a follow-up of 14–21 years based on radiographs, Grobbelaar *et al.*[139] reported a 'lack of measurable wear' in 56 of 64 cases and only two revisions due to osteolysis.

Oonishi *et al.*[140] induced very high levels of cross-linking by exposing finished cups to 100 Mrad of gamma radiation in air. As with Grobbelaar's method, there was no thermal treatment to extinguish free radicals. In a clinical follow-up of 6–8 years, they reported steady state wear rates of 247 μm and 98 μm per year for non-cross-linked polyethylene cups bearing against cobalt–chrome and alumina heads respectively, and 76 μm and 72 μm per year for 100 Mrad cross-linked polyethylene cups bearing against stainless steel and alumina balls respectively.[141] Subsequently, Oonishi *et al.*[142] reported that the long-term wear rates averaged 290 μm and 60 μm per year for the non-irradiated cups and cross-linked cups respectively. While this represented about a 79 per cent reduction, the average wear rate for the non-cross-linked cups was substantially above the range of 100–200 μm per year that has typically reported for gamma–air sterilized polyethylene cups in clinical studies.[106]

More recently, Wroblewski *et al.*[143] chemically cross-linked polyethylene cups using a silane process. After an initial higher rate of penetration (possibly due to greater creep), the average steady state wear rate in 19 patients with up to 8.3 years follow-up was only 22 μm per year for cross-linked cups bearing against alumina ceramic heads. While this was well below the clinical range for gamma–air cups, as with the study by Oonishi and colleagues, it was not clear how much of the advantage was due to cross-linking rather than ball material. Nevertheless, the results of these three clinical studies are encouraging in that, despite any reduction in strength relative to non-cross-linked polyethylene caused by the high levels of cross-linking and the absence of thermal treatment to extinguish free radicals in the gamma-cross-linked materials,[139,140] neither of the groups reported fractures or other mechanical failures in the cross-linked cups.

Intentionally cross-linked–thermally stabilized polyethylenes

Over the past few years, a number of laboratory wear simulations have demonstrated that the wear rate of UHMWPE cups decreases markedly with increasing level of radiation-induced cross-linking.[120–122] Although the baseline wear rate differed among various wear-testing machines because of systematic differences in the load, sliding distance per cycle, and other factors, the dose–wear curves obtained by different laboratories and with different cross-linking techniques were remarkably consistent. The greatest reduction per unit dose occurred as the dose increased from zero to about 5 Mrad, with progressively less improvement at higher doses, and no additional benefit after 15–20 Mrad (Fig. 10.4). While this dose–wear relationship was the basis for the recent development of a variety of intentionally cross-linked polyethylenes, the developers have arrived at very different opinions regarding the appropriate dose and other processing parameters for optimizing the clinical performance of a polyethylene implant. The fabrication and characteristics of these new intentionally cross-linked polyethylenes are described below and are summarized in Table 10.3.

Marathon™ gamma cross-linked and remelted polyethylene

In the Marathon™ process,[121,144–146] extruded bars of UHMWPE are cross-linked by exposing them to 5 Mrad of gamma radiation. The bars are then heated to 155 °C for 24 hours, followed by slow cooling to room temperature. When polyethylene is heated above the melt temperature, it is transformed from a partially crystalline solid to a totally amorphous solid. Since the uncombined free radicals generated during the gamma irradiation are trapped primarily in the crystalline regions,[147] heating above the melt temperature

261

Table 10.3 Comparison of new cross-linked thermally stabilized polyethylenes

Name (manufacturer)	FDA approved? (June 2000)	Radiation type and dose	Thermal stabilization	Final sterilization	Manufacturer's rationale
Marathon™ (DePuy Inc.)	Yes	Gamma radiation to 5 Mrad at room temperature	Remelted at 155°C for 24h	Gas plasma	5 Mrad gamma cross-linking provides about 85 per cent wear reduction (well below the threshold for lysis) while preserving other mechanical properties. Remelting eliminates free radicals and prevents oxidative degradation
XLPE™ (Smith & Nephew– Richards Inc.)	Yes	Gamma radiation to 10 Mrad at room temperature	Remelted at 150°C for 2h	Ethylene oxide	5 Mrad gamma to provide wear reduction (wear data not yet available) while preserving other mechanical properties. Remelting eliminates free radicals and prevents oxidation
Longevity™ (Zimmer Inc.)	Yes	Electron beam radiation to 10 Mrad at warm room temperature	Remelted at 150°C for about 6h	Gas plasma	10 Mrad provides about 89 per cent wear reduction. Remelting eliminates free radicals and prevents oxidation
Durasul™ (Sulzer Inc.)	Yes	Electron beam radiation to 9.5 Mrad at 125°C	Remelted at 150°C for about 2h	Ethylene oxide	9.5 Mrad provides >95 per cent wear reduction. Electron-beam cross-linking at elevated temperature provides more wear reduction than when performed at room temperature. Remelting eliminates free radicals and prevents oxidation

Crossfire™ (Stryker–Osteonics–Howmedica Inc.)	Yes	Gamma radiation to 7.5 Mrad at room temperature	Annealed at about 120°C for a proprietary duration	Gamma radiation at 2.5–3.5 Mrad while packaged in nitrogen	Depending on actual sterilization dose, total gamma cross-linking dose may vary from 10 to 11 Mrad, providing about 90 per cent wear reduction. Annealing provides a different balance of material properties than remelting. Resultant material has substantial free radicals, but oxidation is limited by sterilization and storage in nitrogen
Aeonian™ (Kyocera Inc.)	Approved in Japan Not yet in USA	Gamma radiation to 3.5 Mrad at room temperature	Annealed at 110°C for 10h	Gamma radiation at 2.5–4 Mrad while packaged in nitrogen	Depending on actual sterilization dose, total gamma cross-linking dose may vary from 6 to 7.5 Mrad. Wear data are not yet available. Annealing provides a different balance of material properties than remelting. Resultant material has substantial free radicals, but oxidation is limited by sterilization and storage in nitrogen

The processing parameters shown in this table were compiled from various publications and from information provided by the manufacturers, and are subject to ongoing modification.

releases them to combine with each other to form additional cross-links and, more importantly, to minimize the potential for long-term oxidative degradation.[121] The acetabular cup is then machined from the central portion of the cross-linked remelted bar (thereby removing the surface-oxidized material) and is sterilized using gas plasma rather than gamma radiation to avoid increasing the level of cross-linking or reintroducing residual free radicals. In addition to reducing wear under ideal clean test conditions by about 85 per cent (Fig. 10.4), Marathon™ has shown less wear than non-cross-linked polyethylene bearing against severely roughened femoral balls (i.e. modelling third-body abrasive wear).[144] Comparable results under morasive conditions have been obtained for two other cross-linked polyethylenes tested in hip simulators,[148,149] although greater wear of a cross-linked polyethyelene was observed in one pin-on-plate test configuration.[150]

XLPE™ gamma cross-linked and remelted polyethylene

XLPE™ is fabricated in much the same manner as Marathon™, except that 10 Mrad of gamma radiation is used and final sterilization is carried out with ethylene oxide.[151]

Longevity™ electron-beam cross-linked and remelted polyethylene

In the Longevity™ process, a compression-moulded sheet of UHMWPE is cross-linked by exposure to a 10-MeV electron beam.[152] After cross-linking, the polyethylene is heated above the melt temperature for about 2 hours to extinguish the free radicals, and is then machined into cups and sterilized with gas plasma.

Durasul™ electron-beam cross-linked and remelted polyethylene

The Durasul™ process is similar to the Longevity™ process, except that the polyethylene is machined into short segments or 'pucks' that are cross-linked from both sides with a 10-MeV electron beam to a total of 9.5 Mrad, in order to increase the uniformity of the cross-linking. In addition, the pucks are preheated to about 125°C while being electron-beam cross-linked since comparative tests have indicated that this provides greater wear resistance (Fig. 10.4) and less reduction of elongation to break and toughness than electron-beam cross-linking at room temperature.[153,154] In both processes, the electron beam drives the cross-linking energy into the polyethylene about 2500 times faster than with gamma radiation (i.e. in seconds rather than hours), which generates substantial heating of the polyethylene.[155] After cross-linking, the Durasul™ cups are remelted to remove free radicals and sterilized with ethylene oxide.[156]

Crossfire™ gamma cross-linked and annealed polyethylene

In the Crossfire™ process,[157] extruded bars of UHMWPE are cross-linked by exposure to 7.5 Mrad of gamma radiation. The bars are then annealed (rather than melted) by heating them to just below the melt temperature for a duration that is proprietary. Cups are then machined from the bars, sealed in nitrogen, and sterilized by exposure to an additional 2.5 Mrad of gamma radiation (i.e. to a total gamma dose of 10 Mrad). No thermal treatment to extinguish free radicals is applied after the final gamma sterilization.

The developers of the Crossfire™ process prefer annealing to remelting of the polyethylene on the grounds that it induces less change in 'material morphology and material properties' than does remelting.[157] However, since melting is used in the moulding or extruding processes to fuse the powder into a solid form, it is not clear that remelting has a deleterious effect on the properties of the polymer. In addition, because crystalline regions remain in the polyethylene unless it is heated above the melt temperature, annealing is not as effective as remelting in extinguishing the residual free radicals. Consequently, Crossfire™ polyethylene that was 'artificially aged' by being heated to 80 °C in air for 3 weeks underwent substantial oxidative degradation of its strength and wear resistance.[158] In contrast, artificial ageing has a negligible effect on radiation cross-linked polyethylenes that have been remelted to extinguish the residual free radicals.[158,159] As with other current gamma-sterilized polyethylenes, however, the manufacturer of Crossfire™ implants recommends that they be stored in the nitrogen-filled package, and for only a limited time prior to implantation. In view of this, the developers argue that any oxidative degradation of Crossfire™ implants will be far less than historically occurred in polyethylene components that were irradiated and stored in air or in artificially aged implants, so that it will have negligible effect on the clinical performance of the implants.[157] Careful clinical follow-up will be required to resolve these issues.

Aeonian™ gamma cross-linked and annealed polyethyene

Except for the use of a lower range of cross-linking dose (Table 10.3), the processing and rationale of Aenoian™ parallels that for Crossfire™.

Optimum method for cross-linking

The optimum amount of cross-linking to use is also a subject of current debate. Since increasing the level of cross-linking causes a progressively greater reduction in some mechanical properties, such as ultimate strength, ductility, fracture toughness, and fatigue strength,[121,123,160] one extreme is to avoid cross-linking altogether (e.g. by simply sterilizing with ethylene oxide or gas plasma) to retain the maximum values of strength, elongation, and fracture toughness, despite the fact that this results in substantially higher wear of the polyethylene.

Among those who advocate cross-linking, the particular dose used represents that manufacturer's approach to balancing reduced wear against the need to maintain other mechanical properties well above the level needed for acceptable clinical performance. Those using the high levels of cross-linking (9.5–11 Mrad, Table 10.3), about three to four times the typical dose used historically to sterilize polyethylene components, maintain that this is justified in order to obtain the additional 5–10 per cent improvement in wear over that provided by a moderate dose (Fig. 10.4), despite the corresponding reduction in other physical properties. In contrast, advocates of a moderate cross-linking dose (5 Mrad, Table 10.3) maintain that the corresponding reduction in wear to 85 per cent below that of a non-cross-linked polyethylene, if realized clinically, will be sufficient to avoid an osteolytic reaction in even the most active patients without unnecessarily reducing other physical properties.

Clearly, it is not desirable to use a dose that will result in mechanical failure of the polyethylene components. However, it is important to recall the following facts when considering the likelihood of failure of a cross-linked cup *in vivo*: (a) the vast majority of polyethylene cups implanted in the past were moderately cross-linked at gamma doses ranging from 2.5 to 4 Mrad; (b) this was done in air and without the benefit of post-irradiation thermal treatment, such that many of these cups were subject to immediate and long-term oxidative degradation; (c) this post-sterilization oxidative degradation caused a much greater loss in strength than the moderate level of cross-linking that was induced by the gamma sterilization.[128,135] Despite their being moderately cross-linked, very few cups used in the past 20–30 years fractured *in vivo* and, when fracture did occur, it was strongly associated with oxidative degradation of the polymer.[161] Therefore it is reasonable to predict that an acetabular cup that is moderately cross-linked *and* adequately stabilized against oxidative degradation will be even *less* likely to fracture than the gamma–air sterilized and oxidized cups that have been the clinical standard for the past three decades.

On the other hand, there is questionable justification for increasing the level of cross-linking substantially above that which is necessary to reduce the wear below the threshold for clinically significant lysis.[162] For example, in a 7-year minimum follow-up, Xenos et al.[163] found that, of the 85 patients without lysis, only 13

(15 per cent) had more than 2 mm of wear, and none exceeded 4 mm, whereas, of the 15 patients with lysis, five (33 per cent) had more than 2 mm of wear and three (20 per cent) exceeded 4 mm. Similarly, Devane et al.[164] reported that, after 4–7.2 years, those patients without lysis averaged a total radiographic wear depth of only 0.8 mm, while patients with lysis averaged 1.2 mm. Consistent with this, Nashed et al.[165] reported no lysis in a group of patients with a hip prosthesis that averaged 0.1 mm per year or less, 31 per cent in a group averaging 0.13 mm per year, 24 per cent in a group averaging 0.17 mm per year, and 87 per cent in a group averaging 0.25 mm per year. Similarly, Moreland and Moreno[166] reported that 'major' lysis was absent in patients without measurable radiographic cup wear, but was present in 3.5 per cent of patients with wear of up to 0.19 mm per year, 9 per cent of those with 0.2–0.39 mm per year, and 27 per cent of those with 0.4 mm per year or more. Wan and Dorr[167] found that osteolysis was more likely to be present in hips with polyethylene wear depths exceeding 0.2 mm per year.

Together, these studies show that clinically significant osteolysis is very rare in patients with polyethylene acetabular cups wearing less than about 0.1 mm (100 μm) per year. As noted above, while the inherent wear rate of UHMWPE (i.e. absent substantial oxidative degradation) may fall in the range of 0.05–0.1 mm per year in a patient with *average* activity, the most active patients walk three to four times times the average,[45] which would be sufficient to increase the wear rate of conventional polyethylene to as much as 0.4 mm per year, well into the range for clinical osteolysis. In contrast, the 85 per cent reduction provided by 5 Mrad of cross-linking (Fig. 10.4) would reduce the wear rate in such active patients to 0.06 mm per year or less, well below the threshold for lysis. Although increasing the dose as high as 10 Mrad provides some additional reduction in wear (Fig. 10.4), it also increases the risk of introducing new problems that were not encountered with the historical maximum of 4 Mrad used for routine sterilization of polyethylene components.

Conclusion

Since the UHMWPE components fabricated by the historical process of gamma sterilization in air are no longer marketed, a surgeon who wishes to continue performing joint replacement surgery must choose from the new polyethylenes or a modern metal–metal or ceramic–ceramic bearing, each of which has its potential advantages and disadvantages (Table 10.4). Ultimately, it is the responsibility of the surgeon to assess the risk–benefit ratios of each of the new bearing combinations and make an informed and wise choice among them.

Table 10.4 Overall advantages and disadvantages of current bearing choices

Bearing combination	Potential Advantages	Potential disadvantages
Alumina on alumina	Usually very low wear High biocompatilbility	Sometimes high wear Component fracture Higher cost Technique-sensitive surgery
Cobalt–chrome on cobalt–chrome	Usually low wear Can self-polish moderate surface scratches	Question of long-term local and systemic reactions to metal debris and/or ions
Hardened cobalt–chrome on polyethylene	Some additional protection against third-body abrasion	Hardened layer can wear off Higher cost
Ceramic on polyethylene	Lower wear of polyethylene than with conventional metal–polyethylene Some additional protection against third-body abrasion	Component fracture Difficulty of revision (i.e. if Morse taper is damaged) Higher cost
Polyethylene sterilized with ethylene oxide or gas plasma Polyethylene sterilized with gamma in low oxygen	No short- or long-term oxidation Some cross-linking Some wear reduction	No cross-linking so does not minimize polyethylene wear Polyethylene wear not minimized Residual free radicals (long-term oxidation?)
Cross-linked thermally stabilized polyethylene	Minimal polyethylene wear rate No short- or long-term oxidative degradation	Newest of low-wear bearing combinations; only early clinical results available Questions remain regarding optimum cross-linking level and optimum method for thermal stabilization (Table 10.3)

References

1 Rostoker W, Chao EYS, Galante J: The appearances of wear on poly-ethylene—a comparison of *in vivo* and *in vitro* wear surfaces. *Journal of Biomedical Materials Research* **12**: 317–35, 1978.
2 Hood RW, Wright TM, Burstein AH: Retrieval analysis of total knee prostheses: a method and its application to 48 total condylar pros-theses. *Journal of Biomedical Materials Research* **17**: 829–42, 1983.
3 McKellop HA: Wear modes, mechanisms, damage, and debris. Separating cause from effect in the wear of total hip replacements. In *Total hip revision surgery* (ed. JO Galante, AG Rosenberg, JJ Callaghan), pp. 21–39. Raven Press, New York, 1995.
4 Cooper JR, Dowson D, Fisher J: Macroscopic and microscopic wear mechanisms in ultra-high molecular weight polyethylene. *Wear* **162**: 378–84, 1993.
5 Jasty M, Bragdon C, Jiranek W *et al.*: Etiology of osteolysis around porous-coated cementless total hip arthroplasties. *Clinical Orthopaedics and Related Research* **308**: 111–26, 1994.

6 McKellop HA, Campbell P, Park SH *et al.*: The origin of submicron polyethylene wear debris in total hip arthroplasty. *Clinical Orthopaedics and Related Research* **311**: 3–20, 1995.

7 Wang A, Stark C, Dumbleton JH: Mechanistic and morphological origins of ultra-high molecular weight polyethylene wear debris in total joint replacement prostheses. *Proceedings of the Institute of Mechanical Engineers Part H: Journal of Engineering in Medicine* **210**: 141–55, 1996.

8 Clarke I, Kabo M: Wear in total hip replacement. In *Total hip arthroplasty* (ed. HC Amstutz), pp. 535–54. Churchill Livingstone, New York, 1992.

9 Willert H, Semlitsch M: Reactions of the articular capsule to wear products of artificial joint materials. *Journal of Biomedical Materials Research* **11**: 157–64, 1977.

10 Goldring SR, Jasty M, Roelke MS, Rourke CM: Formation of a synovial-like membrane at the bone–cement interface. Its role in bone resorption and implant loosening after total hip replacement. *Arthritis and Rheumatism* **29**: 836–42, 1986.

11 Howie DW, Vernon-Roberts B, Oakeshott R, Manthey B: A rat model of resorption of bone at the cement-bone interface in the presence of polyethylene wear particles. *Journal of Bone and Joint Surgery* [Am] **70**: 257–63, 1988.

12 Schmalzried TP, Jasty M, Harris WH: Periprosthetic bone loss in total hip arthroplasty. Polyethylene wear debris and the concept of the effective joint space. *Journal of Bone and Joint Surgery* [Am] **74**: 849–63, 1992.

13 Amstutz HC, Campbell P, Kossovsky N, Clarke I: Mechanisms and clinical significance of wear debris induced osteolysis. *Clinical Orthopaedics and Related Research* **276**: 7–18, 1992.

14 McKee GK, Watson-Farrar J: Replacement of arthritic hips by the McKee–Farrar prosthesis. *Journal of Bone and Joint Surgery* [Br] **48**: 245–59, 1966.

15 Amstutz HC, Grigoris P: Metal on metal bearings in hip arthroplasty. *Clinical Orthopaedics and Related Research* **329** (Supplement): S11–34, 1996.

16 Schmidt M, Weber H, Schon R: Cobalt chromium molybdenum metal combination for modular hip prostheses. *Clinical Orthopaedics and Related Research* **329** (Supplement): S35–47, 1996.

17 Willert HG, Buchhorn GH, Gobel D *et al.*: Wear behavior and histopathology of classic cemented metal on metal hip endoprostheses. *Clinical Orthopaedics and Related Research* **329** (Supplement): S160–86, 1996.

18 Scott ML, Lemons JE: The wear characteristics of Sivash/SRN Co-Cr-Mo THA articulating surfaces. In *Alternative bearing surfaces in total joint arthroplasty* (ed. JJ Jacobs, TL Craig), STP 1346, pp. 159–72. ASTM, West Conshohocken, PA, 1998.

19 Chamley J, Cupric Z: The nine and ten year results of the low-friction arthroplasty of the hip. *Clinical Orthopaedics and Related Research* **95**: 9–25, 1973.

20 Walker PS, Salvati E, Hotzler RK: The wear on removed McKee–Farrar total hip prostheses. *Journal of Bone and Joint Surgery* [Am] **56**: 92–100, 1974.

21 Semlitsch M, Streicher RM, Weber H: Long-term results with meta/metal pairings in artificial hip joints. In *Technical principles, design and safety of joint implants* (ed. GH Buchhorn, HG Willert), pp. 62–7. Hogrefe & Huber, Seattle, WA, 1994.

22 Poggie RA: A review of the effects of design, contact stress, and materials on the wear of metal-on-metal hip prostheses. In *Alternative*

bearing surfaces in total joint arthroplasty (ed. JJ Jacobs, TL Craig), STP 1346, pp. 47–54. ASTM, West Conshohocken, PA, 1998.

23 Jacobsson S-A, Kjerf K, Wahlstrom O: A comparative study between McKee–Farrar and Charnley arthroplasty with long term follow-up periods. *Journal of Arthroplasty* **5**: 9–14, 1990.

24 Schmalzried TP, Szuszczewicz ES, Akizuki KH, Petersen TD, Amstutz HC: Factors correlating with long term survival of McKee–Farrar total hip prostheses. *Clinical Orthopaedics and Related Research*: **329** (Supplement): S48–59, 1996.

25 Kothari M, Bartel DL, Booker JF: Surface geometry of retrieved McKee–Farrar total hip replacements. *Clinical Orthopaedics and Related Research* **329** (Supplement): S141–7, 1996.

26 McKellop H, Park S-H, Chiesa, R *et al*.: *In vivo* wear of 3 types of metal on metal hip prostheses during 2 decades of use. *Clinical Orthopaedics and Related Research* **329** (Supplement):128–40, 1996.

27 Griffith MJ, Seidenstein MK, Williams D, Charnley J: Socket wear in Charnley low friction arthroplasty of the hip. *Clinical Orthopaedics and Related Research* **137**: 37–47, 1978.

28 Rimnac CM, Wilson PD, Fuchs MD, Wright TM: Acetabular cup wear in total hip arthroplasty. *Orthopedic Clinics of North America* **19**: 631–6, 1988.

29 Shih CH, Lee PC, Chen JH *et al*: Measurement of polyethylene wear in cementless total hip arthroplasty. *Journal of Bone and Joint Surgery* 1997; 79-B: 361–5, 1997.

30 Schmalzried TP, Dorey FJ, McKellop H: The multifactorial nature of polyethylene wear *in vivo*. *Journal of Bone and Joint Surgery* [Am] **80**: 1234–43.

31 Sochart D: Relationship of acetabular wear to osteolysis and loosening in total hip arthroplasty. *Clinical Orthopaedics and Related Research* **363**: 135–50, 1999.

32 Yamaguchi M, Hashimoto Y, Akisue T, Bauer TW: Polyethylene wear vector *in vivo*: a three-dimensional analysis using retrieved acetabular components and radiographs. *Journal of Orthopaedic Research* **17**: 695–702, 1999.

33 Wagner M, Wagner H: Preliminary results of uncemented metal on metal stemmed and resurfacing hip replacement arthroplasty. *Clinical Orthopaedics and Related Research* **329** (Supplement): S78–88, 1996.

34 Schmalzried TP, Fowble VA, Ure KJ, Amstutz HC: Metal on metal surface replacement of the hip. Technique, fixation, and early results. *Clinical Orthopaedics and Related Research* **329** (Supplement): S106–14, 1996.

35 McMinn D, Treacy R, Lin K, Pynsent P: Metal on metal surface replacement of the hip. Experience of the McMinn prothesis. *Clinical Orthopaedics and Related Research* **329** (Supplement): 89–98, 1996.

36 Rieker C, Windler M, Wyss UE (ed.): *Metasul A metal-on-metal bearing*. Huber, Bern, 1999.

37 Weber BG: Experience with the Metasul total hip bearing system. *Clinical Orthopaedics and Related Research* **329** (Supplement): S69–77, 1996.

38 Dorr LD, Hilton KR, Wan Z, Markovich GD, Bloebaum R: Modern metal on metal articulation for total hip replacements. *Clinical Orthopaedics and Related Research* **333**: 108–17, 1996.

39 Streicher RM, Semlitsch M, Schon R, Weber H, Rieker C: Metal-on-metal articulation for artificial hip joints: laboratory study and

clinical results. *Proceedings of the Institution of Mechanical Engineers Part H: Journal of Engineering in Medicine* **210**: 223–32, 1996.

40 Medley JB, Chan FW, Krygier JJ, Bobyn JD: Comparison of alloys and designs in a hip simulator study of metal on metal implants *Clinical Orthopaedics and Related Research* **329** (Supplement): S148–59, 1996. [Published erratum appears in *Clinical Orthopaedics and Related Research*: **335**: 335–6, 1997.]

41 Chan FW, Bobyn JD, Medley JB, Krygier JJ, Tanzer M: The Otto Aufranc Award. Wear and lubrication of metal-on-metal hip implants. *Clinical Orthopaedics and Related Research* **369**: 10–24, 1999.

42 Rieker CB, Weber H, Schon R, Windler M, Wyss UP: Development of the Metasul articulations. In *Metasul A metal-on-metal bearing* (ed. C Rieker, M Windler, U Wyss), pp. 15–21. Huber, Bern, 1999.

43 Rieker C, Kottig P, Schon R, Windler M, Wyss UP: Clinical tribological performance of 144 metal-on-metal hip articulations. In *Metasul A metal-on-metal bearing* (ed. C Rieker, M Windler, U Wyss), pp. 83–91. Huber, Bern, 1999.

44 Campbell P, McKellop H, Alim R *et al.*: Metal-on-metal hip replacements: wear performance and cellular response to wear particles. In *Cobalt-based alloys for biomedical applications* (ed. JA Disegi, RL Kennedy, R Pilliar), STP 1365. ASTM, West Conshohocken, PA, 1998.

45 Schmalzried TP, Szuszczewicz ES, Northfield MR *et al*: Quantitative assessment of walking activity after total hip or knee replacement. *Journal of Bone and Joint* Surgery [Am] **80**: 54–9, 1998.

46 Park S-H, McKellop H, Lu B, Chan F, Chiesa R: Wear morphology of metal–metal implants: hip simulator tests compared with clinical retrievals. In *Alternative bearing surfaces in total joint arthroplasty* (ed. JJ Jacobs, TL Craig), STP 1346, pp. 129–43. ASTM, West Conshohocken, PA, 1998.

47 Dorr LD, Wan Z, Longjohn DB, Dubois B, Murken R: Total hip arthroplasty with use of the Metasul metal-on-metal articulation. Four to seven-year results. *Journal of Bone and Joint Surgery* [Am] **82**: 789–98, 2000.

48 Walker PS: Friction and wear of artificial joints. In *Human joints and their artificial replacements*, pp. 368–442. CC Thomas, Springfield, IL.

49 Boutin P, Christel P, Dorlot JM *et al.*: The use of dense alumina–alumina ceramic combination in total hip replacement. *Journal of Biomedical Materials Research* **22**: 1203–32, 1988.

50 Mittelmeier H, Heisel J: Sixteen years experience with ceramic hip prostheses. *Clinical Orthopaedics and Related Research* **282**: 64–72, 1992.

51 Nizard RS, Sedel L, Christel P *et al.*: Ten-year survivorship of cemented ceramic–ceramic total hip prosthesis. *Clinical Orthopaedics and Related Research* **282**: 53–63, 1992.

52 Clarke IC: Role of ceramic implants. Design and clinical success with total hip prosthetic ceramic-to-ceramic bearings. *Clinical Orthopaedics and Related Research* **282**:19–30, 1992.

53 Clarke I, Willmann G: Structural ceramics in orthopaedics. In *Bone implant interface* (ed. H Cameron), pp. 203–52. Mosby, St. Louis, MO, 1994.

54 Garcia-Cimbrelo E, Martinez-Sayanes JM, Minuesa A, Munuera L: Mittelmeier ceramic–ceramic prosthesis after 10 years. *Journal of Arthroplasty* **11**: 773–81, 1996.

55 Meunier A, Nizard R, Bizot P, Sedel L: Clinical results of alumina-on-alumina couple in total hip replacement. In *Alternative bearing*

    surfaces in total joint arthroplasty (ed. JJ Jacobs, TL Craig), STP 1346, pp. 213–34. ASTM, West Conshohocken, PA, 1998.

56 Mahoney OM, Dimon JH, III: Unsatisfactory results with a ceramic total hip prosthesis. *Journal of Bone and Joint Surgery* [Am] **72**: 663–71, 1990.

57 Walter A: On the material and the tribology of alumina–alumina couplings for hip joint prostheses. *Clinical Orthopaedics and Related Research* **282**: 31–46, 1992.

58 Richter HG, Willmann G, Weick K: Improving the reliability of the ceramic-on-ceramic wear couple in THR. In *Alternative bearing surfaces in total joint arthroplasty* (ed. JJ Jacobs, TL Craig), STP 1346. ASTM, West Conshohocken, PA, 1998.

59 Ueno M, Amino H, Okimatu H, Oonishi H: Wear, friction, and mechanical investigation and development of alumina-to-alumina combination total hip joint. In *Joint arthroplasty* (ed. S Imura, M Wada, H Omori), pp. 119–31. Springer-Verlag, Tokyo, 1999.

60 Willmann G: Ceramics for total hip replacement—what a surgeon should know. *Orthopedics* **21**: 173–7, 1998.

61 Willmann G, Brodbeck A, Effenberger H *et al.*: Investigation of 87 retrieved ceramic femoral heads. In *Bioceramics in orthopaedics—new applications* (ed. W Puhl), pp. 13–18. Enke, Stuttgart, 1998.

62 Taylor SK: *In-vitro* wear performance of a contemporary alumina: alumina bearing couple under anatomically-relevant hip joint simulation. In *Reliability and long-term results of ceramics in orthopaedics* (ed. S Sedel, G Willmann), pp. 85–90. Thieme, Stuttgart, 1999.

63 Fisher J, Ingham E, Stone MH *et al*: Wear and debris generation in artificial hip joints. In *Reliability and long-term results of ceramics in orthopaedics* (ed. S Sedel, G Willmann), pp. 78–81. Thieme, Stuttgart, 1999.

64 Oonishi H, Nishida M, Kawanabe K *et al.*: *In-vitro* wear of A1203/A1203 implant combination with over 10 million cycles duration. *Transactions of the 45th Annual Meeting, Orthopaedic Research Society*, p. 50, 1999.

65 Winter M, Griss P. Scheller G, Moser T: Ten- to 14-year results of a ceramic hip prosthesis. *Clinical Orthopaedics and Related Research* **282**: 73–80, 1992.

66 Nevelos JE, Fisher J, Ingham E, Doyle C, Nevelos AB: Examination of alumina ceramic components from Mittelmeier total hip arthroplasties. *Transactions of the 44th Annual Meeting of the Orthopaedic Research Society*, p. 219, 1998.

67 Bergman NR, Young DA: The rationale, short-term outcome and early complications of a ceramic couple in total hip arthroplasty. In *Reliability and long-term results of ceramics in orthopaedics* (ed. S Sedel, G Willmann), pp. 52–6. Thieme, Stuttgart, 1999.

68 Yoon TR, Rowe SM, Jung ST, Seon KJ, Maloney WJ: Osteolysis in association with a total hip arthroplasty with ceramic bearing surfaces. *Journal of Bone and Joint Surgery* [Am] **80**: 1459–68, 1998.

69 Boehler M, Knahr K, Plenk H Jr *et al.*: Long-term results of uncemented alumina acetabular implants. *Journal of Bone and Joint Surgery* [Br] **76**: 53–9, 1994.

70 Fuchs GA: 2–4 year clinical results with a ceramic-on-ceramic articulation in a new modular THRsystem. In *Bioceramics in hip joint replacement. Proceedings of the 5th International CeramTec Symposium* (ed. G Willmann, K Zweymuller), pp. 39–46. Thieme, Stuttgart, 2000 (in German).

71 Allain J, Goutallier D, Voisin MC, Lemouel S: Failure of a stainless-steel femoral head of a revision total hip arthroplasty performed

after a fracture of a ceramic femoral head. *Journal of Bone and Joint Surgery* **80**: 1355–60, 1998.

72 Sedel L: Revision strategy for ceramic implant failures. In *Reliability and long-term results of ceramics in orthopaedics* (ed. S Sedel, G Willmann), pp. 75–6. Thieme, Stuttgart, 1999.

73 Kempf I, Semlitsch M: Massive wear of a steel ball head by ceramic fragments in the polyethylene acetabular cup after revision of a total hip prosthesis with fractured ceramic ball. *Archives of Orthopaedic and Traumatic Surgery* **109**: 284–7, 1990.

74 Frohling M, Zichner L, Koch R: Revisionsstrategie bei der Verwendung von Keramikkopfen. In *Reliability and long-term results of ceramics in orthopaedics* (ed. S Sedel, G Willmann), pp. 72–4. Thieme, Stuttgart, 1999.

75 Fritsch EW, Gleitz M: Ceramic femoral head fractures in total hip arthroplasty *Clinical Orthopaedics and Related Research* **328**: 129–36, 1996.

76 Piconi C, Labanti M, Magnani G *et al*: Analysis of a failed alumina THR ball head. *Biomaterials* **20**: 1637–46, 1999.

77 Christel P, Meunier A, Heller M, Torre JP, Peille CN: Mechanical properties and short-term *in-vivo* evaluation of yttrium-oxide-partially-stabilized zirconia. *Journal of Biomedical Materials Research* **23**: 45–61, 1989.

78 Drouin JM, Gales B, Chevalier J, Fantozzi G: Fatigue behavior of zirconia hip joint heads: experimental results and finite element analysis. *Journal of Biomedical Materials Research* **34**: 149–55, 1997.

79 Gales B, Stefani Y: Yttria-stabilized zirconia for improved orthopaedic prostheses. In *Encyclopedic handbook of biomaterials and bioengineering* (ed. DL Wise, DJ Trantolo, MJ Yaszemski, JD Gresser, ER Schwartz). Dekker, New York, 1995.

80 Piconi C, Maccauro G: Zirconia as a ceramic biomaterial. *Biomaterials* **20**: 1–25, 1999.

81 Birkby I, Harrison P, Stevens R: The effect of surface transformation on the wear behavior of zirconia TZP ceramics. *Journal of the European Ceramics Society* **5**: 37–45, 1989.

82 Piconi C, Burger W, Richter HG *et al*.: Y-TZP ceramics for artificial joint replacements. *Biomaterials* **19**: 1489–94, 1998.

83 Allain J, Le Mouel S, Goutallier D, Voison McAllain J: Poor eight-year survival of cemented zirconia–polyethylene total hip replacements. *Journal of Bone and Joint Surgery* [Br] **81**: 835–42, 1999.

84 Gales B, Stefani Y, Lilley E: Long-term *in vivo* and *in vitro* aging of a zirconia ceramic used in orthopaedy. *Journal of Biomedical Materials Research* **28**: 619–24, 1994.

85 Früh HJ, Willmann G, Pfaff HG: Wear characteristics of ceramic-on-ceramic for hip endoprostheses. *Biomaterials* **18**: 873–6, 1997.

86 Willmann G, Früh HJ, Pfaff HG: Wear characteristics of sliding pairs of zirconia (Y-TZP) for hip endoprostheses. *Biomaterials* **17**: 2157–62, 1996.

87 Cales B, Chevalier J: Wear behavior of ceramic pairs compared on different testing configurations. In *Alternative bearing surfaces in total joint arthroplasty* (ed. JJ Jacobs, TL Craig), STP 1346, pp. 186–96. ASTM, West Conshohocken, PA, 1998.

88 Clarke IC, Good V, Schuldies J, Schroeder DAG: Zirconia simulated performance up to 15 Mc in serum lubricant. Presented at the 6th World Biomaterials Congress, 2000.

89 Affatato S, Testoni M, Cacciari GL, Toni A: Mixed-oxides prosthetic ceramic ball heads. Part 2: Effect of the ZrO_2 fraction on the wear of ceramic on ceramic joints. *Biomaterials* **20**: 1925–9, 1999.

90 Affatato S, Testoni M, Cacciari GL, Toni A: Mixed oxides prosthetic ceramic ball heads. Part 1: Effect of the ZrO$_2$ fraction on the wear of ceramic on polythylene joints. *Biomaterials* **20**: 971–5, 1999.

91 Kaddick C, Pfaff HG: Wear study in the alumina–zirconia system. In *Reliability and long-term results of ceramics in orthopaedics* (ed. S Sedel, G Willmann), pp. 96–101. Thieme, Stuttgart, 1999.

92 McKellop H, Clarke IC, Markolf K, Amstutz H: Friction and wear properties of polymer, metal, and ceramic prosthetic joint materials evaluated on a multichannel screening device. *Journal of Biomedical Materials Research* **15**: 619–53, 1981.

93 Lancaster JG, Dowson D, Isaac GH, Fisher J: The wear of ultra-high molecular weight polyethylene sliding on metallic and ceramic counterfaces representative of current femoral surfaces in joint replacement. *Proceedings of the Institution of Mechanical Engineers Part H: Journal of Engineering in Medicine* **211**: 17–24, 1997.

94 Bankston AB, Faris PM, Keating EM, Ritter MA: Polyethylene wear in total hip arthroplasty in patient-matched groups. *Journal of Arthroplasty* **8**: 315–22, 1993.

95 Wroblewski BM: Wear of the high-density polyethylene socket in total hip arthroplasty and its role in endosteal cavitation. *Proceedings of the Institution of Mechanical Engineers Part H: Journal of Engineering in Medicine* **211**: 109–18, 1997.

96 Furman BD, Lee CL, Block A, Lefebvre FK, Li S: A comparison of directly molded and machined retrieved acetabular cups of a single design. *Transactions of the 44th Annual Meeting of the Orthopaedic Research Society* 50, 1998.

97 Devane PA, Horne JG: Assessment of polyethylene wear in total hip replacement. *Clinical Orthopaedics and Related Research* **369**: 59–72, 1999.

98 McKellop HA, Sarmiento A, Schwinn CP, Ebramzadeh E: *In vivo* wear of titanium-alloy hip prostheses. *Journal of Bone and Joint Surgery* [Am] **72**: 512–17, 1990.

99 McKellop H, Rostlund T, Ebramzadeh E, Sarmiento A: Wear of titanium alloy in laboratory tests and in retrieved human joint replacements. In *Medical applications of titanium and its alloys* (ed. SA Brown, JE Lemons), STP 1272, pp. 266–93. ASTM, West Conshohocken, PA, 1996.

100 Agins HJ, Alcock NW, Bansal M *et al.*: Metallic wear in failed titanium-alloy total hip replacements. A histological and quantitative analysis. *Journal of Bone and Joint Surgery* [Am] **70**: 347–56, 1988.

101 Lombardi AV, Jr, Mallory TH, Vaughn BK, Drouillard P: Aseptic loosening in total hip arthroplasty secondary to osteolysis induced by wear debris from titanium-alloy modular femoral heads. *Journal of Bone and Joint Surgery* [Am] **71**: 1337–42, 1989.

102 McKellop HA, Rostlund TV: The wear behavior of ion-implanted Ti–6Al–4V against UHMW polyethylene. *Journal of Biomedical Materials Research* **24**: 1413–26, 1990.

103 Semlitsch M, Willert HG: Clinical wear behaviour of UHMW polyethylene cups paired with metal and ceramic ball heads in comparison to metal-on-metal pairings of hip joint replacements. *Proceedings of the Institution of Mechanical Engineers Part H: Journal of Engineering in Medicine* **211**: 73–88, 1997.

104 Davidson JA, Poggie RA, Mishra AK: Abrasive wear of ceramic, metal, and UHMWPE bearing surfaces from third-body bone, PMMA bone cement, and titanium debris. *Biomedical Materials Engineering* **4**: 213–29, 1994.

105 Mishra AK, Davidson JA, Poggie RA, Kovacs P, FitzGerald TJ: Mechanical and tribological properties and biocompatibility of diffusion hardened Ti–13Nb–13Zr: a new titanium alloy for surgical implants. In *Medical applications of titanium and its alloys* (ed. SA Brown, JE Lemons), STP 1272, pp. 96–112. ASTM, West Conshohocken, PA, 1996.

106 Sauer WL, Anthony ME: Predicting the clinical wear performance of orthopaedic bearing surfaces. In *Alternative bearing surfaces in total joint arthroplasty* (ed. JJ Jacobs, TL Craig), STP 1346, pp. 1–29. ASTM, West Conshohocken, PA, 1998.

107 Schmalzried TP, Dorey FJ, McKellop H: The multifactorial nature of polyethylene wear *in vivo* [comment]. *Journal of Bone and Joint Surgery* [Am] 80: 1234–43, 1998.

108 Willmann G: New generation ceramics. In *Bioceramics in hip joint replacement. Proceedings of the 5th International CeramTec Symposium* (ed. G Willmann, K Zweymuller), pp. 127–35. Thieme, Stuttgart, 2000.

109 Bragdon CR, Jasty M, Kawate K *et al*: Wear of retrieved cemented polyethylene acetabula with alumina femoral heads. *Journal of Arthroplasty* 12: 119–25, 1997.

110 McKellop HA, Lu B, Benya P:Friction, lubrication and wear of cobalt–chromium, alumina and zirconia hip prostheses compared on a joint simulator. *Transactions of the 38th Annual Meeting of the Orthopaedic Research Society*, p. 402, 1992.

111 Li S, Burstein AH: Ultra-high molecular weight polyethylene. The material and its use in total joint implants. *Journal of Bone and Joint Surgery* [Am] 76: 1080–90, 1994.

112 Lewis G: Polyethylene wear in total hip and knee arthroplasties. *Journal of Biomedical Materials Research* 38: 55–75, 1997.

113 Kurtz SM, Muratoglu OK, Evans M, Edidin AA: Advances in the processing, sterilization, and cross-linking of ultra-high molecular weight polyethylene for total joint arthroplasty. *Biomaterials* 20: 1659–88, 1999.

114 Fisher J, Reeves EA, Isaac GH, Saumm KA, Sanford WM: Comparison of the wear of aged and non-aged ultrahigh molecular weight polyehtylene sterilized by gamma irradiation and by gas plasma. *Transactions of the 5th World Biomaterials Congress*, p. 971, 1996.

115 Goldman M, Pruitt L: Comparison of the effects of gamma radiation and low temperature hydrogen peroxide gas plasma sterilization on the molecular structure, fatigue resistance, and wear behavior of UHMWPE. *Journal of Biomedical Materials Research* 40: 378–84, 1998.

116 McNulty DE, Hastings RS, Swope SW, Huston DE: Sterilization methods and artificial aging of UHMWPE resins: the relationship between resilience and oxidation. *Transactions of the 45th Annual Meeting of the Orthopaedic Research Society*, p. 821, 1999.

117 Sutula LC, Collier JP, Saum KA *et al*: Impact of gamma sterilization on clinical performance of polyethylene in the hip. *Clinical Orthopaedics and Related Research* 319: 28–40, 1995.

118 Furman BD, Reish T, Li S: The effect of implantation on the oxidation of ultra high molecular weight polyethylene. *Transactions of the Society for Biomaterials*, p. 427, 1997.

119 Pienkowski D, Patel A, Lee KY *et al*.: Solubility changes in shelf-aged ultra-high molecular weight polyethylene acetabular liners. *Journal of the Long Term Effects of Medical Implants* 9: 273–88, 1999.

120 Wang A, Essner A, Polineni VK, Stark C, Dumbleton JH: Lubrication and wear of ultra-high molecular weight polyethylene in total joint replacements. *Tribology International* 31: 17–33, 1998.

275

121 McKellop HA, Shen FW, Lu B, Campbell P, Salovey R: Development of an extremely wear resistant UHMW polyethylene for total hip replacements. *Journal of Orthopaedic Research* **17**: 157–67, 1999.

122 Muratoglu OK, Bragdon CR, O'Connor DO *et al.*: Unified wear model for highly cross-linked ultrahigh molecular weight polyethylenes (UHMWPE). *Biomaterials* **20**: 1463–70, 1999.

123 Gillis AM, Schmieg JJ, Bhattacharyya S, Li S: An independent evaluation of the mechanical, chemical and fracture properties of UHMWPE cross-linked by 34 different conditions. *Transactions of the Society for Biomaterials*, p. 216, 1999.

124 Roe RJ, Grood ES, Shastri R, Gosselin CA, Noyes FR: Effect of radiation sterilization and ageing on ultrahigh molecular weight polyethylene. *Journal of Biomedical Materials Research* **15**: 209–30, 1981.

125 Eyerer P, Ke YC: Property changes of UHMW polyethylene hip cup endoprostheses during implantation. *Journal of Biomedical Materials Research* **18**: 1137–51, 1984.

126 Premnath V, Harris WH, Jasty M, Merrill EW: Gamma sterilization of UHMWPE articular implants: an analysis of the oxidation problem. *Biomaterials* **17**: 1741–53, 1996.

127 Gillis A, Furman B, Li S: Influence of ultra high molecular weight polyethylene resin type and manufacturing method on real time oxidation. *Transactions of the 44th Annual Meeting of the Orthopaedic Research Society*, p. 360, 1998.

128 Collier JP, Bargmann LS, Currier BH *et al*: An analysis of Hylamer and polyethylene bearings from retrieved acetabular components. *Orthopedics* **21**: 865–71, 1998.

129 Edidin A, Muth J, Spiegelberg S, Schaffner S: Sterilization of UHMWPE in nitrogen prevents oxidative degradation for more than ten years. *Transactions of the 46th Annual Meeting of the Orthopaedic Research Society*, p. 1, 2000.

130 Greer KW, Schmidt MB, Hamilton JV: The hip simulator wear of gamma-vacuum, gamin-air, and ethylene oxide sterilized UHMWPE following a severe oxidative challenge. *Transactions of the 44th Annual Meeting of the Orthopaedic Research Society*, p. 52, 1998.

131 Streicher RM: Influence of ionizing irradiation in air and nitrogen for sterilization of surgical grade polyethylene for implants. *Radiation Physics and Chemistry* **31**: 693–8, 1988.

132 Bapst JM, Valentine RH, Vasquez R: Wear simulation testing of direct compression molded UHMWPE irradiated in oxygenless packaging. *Transactions of the Society for Biomaterials*, p. 72, 1997.

133 Sun DC, Wang A, Stark C, Dumbleton JH: The concept of stabilization in UHMWPE. *Transactions of the 5th World Biomaterials Congress*, p. 195, 1996.

134 McKellop H, F.W. S, Lu B, Campbell P, Salovey R: The effect of sterilization method and other modifications on the wear resistance of acetabular cups of ultra-high molecular weight polyethylene—a hip simulator study. *Journal of Bone and Joint Surgery* [Am] **82**: 1708–25.

135 Currier BH, Currier JH, Collier JP, Mayor MB: Effect of fabrication method and resin type on performance of tibial bearings. *Journal of Biomedical Materials Research* **53**: 143–51, 2000.

136 *Arcom® processed polyethylene. A technical report.* Biomet Inc., Warsaw, IN, 1996.

137 Walsh H, Gillis A, Furman B, Li S: Factors that determine the oxidation resistance of molded 1900: Is it the resin or the molding? *Transactions of the 46th Annual Meeting of the Orthopaedic Research Society*, p. 543, 2000.

138 Grobbelaar CJ, Plessis TAD, Marais F: The radiation improvement of polyethylene prostheses. *Journal of Bone and Joint Surgery* [Br] **60**: 370–4, 1978.

139 Grobbelaar CJ, Weber FA, Spirakis A *et al*.: Clinical experience with gamma irradiation-cross-linked polyethylene—a 14 to 20 year follow-up report. *South African Bone and Joint Surgery* **9**: 140–7, 1999.

140 Oonishi H, Takayama Y, Tsuji E: Improvement of polyethylene by irradiation in artificial joints. *Radiation Physics and Chemistry* **39**: 495–504, 1992.

141 Oonishi H, Takayama Y, Tsuji E: The low wear of cross-linked polyethylene socket in total hip prostheses. In *Encyclopedic Handbook of Biomaterials and Bioengineering. Part A: Materials* (ed. DL Wise, DJ Trantolo, DE Altobelli *et al*.), pp. 1853–68. Dekker, New York, 1995.

142 Oonishi H, Saito M, Kadoya Y: Wear of high-dose gamma irradiated polyethylene in total joint replacement—long term radiological evaluation. *Transactions of the 44th Annual Meeting of the Orthopaedic Research Society*, p. 97, 1998.

143 Wroblewski BM, Siney PD, Fleming PA: Low-friction arthroplasty of the hip using alumina ceramic and cross-linked polyethylene. A ten-year follow-up report. *Journal of Bone and Joint Surgery* [Br] **81**: 54–5, 1999.

144 McKellop H, Shen F-W, DiMaio W, Lancaster J: Wear of gamma-cross-linked polyethylene acetabular cups against roughened femoral balls. *Clinical Orthopaedics and Related Research* **369**: 73–82, 1999.

145 DiMaio WG, Lilly WB, Moore WC, Saum KA: Low wear, low oxidation radiation cross-linked UHMWPE. *Transactions of the 44th Annual Meeting of the Orthopaedic Research Society*, p. 363, 1998.

146 Hastings RS, Huston DE, Reber EW, DiMaio WG: Knee wear testing of a radiation cross-linked and remelted UHMWPE. *Transactions of the Society for Biomaterials*, p. 328, 1999.

147 Bhateja SK, Duerst RW, Martens JA, Andrews EH: Radiation-induced enhancement of crystallinity in polymers. *Journal of Macromolecular Science. Part C: Reviews in Macromolecular Chemistry* **C35**: 581–659, 195.

148 Essner A, Polineni VK, Wang A, Stark C, Dumbleton JH: Effect of femoral head surface roughness and cross-linking on the wear of UHMWPE acetabular cups. *Transactions of the Society for Biomaterials*, p. 4, 1998.

149 Laurent MP, Yao JQ, Gilbertson LN, Swarts DF, Crowninshield Rd: Wear of highly cross-linked UHMWPE acetabular liners under adverse conditions. *Transactions of the 6th World Biomaterials Congress*, p. 874, 2000.

150 Endo MM, Barbour PSM, Barton DC *et al*: Comparative wear and debris generation of cross-linked and non-cross-linked ultrahigh molecular weight polyethylene under three different femoral counterface conditions. *Transactions of the 6th World Biomaterials Congress*, 2000.

151 Greenwald AS, Bauer TW, Ries MW: New polys for old: contribution or caveat. Scientific Exhibit at 67th Annual Meeting, American Academy of Orthopaedic Surgeons, 2000.

152 Laurent M, Yao JQ, Bhambri SK *et al.*: High cycle wear of highly cross-linked UHMWPE acetabular liners evaluated in a hip simulator. *Transactions of the 46th Annual Meeting of the Orthopaedic Research Society*, p. 567, 2000.

153 Muratoglu OK, Bragdon CR, O'Connor DO *et al.*: The effect of temperature and radiation cross-linking on UHMWPE for use in total hip arthroplasty. *Transactions of the 46th Annual Meeting of the Orthopaedic Research Society*, p. 547, 2000.

154 Muratoglu OK:Cross-linked polyethylenes: A promising technology for total joint replacements in the 21st century. Presented at Workshop: Polyethylene 2001, Orthopaedic Research Society, 2000.

155 Harris WH: The advantages and disadvantages of using electron beam radiation for cross-linked UHMWP. *Hip Society, 31st Summer Meeting*, p. 13, 1999.

156 Muratoglu OK, Harris WH, Delaney H *et al*:The development of an *in vitro* hip simulator model for fatigue failure: application to conventional and highly cross-linked UHMWPE. *Transactions of the 46th Annual Meeting of the Orthopaedic Research Society*, p. 548, 2000.

157 Manley MT, Capello WN, D'Antonio JA, Edidin AA: Highly cross-linked polyethylene acetabular liners for reduction in wear in total hip replacement. Scientific Exhibit SE 022, American Academy of Orthopaedic Surgeons, 2000.

158 Muratoglu OK, Bragdon CR, O'Connor DO *et al.*: The comparison of the wear behavior of four different types of cross-linked acetabular components. *Transactions of the 46th Annual Meeting of the Orthopaedic Research Society*, p. 566, 2000.

159 DiMaio WG, Lilly WB, Moore WC, Saum KA:Low wear, low oxidation radiation cross-linked UHMWPE. *Transactions of the 44th Annual Meeting of the Orthopaedic Research Society*, p. 363, 1998.

160 Streicher RM: Ionizing irradiation for sterilization and modification of high molecular weight polyethylenes. *Plastics and Rubber Processing and Applications* 10: 221–9, 1988.

161 Walsh HA, Furman BD, Naab L, Li S: Role of oxidation in the clinical fracture of acetabular cups. *Transactions of the 45th Annual Meeting of the Orthopaedic Research Society*, p. 845, 1999.

162 McKellop H: Assessment of wear of materials for artificial joints. In *The adult hip* (ed. J Callaghan, A Rosenberg, H Rubash), pp. 231–46. Lippincott–Raven, New York, 1998.

163 Xenos JS, Hopkinson WJ, Callaghan JJ, Heekin RD, Savory CG: Osteolysis around an uncemented cobalt chrome total hip arthroplasty. *Clinical Orthopaedics and Related Research* 317: 29–36, 1995.

164 Devane PA, Bourne RB, Rorabeck CH, MacDonald S, Robinson EJ: Measurement of polyethylene wear in metal-backed acetabular cups. *Clinical Orthopaedics and Related Research* 319: 317–26, 1995.

165 Nashed RS, Becker DA, Gustilo RB: Are cementless acetabular components the cause of excess wear and osteolysis in total hip arthroplasty? *Clinical Orthopaedics and Related Research* 317: 19–28, 1995.

166 Moreland JR, Moreno MA: Results of primary AML hip replacements. Presented at The Hip Society Summer Meeting 1995.

167 Wan Z, Dorr LD: Natural history of femoral focal osteolysis with proximal ingrowth smooth stem implant. *Journal of Arthroplasty* 11: 718–25, 1996.

11

Controversies in deep vein thrombosis prophylaxis following total hip arthroplasty: a North American perspective

Clifford W. Colwell and Mary E. Hardwick

Evidence-based medicine, which seeks to integrate individual clinical expertise and the best external evidence derived from scientific research, provides an argument for prescribing thrombosis prophylaxis for all total hip arthroplasty (THA) patients. THA patients treated prophylactically as controls or with placebo have a total deep vein thrombosis (DVT) rate of 45–57 per cent and a proximal DVT prevalence of 23–36 per cent when examined by venography at 7–14 days. Prevalence of pulmonary embolism is less certain, but clinical studies have reported a range of 0.7–30 per cent for total pulmonary embolism and 0.34–6 per cent for fatal pulmonary embolism for control or placebo patients.[1] Studies performing routine ventilation–perfusion lung scans reported a prevalence of 7–11 per cent with high probability scans within 7–14 days of THA.[2,3] Venography studies show that, without prolonged out-of-hospital prophylaxis, 20–25 per cent of patients develop new evidence of DVT within 4–5 weeks of hospital discharge[3,4] and about 6 per cent develop an intermediate or high probability lung scan.[3]

Many clinicians rely on clinical signs and symptoms in THA patients as the initial presentation of DVT or pulmonary embolism. However, the accuracy of diagnosis by signs and symptoms is considered to be low. Most symptomatic patients do not have venous thrombosis and many asymptomatic patients have been shown by objective testing to have DVT. Controversy remains as to whether asymptomatic patients should be screened by objective testing and treated on these results in the same manner as symptomatic patients are treated at this time.

Duplex ultrasound is used in the clinical setting for both screening and diagnosis. Reports of its accuracy and sensitivity vary from high in some institutions[5] to low in others[6] because the results are in part dependent on the technician performing the test.[7] Some clinicians use duplex ultrasound to screen patients at time of discharge in combination with prophylaxis, but studies indicate that this does not decrease the occurrence of DVT during the period following discharge[8] and is not cost effective.[9] Venography remains the standard method of screening and diagnosis for scientific studies accepted by the United States Food and Drug Administration. Because of the invasive nature and increased risk to the patient, venography is seldom used in clinical practice for screening and diagnosis.

The majority of clinicians agree that THA patients should receive prophylaxis for DVT and pulmonary embolism; however, the prophylactic agent of choice remains controversial. Several non-pharmacological prophylaxis methods have been studied, including elastic stockings,[10,11] intermittent pneumatic compression,[12–16] and pneumatic plantar compression.[17–19] Although all appear to be of some benefit with reductions of 25–57 per cent DVT risk,[1] none appear to equal pharmacological prophylaxis in THA or to provide an additive effect. The obvious advantage of minimum side effects is appealing to clinicians, but the patient tolerance of these devices and the actual length of time they remain in place is questionable. There are few randomized controlled studies utilizing these devices, and further studies could provide clearer information on their effectiveness.

Pharmacological agents used in clinical practice to decrease venous thromboembolism in THA include aspirin, dextran, unfractionated heparin, warfarin, and low molecular weight heparins (LMWHs). Although a minority of clinicians continue to use aspirin as a prophylactic, several randomized trials were unable to demonstrate any reduction in venous thromboembolic rate.[1] Dextran appeared to be a good prophylactic agent because of its ability to decrease platelet aggregation and blood viscosity and to stabilize endothelium. However, clinical trials using dextran[20–22] were associated with problems related to intravenous access, fluid overload, and anaphylaxis which have limited its use for prophylaxis despite a relative risk reduction of 41 per cent.[1]

Low-dose unfractionated heparin prophylaxis, although better than placebo, is relatively ineffective when compared with other prophylaxis regiments.[23,24] The American College of Chest Physicians analysis of 10 trials demonstrated a 39 per cent risk reduction using low-dose unfractionated heparin after THA.[1] Postoperative use of adjusted-dose heparin to maintain the activated partial thromboplastin time in the upper range of normal appears to be safe and effective.[25–27] This prophylaxis may be considered for patients at extremely high risk; however, most surgeons consider adjusted-dose heparin impractical for routine use in THA.

Warfarin sodium, a vitamin K antagonist, is used by many clinicians in the United States as an anticoagulant agent in hip surgery. A recent American survey[28] indicated that 47 per cent of 466 surgeons used warfarin as prophylaxis during hospitalization, and a Canadian survey[29] reported the use of warfarin prophylaxis by 46 per cent of 397 surgeons.[29] Since the observed anticoagulant effect of warfarin is delayed by 24–36 hours, the most appropriate time to administer the initial dose is uncertain. It may be given the day before surgery, started immediately after surgery, or started on the first day following surgery. Even with these dosing schedules, the therapeutic range of the international normalized ratio (INR) is not reached until the second or third day after surgery.[30-32]

Adjusted-dose warfarin prophylaxis administered at a dose sufficient to maintain the INR at between 2.0 and 3.0 appears to be the most common practice. A compilation of seven studies using adjusted-dose warfarin with a combined enrollment of 1337 THA patients indicated a 22 per cent prevalence of venous thromboembolism, with a relative risk reduction of 53 per cent.[33] Adjusted-dose warfarin is often prescribed as continued prophylaxis after discharge, although there are few studies demonstrating the effectiveness of continued warfarin prophylaxis.

Two-step warfarin prophylaxis is another regimen that has been used in trials, but is not widely used in practice. Warfarin is begun at a very low dose 14 days prior to surgery, which prolongs the prothrombin time to 1-2 seconds over baseline. Immediately after surgery, the warfarin dose is adjusted upwards to maintain the INR at between 2.0 and 3.0.[34,35] Although it appears safe and marginally effective with a relative risk reduction of 37 per cent,[1] this 'two-step' warfarin prophylaxis regimen is complicated and has not been widely adopted by orthopaedic surgeons.

LMWHs were approved for prophylactic use for THA in 1993 and have been adopted in practice by many clinicians. In an American study[28] 36 per cent of 466 surgeons reported use of LMWHs for prophylaxis of THA patients in the hospital, and similarly a Canadian study[29] reported LMWH prophylaxis by 36 per cent of 397 surgeons. Pharmacologically, LMWHs are substantially different from unfractionated heparin. They have highly predictable pharmacokinetic properties and high bioavailability, as well as a lower associated incidence of thrombocytopenia and ability to target factor Xa while affecting factor IIa to a lesser extent than unfractionated heparin. The favourable pharmacokinetics of LMWHs allow them to be administered subcutaneously once or twice daily with no requirement to follow drug levels or activity.[36]

LMWHs have been studied extensively. Twenty-six studies using LMWH prophylaxis on 5905 THA patients showed a total DVT prevalence of 17 per cent with a relative risk reduction of 67 per cent.[33] However, concern remains about the possibility of increased bleeding with LMWH prophylaxis. One trial[30] has shown an increase in bleeding complications, and another[37] has reported greater blood loss.[37] Three meta-analyses[38-40] of different prophylaxis regimens concluded that LMWH was most effective, although the differences in efficacy between LMWH and either adjusted-dose warfarin or adjusted-dose heparin prophylaxis were small.

The optimal duration of postoperative prophylaxis after THA has been subject to debate in recent years and remains uncertain.

Previous trials have continued prophylaxis for the duration of hospitalization and ranged from 7 to 10 days. Currently, duration of hospital stay is 4 days or less, which may provide inadequate duration of prophylaxis. Studies have suggested that the risk for DVT may persist for up to 2 months after THA.[41-44]

Using venographic DVT as the efficacy outcome, six double-blind randomized trials[3,4,42-45] have examined the need for extended prophylaxis beyond the hospital stay. These trials compared in-hospital prophylaxis of 6–14 days with 30–35 days of prophylaxis with LMWH. All the studies reported a range of 12–37 per cent asymptomatic DVT after hospital discharge and a significant reduction in a range of 4–19 per cent with out-of-hospital prophylaxis with LMWH. Extended prophylaxis reduced total and proximal DVT by more than 50 per cent.

The question of extended treatment remains controversial. Four studies,[46-49] including 4989 THA patients, treated from 7 to 9.8 days with either warfarin or LMWH prophylaxis experienced a range of 1.2–4.3 per cent symptomatic venous thromboembolic events (VTEs) confirmed by ultrasound or venography. Fatal pulmonary embolism was reported in a range of 0–0.1 per cent. In a large clinical study ($n = 3011$), where THA patients were treated with either enoxaparin or warfarin for a mean of 7.3 days, the overall rate of symptomatic venous thrombosis was 3 per cent with no difference in occurrence between the two groups after treatment.[48] THA studies of both means of prophylaxis during hospitalization with about 10 days of treatment and followed for 84–90 days after surgery have shown similar results of symptomatic venous thrombosis.

Despite the low incidence of symptomatic VTE seen in these follow-up studies, 45–80 per cent of all symptomatic DVT and pulmonary embolisms seen in hip and knee arthroplasty patients occur after hospital discharge.[48-51] The estimated median time from arthroplasty to VTE was 17 days for THA patients.[51] Few studies of extended or out-of-hospital treatment examine symptomatic venous thrombosis prevalence; more controlled studies of this type are needed to make an educated decision to extend treatment.

The orthopaedic clinician certainly knows and understands more about venous thromboembolism and the use of prophylaxis because of the investigations and clinical studies that have been done. Using evidence-based medicine to incorporate clinical study information into practice provides patients with treatment using current knowledge to provide the best care possible (Table 11.1). However, many controversies remain, requiring continual examination of practice and tools for DVT prevention through controlled prospective randomized studies. Although venographic studies are needed, more studies based on clinical outcomes are necessary.

New information is available every year to allow improvements in practice and patient care. A new nuclear medicine test using

Table 11.1 Current North American recommendations for thrombosis prophylaxis after THA

Patients undergoing THA	Recommendations
Recommended prophylactic therapy	LMWH or warfarin (goal INR 2.5; range, 2.0–3.0), or adjusted-dose unfractionated heparin; possible adjuvant use of elastic stockings or intermittent pneumatic compression devices*
Optimal initiation time for prophylaxis	LMWH started 12–24 h after surgery, or warfarin started before or immediately after surgery, or adjusted-dose unfractionated heparin started preoperatively
Optimal duration of prophylaxis	7–10 days with LMWH or warfarin; 29–35 days with LMWH may offer additional protection
High-risk patients	Inferior vena cava filter placement if other forms of anticoagulant-based prophylaxis are not effective or have unacceptable risks; this should rarely be necessary
Routine screening for DVT	Not recommended in lieu of prophylaxis

*Low-dose unfractionated heparin, aspirin, dextran, and intermittent pneumatic compression devices reduce the overall incidence of venous thromboembolism but are less effective.
Adapted from Clagett *et al.* 1998.

AcuTect® to ascertain DVT is currently being studied for accuracy, specificity, and sensitivity. This may provide a new tool in the clinician's arsenal to determine thrombosis. With genetic research in its infancy, new tests may become available to screen patients for genetic factors which make them more susceptible to DVT. A factor which is currently known to affect clotting is activated protein-C resistance (APC-R) which can increase the probability of thrombosis.

New pharmacological substances being tested may impact the prophylaxis and treatment of patients. A synthetic pentasaccharide is currently under investigation and new oral compounds are being studied. Huridin compounds, which are direct thrombin inhibitors, may provide an alternative method of prophylaxis. Some of the synthetic thrombin inhibitors are also being developed for oral prophylaxis of DVT in surgical patients. Direct thrombin inhibitors potentially provide a useful alternative to heparin anticoagulation and may prove to be useful in validated clinical use.

The benefits of evidence-based medicine, which defines the value of medical interventions in terms of empirical evidence from clinical trials, are enormous. The promise of evidence-based medicine is a more systematic and scientific practice of clinical medicine. The search for new methods of prophylaxis is continually expanded and explored by questioning current practice and conducting clinical studies that provide information on which to base practice.

References

1 Clagett GP, Anderson FA, Geerts W *et al.*: Prevention of venous thromboembolism. *Chest* **114** (Supplement): 513–60, 1998.
2 Eriksson BI, Kalebo P, Anthymyr BA *et al.*: Prevention of deep-vein thrombosis and pulmonary embolism after total hip replacement. Comparison of low-molecular-weight heparin and unfractionated heparin. *Journal of Bone and Joint Surgery* [Am] **73**: 484–93, 1991.
3 Dahl OE, Andreassen G, Aspelin T *et al.*: Prolonged thromboprophylaxis following hip replacement surgery—results of a double-blind, prospective, randomised, placebo-controlled study with dalteparin. *Thrombosis and Haemostasis* **77**: 26–31, 1997.
4 Planes A, Vochelle N, Darmon J-Y *et al.*: Risk of deep-venous thrombosis after hospital discharge in patients having undergone total hip replacement: double-blind randomized comparison of enoxaparin and placebo. *Lancet* **348**: 28–31, 1996.
5 Grady-Benson JC, Oishi CS, Hanson PB *et al.*: Postoperative surveillance for deep venous thrombosis with duplex ultrasonography after total knee arthroplasty. *Journal of Bone and Joint Surgery* [Am] **76**: 1658–63, 1994.
6 Ciccone WJ, Fox PS, Neumyer M *et al.*: Ultrasound surveillance for asymptomatic deep venous thrombosis after total joint replacement. *Journal of Bone and Joint Surgery* [Am] **80**: 1167–74, 1998.
7 Garino JP, Lotke PA, Kitziger KJ *et al.*: Deep venous thrombosis after total joint arthroplasty. The role of compression ultrasonography and the importance of the experience of the technician. *Journal of Bone and Joint Surgery* [Am] **78**: 1359–65, 1996.
8 Anderson DR, Gross M, Robinson KS *et al.*: Ultrasonographic screening for deep vein thrombosis following arthroplasty fails to reduce posthospital thromboembolic complications. *Chest* **114**: 119S–22S, 1998.
9 Brothers TC, Frank CE, Frank B *et al.*: Is duplex venous surveillance worthwhile after arthroplasty? *Journal of Surgery Research* **67**: 72B, 1997.
10 Ishak M, Morley KD: Deep venous thrombosis after total hip arthroplasty: a prospective controlled study to determine the prophylactic effect of graded pressure stockings. *British Journal of Surgery* **68**: 429–32, 1981.
11 Barnes RW, Brand RA, Clarke W *et al.*: Efficacy of graded-compression antiembolism stockings in patients undergoing total hip arthroplasty. *Clinical Orthopaedics and Related Research* **132**: 61–7, 1978.
12 Gallus A, Raman K, Darby T: Venous thrombosis after elective hip replacement—the influence of preventive intermittent calf compression and of surgical technique. *British Journal of Surgery* **70**: 17–19, 1983.
13 Hull RD, Raskob GE, Gent M *et al.*: Effectiveness of intermittent pneumatic leg compression for preventing deep vein thrombosis after total hip replacement. *Journal of the American Medical Association* **263**: 2313–17, 1990.

14 Paiement G, Wessinger SJ, Waltman AC *et al.*: Low-dose warfarin versus external pneumatic compression for prophylaxis against venous thromboembolism following total hip replacement. *Journal of Arthroplasty* **2**: 23–6, 1987.

15 Woolson ST, Watt JM: Intermittent pneumatic compression to prevent deep benous thrombosis during and after total hip replacement. *Journal of Bone and Joint Surgery* [Am] **73**: 507–9, 1991.

16 Hooker JA, Lachiewicz PF, Kelley SS: Efficacy of prophylaxis against thromboembolism with intermittent pneumatic compression after primary and revision total hip arthroplasty. *Journal of Bone and Joint Surgery* [Am] **81**: 690–6, 1999.

17 Bradley JG, Krugener GH, Jager HJ: The effectiveness of intermittent plantar venous compression in prevention of deep venous thrombosis after total hip arthroplasty. *Journal of Arthroplasty* **8**: 57–61, 1993.

18 Stannard JP, Harris RM, Bucknell AL *et al.*: Prophylaxis of deep venous thrombosis after total hip arthroplasty by using intermittent compression of the plantar venous plexus. *American Journal of Orthopedics* **25**: 127–34, 1996.

19 Warwick D, Williams MH, Bannister GC: Death and thromboembolic disease after total hip replacement. A series of 1162 cases with no routine chemical prophylaxis. *Journal of Bone and Joint Surgery* [Br] **77**: 6–10, 1995.

20 Francis CW, Pellegrini VD, Marder VJ *et al.*: Prevention of venous thrombosis after total hip arthroplasty. Antithrombin III and low-dose heparin compared with dextran 40. *Journal of Bone and Joint Surgery* [Am] **71**: 327–35, 1989.

21 Harris WH, Athanasoulis CA, Waltman AC *et al.*: Prophylaxis of deep-vein thrombosis after total hip replacement. Dextran and external pneumatic compression compared with 1.2 or 0.3 gram of aspirin daily. *Journal of Bone and Joint Surgery* [Am] **67**: 57–62, 1985.

22 Salvati EA, Lachiewicz P: Thromboembolism following total hip replacement arthroplasty: The efficacy of dextran–aspirin and dextran–warfarin in prophylaxis. *Journal of Bone and Joint Surgery* [Am] **58**: 921–5, 1976.

23 Planes A, Vochelle N, Darmon JY *et al.*: Prevention of postoperative venous thrombosis: a randomized trial comparing unfractionated heparin with low molecular weight heparin in patients undergoing total hip replacement. *Thrombosis and Haemostasis* **60**: 407–10, 1989.

24 Hoek J, Nurmohamed MT, Hamelynck KJ *et al.*: Prevention of deep vein thrombosis following total hip replacement by low molecular weight heparinoid. *Thrombosis and Haemostasis* **67**: 28–32, 1992.

25 Leyvraz PF, Richard J, Bachmann F.: Adjusted versus fixed-dose subcutaneous heparin in prevention of deep vein thrombosis after total hip replacement. *New England Journal of Medicine* **309**: 954–8, 1983.

26 Leyvraz PF, Bachmann F, Hoek J *et al.*: Prevention of deep vein thrombosis after hip replacement: randomized comparison between unfractionated heparin and low molecular weight heparin. *British Medical Journal* **303**: 543–8, 1991.

27 Dechavanne M, Ville D, Berruyer M *et al.*: Randomized trial of a low-molecular-weight heparin (Kabi 2165) versus adjusted-dose subcutanteous standard heparin in the prophylaxis of deep-vein thrombosis after elective hip surgery. *Haemostasis* **19**: 5–12, 1989.

28 Hip and Knee Registry: *Aggregate Report, 1999, Quarter 3*. University of Massachusetts Medical School Center for Outcomes Research, Worcester, MA.

29 Gross M, Anderson DR, Nagpal S *et al.*: Venous thromboembolism prophylaxis after total hip or knee arthroplasty: a survey of Canadian orthopedic surgeons. *Canadian Journal of Surgery* **42**: 457–61, 1999.

30 RD Heparin Arthroplasty Group: RD heparin compared with warfarin for prevention of venous thromboembolic disease following total hip or knee arthroplasty. *Journal of Bone and Joint Surgery* [Am] **76**: 1174–85, 1994.

31 Heit JA, Berkowitz SD, Bona R *et al.*: Efficacy and safety of low molecular weight heparin (ardeparin sodium) compared to warfarin for the prevention of venous thromboembolism after total knee replacement surgery: a double-blind, dose-ranging study. *Thrombosis and Haemostasis* **77**: 32–8, 1997.

32 Francis CW, Pelegrini VD, Trotterman S *et al.*: Prevention of deep-vein thrombosis after total hip arthroplasty. Comparison of warfarin and dalteparin. *Journal of Bone and Joint Surgery* [Am] **79**: 1365–72, 1997.

33 Geerts WH, Heit JA, Clagett P *et al.*: Prevention of venous thromboembolism. *Chest* **119** (Supplement 1): 132S–75S, 2001.

34 Francis CW, Marder VJ, Evarts CM *et al.*: Two-step warfarin therapy. Prevention of postoperative venous thrombosis without excessive bleeding. *Journal of the American Medical Association* **249**: 374–8, 1983.

35 Francis CW, Pelegrini VD, Marder VJ *et al.*: Comparison of warfarin and external pneumatic compression in prevention of venous thrombosis after total hip replacement. *Journal of the American Medical Association* **267**: 2911–15, 1992.

36 Leizorovicz A, Haugh MC, Chapuis FR: Low molecular weight heparin in prevention of perioperative thrombosis. *British Medical Journal* **305**: 913–20, 1992.

37 Hull RD, Raskob GE, Pineo GF *et al.*: A comparison of subcutaneous low-molecular-weight heparin with warfarin sodium for prophylaxis against deep-vein thrombosis after hip or knee implantation. *New England Journal of Medicine* **329**: 1370–6, 1993.

38 Palmer AJ, Koppenhagen K, Kirchhof B *et al.*: Efficacy and safety of low molecular weight heparin, unfractionated heparin and warfarin for thrombo-embolism prophylaxis in orthopaedic surgery: a meta-analysis of randomised clinical trials. *Haemostasis* **27**: 75–84, 1997.

39 Imperiale TF, Speroff T: A meta-analysis of methods to prevent venous thromboembolism following total hip replacement. *Journal of the American Medical Association* **271**: 1780–5, 1994.

40 Mohr DN, Silverstein MD, Murtaugh PA *et al.*: Prophylactic agents for venous thrombosis in elective hip surgery. Meta-analysis of studies using venographic assessment. *Archives of Internal Medicine* **153**: 2221–8, 1993.

41 Pellegrini VD, Clement D, Lush-Ehmann C *et al.*: Natural history of thromboembolic disease after total hip arthroplasty. *Clinical Orthopaedics and Related Research* **333**: 27–40, 1996.

42 Bergqvist D, Benoni G, Björgell O *et al.*: Low-molecular-weight heparin (enoxaparin) as prophylaxis against venous thromboembolism after total hip replacement. *New England Journal of Medicine* **335**: 696–700, 1996.

43 Spiro TE, Enoxaparin Clinical Trial Group: A double blind multicenter clinical trial comparing long term enoxaparin and placebo treatments in the prevention of venous thromboembolic disease

after hip and knee replacement surgery. *Blood* **90** (Supplement 1): 295a, 1997 (abstract).

44 Lassen MR, Borris LC, Anderson BS *et al.*: Efficacy and safety of prolonged thromboprophylaxis with a low molecular weight heparin (dalteparin) after total hip arthroplasty—the Danish Prolonged Prophylaxis (DAPP) Study. *Thrombosis Research* **89**: 281–7, 1998.

45 Hull RD, Pineo GF, Francis CW *et al.*: A double-blind comparison of low-molecular-weight heparin prophylaxis using dalteparin in close proximity to surgery versus warfarin in hip-arthroplasty patients: a double-blind, randomized comparison. *Archives of Internal Medicine* **160**: 2199–207, 2000.

46 Robinson KS, Anderson DR, Gross M *et al.* Ultrasonographic screening before hospital discharge for deep venous thrombosis after arthroplasty: the Post-Arthroplasty Screening Study. A randomized, controlled trial. *Annals of Internal Medicine* **127**: 439–45, 1997.

47 Leclerc JR, Gent M, Hirsh J *et al.*: The incidence of symptomatic venous thromboembolism during and after prophylaxis with enoxaparin: a multi-institutional cohort study of patients who underwent hip or knee arthroplasty. *Archives of Internal Medicine* **158**: 873–8, 1998.

48 Colwell CW, Collis DK, Paulson R *et al.*: Comparison of enoxaparin and warfarin for the prevention of venous thromboembolic disease after total hip arthroplasty: evaluation during hospitalization and three months after discharge. *Journal of Bone and Joint Surgery* [Am] **81**: 932–40, 1999.

49 Heit JA, Elliott CG, Trowbridge AA *et al.*: Extended out-of-hospital LMWH venous thromboembolism prophylaxis after total hip or knee replacement surgery. *Blood* **92** (Supplement 1): 500a, 1998 (abstract).

50 Warwick D, Harrison J, Glew D *et al.*: Comparison of the use of a foot pump with the use of low-molecular-weight heparin for the prevention of deep-vein thrombosis after total hip replacement. *Journal of Bone and Joint Surgery* [Am] **80**: 1158–66, 1998.

51 White RH, Romano PS, Zhou H *et al.*: Incidence and time course of thromboembolic outcomes following total hip or knee arthroplasty. *Archives of Internal Medicine*, **158**: 1525–31, 1998.

12

Management of the infected total hip arthroplasty: a North American perspective

M. Gavan McAlinden, Bassam A. Masri, and
Clive P. Duncan

Introduction

Total hip arthroplasty (THA) is recognized as one of the great successes of orthopaedic surgery. However, when infection occurs, it remains one of the most devastating complications of this operation. Despite early reports of an unacceptably high infection rate (nine out of 109 patients (9 per cent)),[1] use of modern prophylactic measures, which may include prophylactic antibiotics, laminar-flow ventilation systems in the operating theatre, and all-enclosing exhaust suits, has led to a fall in the rate of infection after primary THA to less than 1.5 per cent in series from specialist centres and state registries.[2–6] Fender et al.[2] reported an infection rate of 1.4 per cent at 5 years in a regional hip register, while Kreder et al.[3] looking at the Washington State Department of Health dataset, reported an infection rate of 0.8 per cent (67/8774 patients) at 1 year. In an MRC trial conducted at 19 British and Swedish hospitals,[4] it was found that the use of laminar-flow ventilation, prophylactic antibiotics, and body exhaust suits could reduce infection to 0.2 per cent in the short term. Josefsson et al.[5] reported infection rates at 2 years of 1.6 per cent (13/812) in patients treated with systemic antibiotics compared with 0.4 per cent (3/821) in patients treated with antibiotic-laden cement. Schutzer and Harris,[3] reporting the experience of a single surgeon, found that 1 per cent of primary THAs became infected by an average of 4.2 years, although four of these patients (out of 103) had undergone complex primary procedures.

Some of the risk factors for infection after hip replacement include medical comorbidities and previous surgery. Some of these medical comorbidities include inflammatory joint disease, particularly rheumatoid arthritis, previous transplant surgery, and diabetes mellitus.[7–11] This effect may often be ascribed to the patients' medications rather than to the disease process itself. Previous surgery to the hip, prior to primary THA, has been associated with a higher subsequent infection rate (2.5 per cent) than that seen in patients with no previous surgery (0.9 per cent).[7] Poss et al.[8] reviewed 2012 primary and revision THAs and found that patients with rheumatoid arthritis had an almost twofold increase in the risk of infection compared with patients with osteoarthritis. This contradicted an earlier report from the same authors,[12] a fact they attributed to the longer follow-up in the latter study. Maderazo et al.[9] found that all of their series of patients with rheumatoid arthritis who became infected were taking steroids, predominantly prednisone. Tannenbaum et al.[10] reported that 19 per cent (5/27) of THAs performed after a renal or liver transplantation became infected at an average of 3.4 years. They noted a high prevalence of infection in patients taking cyclosporin A. Espehaug et al. (1997)[11] found an increased infection risk in patients taking antidiabetic medication, regardless of whether this was insulin or oral hypoglycaemics.

Revision THA in patients without other complicating medical conditions has also been associated with higher infection rates than primary procedures. James et al.[13] reviewed several series of revision THAs and reported an infection rate of 12 per cent (79/661 cases), initially in the absence of sepsis, with a *maximum* follow-up of 10 years. Fortunately, more recent studies, such as that of Katz et al.[14] report infection rates which are little higher (2/82 (2.5 per cent)) than those achieved at primary procedures.

Periprosthetic infections are a significant problem for the patient. Buchholz et al.[15] reported that nine of their series of 583 patients died as a result of the surgical treatment of their infection, and Nelson et al.[16] in a small series, reported that six of 13 patients died for reasons which were 'in some way related to the hip infection'. As well as the cost to the patient, the cost to the community is not inconsiderable. The cost of treating infection after arthroplasty has been estimated at $50 000 per case.[9,17]

Interpretation of the literature dealing with the issue of infection after THA is fraught with difficulty, reflecting the clinical complexities of dealing with these challenging cases. Each case of an infected THA presents particular challenges to the surgeon, making an individualized approach essential. Consideration needs to be given to the chronicity of the infection, the patient's bone stock, and the patient's general health and suitability for surgery. The basic tenet guiding treatment is eradication of infection, with the secondary aims of pain reduction and restoration of function.[18] It has been highlighted that many of the 'principles' of managing infection are based on early papers, which dealt with THA following septic arthritis, internal fixation of hip fractures, and endoprostheses.[19] The outcome of treatment for infection involving hip screws and plates, endoprostheses, and resurfacing arthroplasties may be quite different from that of an infected THA in both one- and two-stage revisions.[20-23] Jupiter et al.[20] reported the results of revision of 18 patients with infected metalwork within the hip joint. Infection was successfully eradicated in all (100 per cent) of nine patients who had infected cup arthroplasties, femoral endoprostheses, or other metalwork with a minimum of 2 years follow-up. Similar success was obtained in only five of nine patients (56 per cent) with an infected THA. Cherney and Amstutz[22] reported recurrence of infection in three of eight patients (37.5 per cent) who had previously undergone THA, while only three of 15 patients who had initially had infected cup arthroplasties, hemi-arthroplasties, or internal fixation became infected at a minimum follow-up of 3 years. Furthermore, many early authors describe their experiences prior to the widespread use of modern adjuncts such as antibiotic-loaded cement, modern organism-specific antibiotics delivered at an adequate dosage by an appropriate route, and active participation by infectious diseases consultants.

Adequate follow-up of patients who have undergone treatment for an infected THA is essential. The importance of long-term follow-up of revision arthroplasty has been stressed, as infection may first present some years after the index procedure.[13,22,24]

In this chapter, we review the North American perspective on the classification and management of infection after THA.

Classification

In order to understand the North American treatment algorithms and their rationale, it is important to classify these infections into similar types. Coventry[25] and Fitzgerald et al.[2] classified periprosthetic infections according to their chronicity. They initially defined phase I infections as those presenting within 3 months of the index procedure, but most commonly within the first 3 weeks of the operation as an acute suppurating infection (phase Ia). These patients may have the stigmata of acute systemic infection (tachycardia, pyrexia, and local signs of acute infection). Patients with haematoma formation, but no overt signs of infection, were also included as part of the phase I group. Phase II infections were defined as low-grade insidious infection, which usually becomes apparent between 2 and 12 months after operation. They were chiefly characterized by increasing pain in a previously painless joint. In the untreated case, loosening of femoral and acetabular components may become apparent with time. Coventry[25] also alluded to late acute haematogenous infection, but contrary to many subsequent citations of his work did not refer to these cases as phase III infections. In his paper, phase III simply referred to reimplantation after a resection arthroplasty.

Tsukayama et al.[26] modified the time-scale and clarified the definitions of Coventry's classification.

Acute infections were defined as those presenting within 4 weeks of the primary procedure. Debridement and component retention with intravenous antibiotic administration for 4 weeks were recommended for these cases. Infection was successfully eradicated in 25 of 35 cases (71 per cent).

Chronic infections were present for more than 4 weeks in patients who, frequently, had not had a pain-free period since their initial surgery. Debridement, removal of the infected hardware, and reconstruction, where appropriate, were recommended. With a two-stage reconstruction, infection was successfully eradicated in 29 of 34 cases (85 per cent).

Acute haematogenous infections were defined as those which had arisen, *de novo*, in a previously asymptomatic joint and may have been associated with a recent invasive surgical or prolonged dental procedure. Debridement and component retention with intravenous antibiotic administration for 6 weeks were recommended for these cases. Infection was eradicated in three out of six cases (50 per cent).

Unsuspected infections or **positive intra-operative cultures** were those in which intra-operative cultures, taken at the time of revision surgery, proved to be positive in a patient where infection was not clinically suspected. Treatment with intravenous antibiotics for 6 weeks, with no further surgical procedure, resulted in 18 out of 20 patients (90 per cent) remaining infection free.

Some authors[9] believe that most late infections are the result of infection from a distant focus. However, most consider that the group of patients presenting with chronic infection include those in whom infection is a result of bacterial colonization at the time of the index procedure as well as those in whom infection arises acutely by haematogenous spread from a distant focus.

Over the years, there has been little debate about the treatment of acute haematogenous infections or early postoperative infections. However, the treatment of chronic infections has been controversial, with the Atlantic Ocean creating not only a geographic but also a philosophical divide in terms of the specific treatment approach to these difficult problems. While one-stage exchange arthroplasty has been popular in Europe,[5,15,27–29] two-stage exchange arthroplasty has become the preferred approach in North America.[19,21,26,30,31]

How should the positive intra-operative culture be managed in 'aseptic' revision THA?

The importance of positive intra-operative cultures in the hip that was not thought to be infected following preoperative investigation has become an increasingly controversial issue. A recent study, in which strict anaerobic bacteriological practice and ultrasonication were used to dislodge bacteria from biofilms, isolated bacteria in

26 of 120 patients (22 per cent) undergoing revision THA.[32] Infection was suspected in only six of these patients. The same authors used immunofluorescent microscopy and 16S ribosomal RNA and identified bacteria or bacterial RNA in 71 of 113 patients (63 per cent) and 85 of 118 patients (72 per cent) respectively. Their findings correlated well with histopathology. The idea of unsuspected infection or colonization of a prosthesis is not new, but the significance is not always clear. Murray[30] reported that 40 per cent (61/151) of culture-positive revision hip arthroplasties were diagnosed only at the time of surgery. It has been suggested that, to be considered positive, cultures should be positive from at least two different sites within the operative field.[33] Tsukayama et al.[26] reported their experience of 31 patients in whom intra-operative cultures were positive, but infection was not suspected preoperatively. These patients represented 11 per cent of the 275 revision arthroplasties performed over the study period. All were treated with a 6-week course of intravenous antibiotics. In three patients (10 per cent) infection was not eradicated at 6 weeks and two had recurrence of infection at a minimum of 2 years. It seems that, in at least some cases, positive cultures represent previously undiagnosed infection and require treatment. Graziani et al.[33] have recommended that all cases of positive intra-operative cultures should be treated with antibiotics.

Can infection be managed with component retention?

Antibiotic suppression

Coventry, writing in 1975, stated that antibiotic suppression 'may control the symptoms and delay another operation, but probably is not strictly curative'.[25] These words are as true today as they were a quarter of a century ago. Goulet et al.[34] followed up 19 patients, most (18 of 19) with acute infections, who were treated with long-term suppressive antibiotics. Eleven patients had a surgical debridement. The group was made up of patients who had refused surgery or who were deemed to be unsuitable for an extensive reconstructive procedure. Seven of these patients (37 per cent) eventually required revision within the follow-up period, although a further two had persistent draining sinuses. Goulet et al. concluded that suppressive antibiotic treatment is an effective option if the preferred surgical reimplantation cannot be achieved. Zimmerli et al.[35] followed up 33 patients with staphylococcal infection of a variety of orthopaedic implants, including eight THAs. All underwent surgical debridement and were randomized to long-term ciprofloxacin with or without rifampin (rifampicin). All 12 of those who completed the course of ciprofloxacin with rifampin were free of infection at 2 years. The authors did not explicitly outline the results for the hip patients. Nevertheless, these results are promising for the treatment of patients who are unable to have extensive surgery. It has been recommended that antibiotic suppression should be reserved for patients with well-fixed components, without systemic symptoms, in whom there is a contraindication to surgery or who refuse surgery. The organism must be sensitive to the antibiotics, which should be available in an oral form and well tolerated.[34,36,37]

Debridement and prosthesis retention

Debridement and prosthesis retention are often used as the initial treatment in cases of acute or acute haematogenous infection, although these cases only represent a small proportion of the total number of periprosthetic infections. The former practice of closed suction–irrigation has now largely been abandoned because of the occurrence of super-infection.[16] In the setting of chronic periprosthetic infection, debridement and prosthesis retention are uniformly associated with a dismal outcome.[7,38,39] Fitzgerald et al.[7] reported that only one of 18 patients retained their hardware at a minimum of 2 years. Canner et al.[38] who grouped patients by time from operation rather than chronicity of infection, reported failure in 22 of 23 cases who were also treated with concomitant antibiotics. Crockarell et al.[39] reported the results of 19 cases with chronic infection. None were successfully treated by debridement and prosthesis retention.

The results of treatment of acute and acute haematogenous infections are somewhat better than those for chronic infections. Tsukayama et al.[26] reported success rates of 71 per cent (25/35) in the treatment of acute infection with debridement and component retention with 4 weeks of intravenous antibiotics, and 50 per cent in the similar treatment of acute haematogenous infection but with 6 weeks of intravenous antibiotics. In a small series, Hyman et al.[40] treated eight patients with acute haematogenous infections with arthroscopic drainage, irrigation, and debridement, followed by prolonged antibiotic suppression. At a mean follow-up of 70 months, no infection recurred. However, even in the selected population of acute and acute haematogenous infections, optimistic expectations must be tempered by success rates as low as 26 per cent (6/23).[39]

The chronicity of symptoms appears to correlate well with success of treatment. Brandt et al. (1997),[41] who investigated patients infected only with *Staphylococcus aureus* (treated between 1980 and 1981), found that 56 per cent (8/18) of those treated within 2 days of onset of symptoms still had successful eradication of disease after 2 years. They did not distinguish between acute and acute haematogenous infections. Crockarell et al.[39] noted that infection was not eradicated in any patient treated by debridement more than 2 weeks after onset of symptoms.

Should infection be treated with a one-stage or a two-stage procedure?

Comparisons of studies comparing one- and two-stage revision procedures are complicated by the fact that some studies are performed in selected patient populations rather than on a consecutive series. For example, Ure et al.[42] in presenting excellent results of surgery on patients who underwent one-stage revision, concede that they 'do not recommend direct exchange for patients who are immunocompromized; for those who have an infection with a known resistant Gram-negative or methicillin-resistant organism; or for those who have a major skin, soft-tissue, or osseous defect that makes it impossible to obtain a closed wound or a stable implant'. Katz et al.[43] also reported excluding patients who had 'no gross purulence with no periprosthetic abscesses or sinus tracts [sic]'. These exclusions, while conveying an important message regarding the role of one-stage revision, may bias the reported results. To date, 'the complexity of the operative procedure and the many factors involved ... have discouraged investigators from performing prospective randomized trials to evaluate the timing [of one-stage or two-stage procedures]'.[44] Nevertheless, Garvin et al.[45] described the results of one-and two-stage revisions of 123 infected hip arthroplasties, as well as a combination of 88 conversion (from infected metalwork or a previously septic joint) arthroplasties, at-risk primary hip arthroplasties, and revision total knee arthroplasties. They used gentamicin-impregnated poly-methylmethacrylate cement. While conceding that 'less severe infections' were more likely to be treated in one stage, they found that these procedures carried a higher recurrence risk (10.1 versus 5.6 per cent), although this was not statistically significant. They recommended that one-stage revision should be reserved for elderly infirm patients, who are ill suited for 3 weeks of skeletal traction, in the presence of sensitive organisms and an adequately debrided joint.

Early results of either one- or two-stage reconstructions for infection after THA were generally poor.[20,24] Hunter and Dandy[24] reported on 30 patients who underwent a two-stage reconstruction for infection; 20 of them became reinfected. Similarly, Jupiter et al.[20] reported the results of a one-stage procedure performed, for infection, in eight patients. Four of the eight became reinfected. The advent of antibiotic-loaded cement and the prolonged use of intravenous antibiotics tailored to organism sensitivities signalled a marked improvement in the results of reconstruction.[15,46] Buchholz et al.[15] reported the experience of treating 583 patients with an infected prosthesis using antibiotic-loaded cement but no adjuvant antibiotics. They were successful in eradicating infection in 448 patients (77 per cent) with a one-stage exchange, with a further 74 patients successfully treated by an additional one to four operations, giving an overall success rate of 90 per cent. Hughes *et al.*[46] treated 13 patients with infected THAs and 13 others with infected fixation hardware or hemiarthroplasties in two stages, giving prolonged antibiotic therapy before surgery and before and after reimplantation. They reported four recurrent infections out of the 26 cases, a success rate of 85 per cent. Combining treatment modalities has been shown to result in excellent results for both one- and two-stage reconstructions. For example, Wroblewski[28] treated 102 infected THAs in one stage with both antibiotic-loaded cement and antibiotics (88 per cent of patients). Infection was eradicated in 93 of the 102 patients at between 27 and 38 months, a success rate of 91 per cent. Our own results,[47–49] using both antibiotic-loaded cement and parenteral antibiotics in a two-stage procedure, showed that only four of 81 patients (a success rate of 95 per cent) became reinfected at a minimum of 2 years. The results of one- and two-stage revision in patients whose treatment regimes included both antibiotic-loaded cement and adjuvant antibiotics are compared in Tables 12.1 and 12.2. It can be seen that a higher infection eradication rate (90 versus 87 per cent) was obtained in the group managed in two stages, even though this group includes two series[54,56] dealing specifically with the issues of use of allograft in reconstruction.

In North America, the current standard of care for the management of the infected hip arthroplasty is two-stage exchange arthroplasty, where the implants are removed in the first stage and the joint is debrided (Fig. 12.1). Antibiotic-loaded cement may or may not be used between stages, and the second stage involves the actual reimplantation.

Table 12.1 Results of one-stage revision with antibiotic-laden cement and adjuvant antibiotics

	Follow-up	No. of THAs	No. reinfected	Percentage eradication
Carlsson *et al.*[27]	>6 months	54	5 (+ some remaining symptomatic)	91
Miley *et al.*[50]	>32 months	47	6	87
Wroblewski[28]	27–38 months	102	9	91
Sanzen *et al.*[51]	>24 months	72	17	76
Katz *et al.*[43]	10–13 years	24	2	92
Raut *et al.*[52]	2–12 years	57	8	86
Garvin *et al.*[53]	2–10 years	10	1	90
Ure *et al.*[42]	6–17 years	20	0	100
Total		332	43	87

Table 12.2 Results of two-stage revision with antibiotic-laden cement and adjuvant antibiotics

	Follow-up	No. of THAs	No. reinfected	Percentage eradication
Murray[30]		51	4	92
Sanzen et al.[51]	>24 months	30	8	73
Berry et al.[54]	2–8.1 years	18	2	89
Garvin et al.[53]	2–10 years	30	1	97
Lieberman et al.[55]	24–74 months	32	3	91
Tsukayama et al.[26]	0.3–11 years	41	6	85
Alexeeff et al.[56]	24–72 months	11	0	100
Haddad et al.[49]	>2 years	81	4	95
Total		294	28	90

Table 12.3 Effect of duration to reimplantation on success of reconstruction

	No. of THAs	Duration to reimplantation	Significance of duration
McDonald et al.[19]	81	6 days–6.2 years'	At <1year 27% (7/25) failed At >1 year 7% (4/56) failed
Colyer and Capello[58]	37	4–214 weeks (26 within 6 weeks)	At >22 weeks 22% (2/9) failed At <6 weeks 14% (4/28) failed
Lieberman et al.[55]	32	20 days–32 months	Not significant
Nestor et al.[31]	34	3–19 months	Not significant
Tsukayama et al.[26]	41	1–24 months	At <60 days 7% (1/15) failed compared with 15% (7/41) for total group

Two-stage exchange: when should reimplantation take place?

Early studies of two-stage revision of infected THA reported a prolonged interval between implant removal and reimplantation. Hunter[57] discussed the results of two-stage reconstruction of 57 infected arthroplasties. The second stage (reimplantation) was performed between 5 weeks and 3 years after the first (excision arthroplasty). Without comparing the results of early and late reconstruction, his stated preference was for reconstruction after 1 year. Support for Hunter's view came from McDonald et al.[19] who noted that 27 per cent (7/25) of reimplantations which took place within 1 year became reinfected compared with only 7 per cent (4/56) reimplanted after 1 year. More recent reports, summarized in Table 12.3, fail to support a lengthy interval. Indeed, Colyer and Capello[58] found that two of nine patients with reimplantation after 22 weeks suffered reinfection compared with four of 28 who were reimplanted within 6 weeks. Tsukayama et al.[26] also noted better results (only one of 15 patients reinfected) in those who were reimplanted early. A subsequent report from Garvin et al.[45] also noted

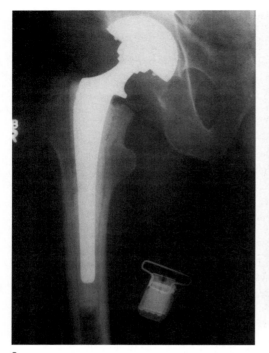

a

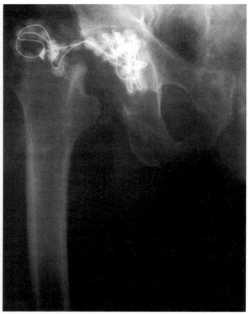

b

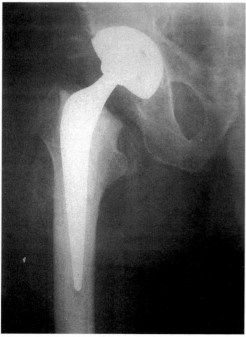

c

Fig. 12.1

An example of two-stage revision of an infected total hip arthroplasty. (a) An infected THA 1 year after primary arthroplasty: lucency is displayed around the cement mantle. (b) Following resection arthroplasty: the interval has been packed with antibiotic-loaded polymethylmethacrylate 'rosary beads'. (c) Final appearance after implantation of a cemented femoral component and a cementless acetabular component.

that earlier reimplantation improved the success rate from 85 to 93 per cent.

In summary, recent evidence indicates greater success when reimplantation takes place at around 3 months rather than at a year or more.

Is the infecting organism important?

In most reports of periprosthetic infection, *Staphylococcus aureus* and *Staphylococcus epidermidis* are the most common infective organisms, although a wide range of Gram-positive and Gram-negative organisms, as well as anaerobic organisms, have also been implicated. Several workers have drawn attention to the importance of the identified bacterial flora when planning treatment of an infected THA. There are good theoretical bases for this approach. Firstly, it has been contended that high-virulence organisms such as Gram-negative organisms are more difficult to eradicate. The definition of virulence differs from paper to paper. Gram-negative organisms and Group D streptococci are considered virulent by all. *Staphylococcus aureus*, both methicillin-sensitive and methicillin-resistant, other streptococci groups, and entero-cocci have been considered as both virulent and less virulent,[19,45] and *Staphylococcus epidermidis* is generally considered to be of low virulence. Secondly, organisms which form a glycocalyx *in vivo* may also be less susceptible to eradication. Implantation of orthopaedic prostheses provides an ideal environment for the colonization and proliferation of micro-organisms, which Gristina and Costerson[59] have described as the 'race for the surface', i.e. the race between bacterial colonization and the host's sealing of the bone–prosthetic interface. Many micro-organisms form a glycocalyx or slime of secreted polysaccharide within which bacteria can exist in a sessile form. In effect, a stable population of these organisms exists, using extracellular signalling, as a multicellular organism. Because the population is stable, bacteria within the glycocalyx have a low rate of replication, rendering them up to 1000 times less susceptible to antibiotics targeted at multiplying organisms.

Reinfection rates have been found to be higher in patients infected with Gram-negative organisms and more virulent Gram-positive organisms (*Staphylococcus aureus* and ß-haemolytic *Streptococcus* species) in some studies.[20,22] For this reason, many have considered these to be more difficult infections to eradicate, a fact which has been attributed, in part, to glycocalyx formation. However, it is now thought that up to 90 per cent of micro-organisms, including the 'low-virulence' *Staphylococcus epidermidis* can form a glycocalyx, given the right conditions.[60] In contrast to the concerns raised regarding Gram-negative and highly virulent organisms, others have recommended that coagulase-negative

Staphylococcus species should be treated with caution because of their tendency to be resistant to multiple antibiotics.[29] Several different multiresistant coagulase-negative *Staphylococcus* species may coexist in a single infected joint.

The concern regarding infection with particular organisms may well have been based on papers which do not reflect current practice. Hunter and Dandy[24] reviewed 135 cases of infected THAs in a Canadian national survey. They found that 20 out of 30 of these patients had failed reimplantation of a prosthetic joint. Of the successful cases, nine grew Gram-positive organisms from the infected joint and one had sterile cultures, while four of the failed cases grew *Escherichia coli*. From this they deduced that eradication of Gram-negative organisms presented a particular problem. Importantly, they also noted that none of these cases involved the use of antibiotic-loaded cement or 'massive antibiotic regimes'. Jupiter *et al.*[20] reported on the reconstruction of nine infected THAs. Four of the nine procedures became reinfected, including both cases infected with Gram-negative organisms. Antibiotic-loaded cement does not appear to have been used in these cases.

Several more recent papers have explicitly addressed the question of difficulty in eradicating particular groups of organisms (Table 12.4). None of these authors have identified a relationship between recurrence of infection and organism type. Only McDonald *et al.*[19] found a significant ($p = 0.055$) increase in reinfection following treatment of Gram-negative bacilli or group D streptococcal organisms, but only when looking at patients who had received less than 4 weeks treatment with antibiotics and reimplantation at less than a year. It is important to note that, in this series, early reimplantation was significantly associated with increased recurrence ($p < 0.001$), independently of all other factors.

Perhaps of more importance than the identity of the organisms is their susceptibility to attack by antimicrobial agents and the ability to deliver antibiotics in appropriate doses to the site of infection. For example, most staphylococci, with the exception of the strains

Table 12.4 The effect of infecting organism(s) on success of reconstruction

	No. of infected THAs	Significance of organism type
Salvati *et al.*[21]	27	Not significant
Poss *et al.*[8]	18	Not significant
Balderson *et al.*[23]	22	Not significant
McDonald *et al.*[19]	82	Not independently significant (see text)
Lieberman *et al.*[55]	42	Not significant
Nestor *et al.*[31]	34	Not significant
Tsukayama *et al.*[26]	106	Gram-negative organisms no more difficult to treat

designated as methicillin or oxacillin resistant, are susceptible to first- or second-generation cephalosporins. There is substantial regional variation in the sensitivity profiles of *Staphylococcus epidermidis* and *Staphylococcus aureus*: in our hospital, more than 95 per cent of the *Staphylococcus aureus* organisms encountered are sensitive to oxacillin (and therefore cephalosporin), while less than 70 per cent of the *Staphylococcus epidermidis* organisms share this sensitivity.[36] Indeed, a range of differing bacterial sensitivities and resistances may be encountered among staphylococci isolated from a single infected joint.[61] Our practice is to identify the infecting organism(s) and their antibiotic sensitivities by synovial biopsy and joint aspiration preoperatively. This guides the antibiotic regime adopted for antibiotic-loaded cement and intravenous antibiotics in the postoperative period, but does not influence the surgical approach or technique.

In summary, the identity of the infecting organism probably does not affect the success or failure of the procedure. However, preoperative identification of the infecting organism continues to be of great importance to ensure that the correct antibiotic regime (local and systemic) is used.

Can bone grafting be used safely in the treatment of an infected THA?

Chronic bone infection around an infected implant may result in femoral or acetabular bone loss, which needs to be addressed as part of the treatment plan for managing infection. A two-stage reconstruction, allowing infection to be eradicated prior to inserting large amounts of foreign material, seems rational. Even the advocates of one-stage reconstruction will concede that dealing with extensive bone loss requires a staged treatment plan.[42] Use of bone grafting in primary THA has been associated with an increased rate of infection even with the use of prophylactic antibiotics, vertical laminar airflow, and a helmet aspirator suit. In a study of 659 hips, four of 125 (3 per cent) who received a structural graft had a subsequent infection compared with one of 534 (0.2 per cent) who did not.[3] It is not clear whether this observation relates to increased complexity, prolonged operating time, or disease transmission by the graft.

A few papers have dealt exclusively or in part with the safety of using bone graft in infection. These are summarized in Table 12.5. A study from Boston of 18 patients, on whom structural and morsellized allograft was used, reported reinfection in two cases out of 18 (12 per cent) at a mean of 4.2 years from implantation in staged reconstructions.[54] Results from the Mayo Clinic[31] reported a higher infection rate (five of 28 cases (17.9 per cent)) at an average of 47 months, although this was no different to the infection rate for patients treated with an identical implant without graft

Table 12.5 Success of bone grafting in reconstruction after infection

	No. of patients with type of graft used (structural/morsellized/both)	Outcome
Berry et al.[54]	8/5/5	Reinfection of one structural allograft and one morsellized (2/18)
Duncan and Beauchamp[62]	3/0/0	One allograft non-union; no infections
Nestor et al.[31]	0/8 autograft; 17 allograft /3	1/3 structural grafts infected; 5/28 grafted patients reinfected; 1/6 non-grafted patients reinfected; no statistical significance
Lieberman et al.[55]	0/0/5	No reinfection
Alexeeff et al.[56]	11/0/0	No reinfection
Wang and Chen[63]	1/17/4	Reinfection of 2 morsellized allografts. No reinfection of structural allograft
Total	23/30/14	9/67 reinfected (86.6% infection free)

(one of 6 cases (17 per cent). The experiences of Toronto, Vancouver, and the Hospital for Special Surgery were somewhat better, with no infections reported from 18 cases.[55,56,62] Wang and Chen[63] reported two reinfections out of 22 cases. Nine of these 67 cases became reinfected, giving an infection rate of 83 per cent, which is not markedly worse than revision without grafting. It is safe, as part of a staged reconstruction, to use allograft following an infected THA where bone loss dictates its necessity.

Segmental bone loss presents a significant technical problem in management of the infected THA. When the initial resection arthroplasty is performed, substantial proximal bone loss may result in considerable shortening of the limb unless a spacer is used.[64] This shortening may make the subsequent reimplantation procedure more difficult.[65] We believe that using a prosthesis coated with antibiotic-loaded acrylic cement (PROSTALAC) may maintain some function in the interval between resection and reimplantation, while creating an infection-free bed for subsequent bone grafting to make good the bone defect.[47]

What treatment alternatives exist?

Excision arthroplasty

As recently as 1984, it was reported that 'only excisional arthroplasty consistently eliminated infection and resulted in a clinically satisfactory result'.[38] The main findings of a number of papers dealing with the use of excisional arthroplasty in the treatment of infection are summarized in Table 12.6. Canner et al.[38] claimed that removal of all cement and infected tissue, production of a dry surgical wound, and adherence to Girdlestone's procedure[69] (excision of infected muscle, superior acetabular rim, femoral neck, and portion of greater trochanter) enhanced the eradication of infection. In their study, they found that adherence to these principles resulted in a good infection-free outcome in all of 10 patients treated in this way, while only 10 of 23 patients who underwent a less radical excisional arthroplasty had a similar result. Bourne et al.[68] reported only one reinfection in a group of 33 patients who had undergone a resection arthroplasty. However, they commented that an additional five patients had prolonged wound discharges. Other authors have highlighted the point that, while excisional arthroplasty may be a reasonably successful means of eradicating infection in the majority of patients, the functional outcome often leaves much to be desired. Six patients who underwent excision arthroplasty were found to have similar pain scores to patients with a reimplanted prosthesis, but functional scores were comparable to their preoperative infected status.[22] Although resection arthroplasty can provide some pain relief and help to control infection, albeit to no greater extent than reconstruction, the poor functional outcome means that it is now rarely indicated as a primary procedure. Its place is as a salvage procedure in patients unsuitable for a more exacting reconstructive program.

Arthrodesis

Arthrodesis has been suggested as a treatment option in selected young patients with an infected prosthesis. Kostuik and Alexander[70] reported on seven patients treated with this procedure for infection.

Table 12.6 Results of excision arthroplasty in controlling infection and improving function in treatment of infected THA

	No. of patients	Infection control	Functional outcome and symptomatic relief
Hunter and Dandy[24]	85	19 required further procedures to eradicate infection; 13 patients still draining at review	Not stated
Nelson et al.[16]	9		Only 2/9 with good function
Petty and Goldsmith[66]	35	7/35 wounds still draining at review	4/35 satisfied with results of surgery
Bittar and Petty[67]			
Bourne et al.[68]	33	One reinfection; 5 patients with 'prolonged wound discharge'	14/33 satisfied with function 30/33 satisfied with pain relief
Canner et al.[38]	33	6/33 reinfected	
Grauer et al.[65]	33	3/33 reinfected	Overall level of activity little better than before surgery; 21/33 only poor or fair pain relief
Lieberman et al.[55]	15	One patient reinfected	1/9 surviving patients able to walk more than six blocks

Four were performed in one stage and three in two stages. There were no recurrent infections and five patients returned to their former work. This technique does not appear to have been used by others.

Reinfection after reconstruction of an infected THA has a poor outlook, particularly if a further reconstruction is envisaged. Pagnano et al.[18] reported on 34 patients who became reinfected after reimplantation. Most were treated by long-term antibiotics with or without debridement or by resection arthroplasty. Of the eight patients who underwent a further reconstruction (three one-stage and five two-stage procedures), three (38 per cent) became reinfected and these had the worst functional outcome of all.

Our preferred treatment

We use a variety of treatment modalities tailored to the individual case. In early postoperative or acute haematogenous infection, with a well-documented brief history and a well-fixed prosthesis, we prefer a thorough open debridement after establishing the diagnosis by ery-throcyte sedimentation rate (ESR), C-reactive protein (CRP) estima-tion, and aspiration and Gram stain of the affected hip. Copious lavage is used at debridement. In the case of an uncemented cup, we exchange the polyethylene liner where appropriate. Postoperatively, patients are treated with intravenous antibiotics for 4–6 weeks under the supervision and guidance of infectious diseases personnel.

We reserve resection arthroplasty for patients who are considered medically unfit for further reconstruction and for those who are mentally impaired and would be unable to co-operate with post-operative restrictions and rehabilitation. We also advocate it for patients who are taking major immunosuppression medication, particularly following solid organ transplantation, and those who have an active history of intravenous abuse because such patients have a tendency toward poor compliance with postoperative instructions and a high risk of reinfection. We also recommend this option in patients with a failed two-stage exchange arthroplasty.

In chronic infections or in cases where a distinction between acute and chronic infection cannot be made with confidence, our preferred approach for reconstruction is a two-stage procedure using the PROSTALAC system between stages (Fig. 12.2). We use the same technique regardless of the infecting organism. The PROSTALAC system consists of a constrained cemented polyethylene acetabular component and a femoral component with a modular head, which is made intra-operatively. A metal shaft and neck are placed into one of a series of moulds with polymethylmethacrylate, to which is added a high dose of heat-stable antibiotics (usually 2.4–3.6 g of tobramycin (Nebcin®, Eli Lilly Canada Inc.) and 1–1.5 g vancomycin (Vancocin®, Eli Lilly Canada Inc)). The implants are cemented in place *without pres-surization* and the wound is closed without suction drainage, to prevent loss of locally high levels of antibiotic. Patients are given

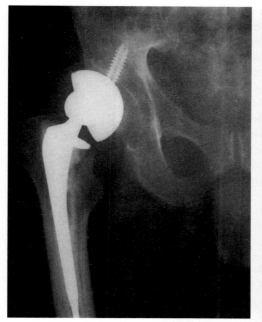

a

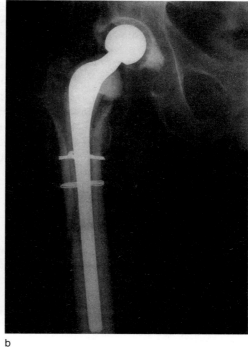

b

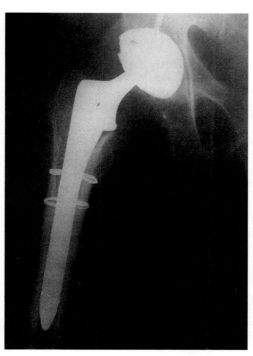

c

Fig. 12.2

An example of two-stage revision of an infected total hip arthroplasty using the PROSTALAC system. (a) An infected total hip arthroplasty, with a loose acetabular component. Demarcation can be seen around the femoral cement mantle. (b) Following an extended trochanteric osteotomy and removal of infected components, a long-stem PROSTALAC stem and cup have been inserted. (c) At the second stage, an extensively porous-coated femoral component and an acetabular component have been inserted without cement.

6 weeks of intravenous antibiotics postoperatively and reassessed by repeat ESR, CRP, and hip aspiration. We do not favour a prolonged interval between stages and therefore reimplantation of the definitive components takes place approximately 3 months after the first stage. We use both cementless and cemented components at this stage, the choice being dictated by the patient's bone stock and any requirement for bone grafting. To date, 81 patients have been followed for a minimum of 2 years after PROSTALAC treatment. The success rate has been 95 per cent (four failures).[47-49] We believe this technique affords a maximal opportunity for eradication of infection, while allowing us the choice of the optimal implant for the patient at the reimplantation stage.

References

1 Charnley J, Eftekhar N: Postoperative infection in total prosthetic replacement arthroplasty of the hip-joint with special reference to the bacterial content of the air of the operating room. *British Journal of Surgery* **56**: 641–9: 1969.

2 Fender D, Harper WM, Gregg PJ: Outcome of Charnley total hip replacement across a single health region in England: the results at five years from a regional hip register. *Journal of Bone and Joint Surgery* [Br] **81**: 577–81, 1999.

3 Schutzer SF, Harris WH: Deep-wound infection after total hip replacement under contemporary aseptic conditions. *Journal of Bone and Joint Surgery* [Am] **70**: 724–7, 1988.

4 Lidwell OM: Clean air at operation and subsequent sepsis in the joint. *Clinical Orthopaedics and Related Research* **211**: 91–102, 1986.

5 Josefsson G, Lindberg L, Wiklander B: Systemic antibiotics and gentamicin-containing bone cement in the prophylaxis of postoperative infections in total hip arthroplasty. *Clinical Orthopaedics and Related Research* **159**:194–200, 1981.

6 Kreder HJ, Deyo RA, Koepsell T, Swiontkowski MF, Kreuter W: Relationship between the volume of total hip replacements performed by providers and the rates of postoperative complications in the State of Washington. *Journal of Bone and Joint Surgery* [Am] **79**: 485–94, 1997.

7 Fitzgerald RH, Nolan DR, Ilstrup DM, Van Scoy RE, Washington JA II, Coventry MB: Deep wound sepsis following total hip surgery. *Journal of Bone and Joint Surgery* [Am] **59**: 847–55, 1977.

8 Poss R, Thornhill TS, Ewald FC, Thomas WH, Batte NJ, Sledge CB: Factors influencing the incidence and outcome of infection following total joint arthroplasty. *Clinical Orthopaedics and Related Research* **182**: 117–26, 1984.

9 Maderazo EG, Judson S, Pasternak H: Late infections of total joint prostheses: a review and recommendations for prevention. *Clinical Orthopaedics and Related Research* **229**: 131–42, 1988.

10 Tannenbaum DA, Matthews LS, Grady-Benson JC: Infection around joint replacements in patients who have a renal or liver transplant. *Journal of Bone and Joint Surgery* [Am] **79**: 36–43, 1997.

11 Espehaug B, Havelin LI, Engesaeter LB, Langelang N, Vollset SE: Patient-related risk factors for early revision of total hip replacements. *Acta Orthopaedica Scandinavica* **68**: 207–15, 1997.

12 Poss R, Ewald FC, Thomas WH, Sledge CB: Complications of total hip replacement arthroplasty in patients with rheumatoid arthritis. *Journal of Bone and Joint Surgery* [Am] **58**: 1130–3, 1976.

13 James ETR, Hunter GA, Cameron HU: Total hip arthroplasty. does sepsis influence the outcome? *Clinical Orthopaedics and Related Research* **170**: 88–94, 1982.

14 Katz RP, Callaghan JJ, Sullivan PM, Johnston RC: Long-term results of revision total hip arthroplasty. *Journal of Bone and Joint Surgery* [Am] **79**: 322–6, 1997.

15 Buchholz HW, Elson RA, Engelbrecht E, Lodenkämper H, Röttger J, Siegel A: Management of deep infection of total hip replacement. *Journal of Bone and Joint Surgery* [Br] **63**: 342–53, 1981.

16 Nelson CL, Evarts CM, Andrish J, Marks K: Results of infected total hip arthroplasty. *Clinical Orthopaedics and Related Research* **147**: 258–61, 1980.

17 Sculco TP: The economic impact of infected total joint arthroplasty. *Instructional Course Lectures* **41**: 349–53, 1993.

18 Pagnano MW, Trousdale RT, Hanssen AD: Outcome after reinfection following reimplantation hip arthroplasty. *Clinical Orthopaedics and Related Research* **338**: 192–204, 1997.

19 McDonald DJ, Fitzgerald RH Jr, Ilstrup DM: Two-stage reconstruction of a total hip arthroplasty because of infection. *Journal of Bone and Joint Surgery* [Am] **71**: 828–34, 1989.

20 Jupiter JB, Karchmer AW, Lowell JD, Harris WH: Total hip arthroplasty in the treatment of adult hips with current or quiescent sepsis. *Journal of Bone and Joint Surgery* [Am] **63**: 194–200, 1981.

21 Salvati EA, Chekofsky KM, Brause BD, Wilson PD Jr: Reimplantation in infection. A 12-year experience. *Clinical Orthopaedics and Related Research* **170**: 62–75, 1982.

22 Cherney DL, Amstutz HC: Total hip replacement in the previously septic hip. *Journal of Bone and Joint Surgery* [Am] **65**: 1256–65, 1983.

23 Balderson RA, Hiller WDB, Ianotti JP *et al.*: Treatment of the septic hip with total hip arthroplasty. *Clinical Orthopaedics and Related Research* **221**: 231–7, 1987.

24 Hunter GA, Dandy D: The natural history of the patient with an infected total hip replacement. *Journal of Bone and Joint Surgery* [Br] **59**: 293–7, 1977.

25 Coventry MB: Treatment of infections occurring in total hip surgery. *Orthopaedic Clinics of North America* **6**: 991–1003, 1975.

26 Tsukayama DT, Estrada R, Gustilo RB: Infection after total hip arthroplasty. *Journal of Bone and Joint Surgery* [Am] **78**: 512–23, 1996.

27 Carlsson AS, Josefsson G, Lindberg L: Revision with gentamicin-impregnated cement for deep infections in total hip arthroplasties. *Journal of Bone and Joint Surgery* [Am] **60**: 1059–62, 1978.

28 Wroblewski BM: One-stage revision on infected cemented total hip arthroplasty. *Clinical Orthopaedics and Related Research* **211**: 103–7, 1986.

29 Elson R: Sepsis: one-stage exchange. In *The adult hip* (ed. JJ Callaghan, AG Rosenberg, HE Rubash), pp. 1307–15. Lippincott-Raven, Philadelphia, PA, 1998.

30 Murray WR: Use of antibiotic-containing bone cement. *Clinical Orthopaedics and Related Research* **190**: 89–95, 1984.

31 Nestor VJ, Hanssen AD, Ferrer-Gonzalez R, Fitzgerald RH Jr: The use of porous-coated prostheses in delayed reconstruction of total hip replacements that have failed because of infection. *Journal of Bone and Joint Surgery* [Am] **76**: 349–59, 1994.

32 Tunney MM, Patrick S, Curran MD *et al.*: Detection of prosthetic hip infection at revision arthroplasty by immunofluorescent microscopy and PCR amplification of the bacterial 16S rRNA gene. *Journal of Clinical Microbiology* **37**: 3281–90, 1999.

33 Graziani AL, Hines JM, Morgan AS, MacGregor RR, Esterhai JL Jr: Infecting organisms and antibiotics. In *Revision total hip arthroplasty* (ed. ME Steinberg, JP Garino), pp. 407–17. Lippincott–Williams and Wilkins, Philadelphia, PA, 1999.

34 Goulet JA, Pellicci PM, Brause BD, Salvati EM: Prolonged suppression of infection in total hip arthroplasty. *Journal of Arthroplasty* **3**: 109–16, 1988.

35 Zimmerli W, Widmer AF, Blatter M, Frei R, Oschner PE: Role of rifampicin for treatment of orthopaedic implant-related staphylococcal infections. *Journal of the American Medical Association*, **279**: 1539–41, 1998.

36 Masterson EL, Masri BA, Duncan CP: Treatment of infection at the site of total hip replacement. *Journal of Bone and Joint Surgery* [Am] **79**: 1740–9, 1997.

37 Masri BA, Salvati EA: Two-stage exchange arthroplasty in the treatment of the infected hip replacement. In *The adult hip* (ed. JJ Callaghan, A Rosenberg, H Rubash), pp. 1317–30. Lippincott-Raven, Philadelphia, PA, 1998.

38 Canner GC, Steinberg ME, Heppenstall RB, Balderston R: The infected hip after total hip arthroplasty. *Journal of Bone and Joint Surgery* [Am] **66**: 1393–9, 1984.

39 Crockarell JR, Hanssen AD, Osmon DR, Morrey BF: Treatment of infection with debridement and retention of the components following hip arthroplasty. *Journal of Bone and Joint Surgery* [Am] **80**: 1306–13, 1998.

40 Hyman JL, Salvati EA, Laurencin CT, Rogers DE, Maynard M, Brause BD: The arthroscopic drainage, irrigation and debridement of late, acute total hip arthroplasty infections. *Journal of Arthroplasty* **14**: 903–10, 1999.

41 Brandt *et al.*: 1997.

42 Ure KJ, Amstutz HC, Nasser S, Schmalzried TP: Direct-exchange arthroplasty for the treatment of infection after total hip replacement. An average ten-year follow-up. *Journal of Bone and Joint Surgery* [Am] **80**: 961–8, 1998.

43 Katz RP, Callaghan JJ, Johnston RC: A minimum ten year follow-up study of one stage reimplantation of the infected total hip. *Orthopaedic Transactions* **18**: 993, 1994.

44 Garvin KL, Hanssen AD: Infection after total hip arthroplasty. past, present and future. *Journal of Bone and Joint Surgery* [Am] **77**: 1576–88, 1995.

45 Garvin KL, Fitzgerald RH, Salvati EA *et al.*: Reconstruction of the infected total hip and knee arthroplasty with gentamicin-impregnated Palacos bone cement. *Instructional Course Lectures* **42**: 293–302, 1993.

46 Hughes PW, Salvati EA, Wilson PD, Blumenfeld EL: treatment of subacute sepsis of the hip by antibiotics and joint replacement: criteria for diagnosis with evaluation of twenty-six cases. *Clinical Orthopaedics and Related Research* **141**: 143–57, 1979.

47 Younger ASE, Duncan CP, Masri BA, McGraw RW: The outcome of two-stage arthroplasty using a custom-made interval spacer to treat the infected hip. *Journal of Arthroplasty* **12**: 615–23, 1997.

48 Younger ASE, Duncan CP, Masri BA: Treatment of infection associated with segmental bone loss in the proximal part of the

femur in two stages with use of an antibiotic-loaded interval prosthesis. *Journal of Bone and Joint Surgery* [Am] **80**: 60–9, 1998.

49 Haddad FS, Masri BA, Garbuz DS, Duncan CP: The treatment of the infected hip replacement. the complex case. *Clinical Orthopaedics and Related Research* **369**: 144–56, 1999.

50 Miley GB, Scheller AD, Turner RH: Medical and surgical treatment of the septic hip with one-stage revision arthroplasty. *Clinical Orthopaedics and Related Research* **170**: 76–82, 1982.

51 Sanzen L, Carlsson AS, Josefsson G, Lindberg LT: Revision operations on infected total hip arthroplasties. *Clinical Orthopaedics and Related Research* **229**: 165–72, 1988.

52 Raut VV, Siney PD, Wroblewski BM: One-stage revision of infected total hip arthroplasty with discharging sinuses. *Journal of Bone and Joint Surgery* [Br] **76**: 721–4, 1994.

53 Garvin KL, Evans BG, Salvati EA, Brause BD: Palacos gentamicin for the treatment of deep periprosthetic hip infections. *Clinical Orthopaedics and Related Research* **298**: 97–105, 1994.

54 Berry DJ, Chandler HP, Reilly DT: The use of bone allografts in two-stage reconstruction after failure of hip replacements due to infection. *Journal of Bone and Joint Surgery* [Am] **73**: 1460–8, 1991.

55 Lieberman JR, Callaway GH, Salvati EA, Pellicci PM, Brause BD: Treatment of the infected total hip arthroplasty with a two-stage reimplantation protocol. *Clinical Orthopaedics and Related Research* **301**: 205–12, 1994.

56 Alexeeff M, Mahomed N, Morsi E, Garbuz D, Gross A: Structural allograft in two-stage revisions for failed septic hip arthroplasty. *Journal of Bone and Joint Surgery* [Br] **78**: 213–16, 1996.

57 Hunter GA: The results of reinsertion of a total hip prosthesis after sepsis. *Journal of Bone and Joint Surgery* [Br] **61**: 422–3, 1979.

58 Colyer and Capello: 1994.

59 Gristina AG, Costerson JW: Bacterial adherence to biomaterials and tissue. The significance of it role in clinical sepsis. *Journal of Bone and Joint Surgery* [Am] **65**: 264–73, 1985.

60 Zavansky DM, Sande MA: Reconsideration of rifampicin: a unique drug for a unique infection. *Journal of the American Medical Association* **279**: 1575–7, 1998.

61 Hope PG, Kristinsson KG, Norman P, Elson RA: Deep infection of cemented total hip arthroplasties caused by coagulase-negative staphylococci. *Journal of Bone and Joint Surgery* [Br] **71**: 851–5, 1989.

62 Duncan CP, Beauchamp C: A temporary antibiotic-loaded joint replacement system for management of complex infections involving the hip. *Orthopaedic Clinics of North America* **24**: 751–9, 1993.

63 Wang J-W, Chen C-E: Reimplantation of infected hip arthroplasties using bone allografts. *Clinical Orthopaedics and Related Research* **335**: 202–10, 1997.

64 Fitzgerald RH Jr: Infected total hip arthroplasty: diagnosis and treatment. *Journal of the American Academy of Orthopaedic Surgeons* **3**: 249–62, 1995.

65 Grauer JD, Amstutz HC, O'Carroll PF, Dorey FJ: Resection arthroplasty of the hip. *Journal of Bone and Joint Surgery* [Am] **71**: 669–78, 1989.

66 Petty W, Goldsmith S. (1980) Resection arthroplasty after total hip arthroplasty. *Journal of Bone and Joint Surgery* [Am] **62**: 889–96, 1980.

67 Bittar ES, Petty W: Girdlestone arthroplasty for infected total hip arthro-
     plasty. *Clinical Orthopaedics and Related Research* **170**: 83–7, 1982.
68 Bourne RB, Hunter GA, Rorabeck CH, Macnab JJ: A six-year follow-
     up of infected total hip replacements managed by Girdlestone's
     arthroplasty. *Journal of Bone and Joint Surgery* [Br] **66**: 340–3,
     1984.
69 Girdlestone GR: Acute pyogenic arthritis of the hip. *Lancet* **i**: 419–21,
     1943.
70 Kostuik J, Alexander D: Arthrodesis for failed arthroplasty of the hip.
     Clinical Orthopaedics and Related Research **188**: 173–82, 1984.

Index

311